"In this beautifully written, authoritative, and accessible book, Alschuler and Gazella offer state-of-the-art advice, direction, and companionship to anyone diagnosed with cancer. *The Definitive Guide to Cancer* is a unique synthesis of information and wisdom, research and loving-kindness. This book is a lighthouse for anyone frightened and adrift in the dark."

—**Rachel Naomi Remen, MD,** clinical professor at UCSF School of Medicine and author of *Kitchen Table Wisdom* and *My Grandfather's Blessings*

"If you or a loved one has heard the words 'you have cancer,' you should read this book. Written in plain English, this book addresses conventional, complementary, and alternative therapies in a way that allows one to make informed decisions about prevention and treatment."

—**Tieraona Low Dog, MD,** director of education for the Program in Integrative Medicine at the University of Arizona

"If knowledge is power, then expect to be empowered by Alschuler and Gazella's thorough and comprehensive review of cancer. They tackle difficult and complex subject matter without losing sight of the fact that each of us is mind, body, and spirit."

—**William T. O'Donnell, Jr.,** founder of Miraval, Life in Balance Resort and Spa and the Sierra Tucson Treatment Center

"This is currently the best book available for cancer patients. It is well researched and well written, with eloquent patient stories and invaluable, easy-to-use information on chemotherapy and herbal contraindications. Alschuler and Gazella provide a concise review and evaluation of popular alternative therapies that should be assigned reading for anyone who has been touched by cancer—and that's all of us."

—**Leanna Standish, ND, PhD, L.Ac.,** research professor at Bastyr University

"This book is a remarkable resource. From helping readers understand cancer prevention, causes, and diagnosis to compiling information about specific cancers and conventional and alternative treatment options, the authors combine compelling science with a compassionate, integrative perspective. This integration of conventional and natural medicine is the hope for the future of both cancer prevention and treatment."

—**Tori Hudson, ND,** author of *Women's Encyclopedia of Natural Medicine* and program director of the Institute of Women's Health and Integrative Medicine

The Definitive Guide to Cancer

The Definitive Guide to Cancer

An Integrative Approach to
Prevention, Treatment, and Healing

THIRD EDITION

Previously published as *Alternative Medicine Magazine's
Definitive Guide to Cancer, Second Edition*

Lise N. Alschuler, ND, FABNO
Karolyn A. Gazella

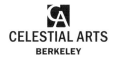
CELESTIAL ARTS
BERKELEY

Published in the United States by Celestial Arts, an imprint of the Crown Publishing Group, a division of Random House, Inc., New York.
www.crownpublishing.com
www.tenspeed.com

Celestial Arts and the Celestial Arts colophon are
registered trademarks of Random House, Inc.

Previous editions of this work were published in the United States as *An Alternative Medicine Definitive Guide to Cancer* by Future Medicine Publishing, Inc., Tiburon, CA, in 1997, and subsequently as *Alternative Medicine Magazine's Definitive Guide to Cancer, Second Edition*, by Celestial Arts, Berkeley, CA, in 2007.

"Screening Guidelines for the Early Detection of Cancer in Average-risk Asymptomatic People" on pages 29–30 used by permission of the American Cancer Society.

Library of Congress Cataloging-in-Publication Data
The definitive guide to cancer : an integrative approach to prevention, treatment, and healing. — 3rd ed. / Lise N. Alschuler, Karolyn A. Gazella.
        p. cm.
Rev. ed. of: Alternative medicine magazine's definitive guide to cancer. 2nd ed., completely rev. and updated. c2007.
Summary: "A comprehensive cancer guide offering an integrative approach that embraces both alternative and conventional therapies for cancer prevention, treatment, and healing"— Provided by publisher.
Includes bibliographical references and index.
1. Cancer—Alternative treatment. I. Gazella, Karolyn A. II. Alschuler, Lise. Alternative medicine magazine's definitive guide to cancer. III. Title.

RC271.A62D53 2010
616.99'406—dc22

2009053541
ISBN 978-1-58761-358-6

Printed in the United States of America

Text design by Chris Hall
Cover design by Colleen Cain

10 9 8 7 6 5 4 3
Third Edition

Contents

About the Authors

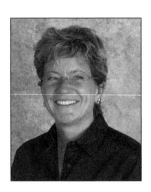

Lise N. Alschuler, ND, FABNO

Dr. Lise Alschuler earned her naturopathic medical doctorate from Bastyr University in 1994, and is a board-certified naturopathic oncologist. She received her BA with honors in anthropology from Brown University in 1988. Dr. Alschuler is the vice president of quality and education at Emerson Ecologics, a distributor of natural products to health-care professionals. She also practices naturopathic oncology with Naturopathic Specialists, LLC, in Scottsdale, Arizona, specializing in prevention and integrated treatment for people who have been affected by cancer. From 2003 to 2008, Dr. Alschuler was the director of naturopathic medicine at Midwestern Regional Medical Center (MRMC), a JCAHO-accredited regional hospital specializing in comprehensive integrative cancer care. MRMC is managed by Cancer Treatment Centers of America and is located in Zion, Illinois. Prior to joining MRMC, she was the clinical medical director at the Bastyr Center for Natural Health in Seattle, Washington. She was an associate professor on the clinical and academic faculty at Bastyr University from 1996 to 2003.

Dr. Alschuler is a published author, has presented at numerous professional conferences and public events internationally, and is very active in promoting naturopathic medicine in the United States. She is the immediate past-president of the American Association of Naturopathic Physicians and on the founding board of directors of the Naturopathic Post-Graduate Association. She has received professional recognition and many awards for her work in integrative medicine. She believes that her job as a naturopathic physician and educator is to stimulate and support the innate healing processes within each individual by applying a scientifically based strategy that utilizes the most natural approaches possible. After her own diagnosis of breast cancer in 2008, she has utilized an integrative approach to support her own wellness. Dr. Alschuler is licensed as a naturopathic physician in New Hampshire, Arizona, and Washington states. She resides in New Hampshire.

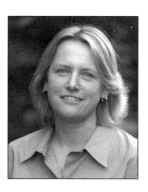

Karolyn A. Gazella

Karolyn A. Gazella is the coauthor of *Return to Beautiful Skin* and *Boost Your Health With Bacteria*. She has been involved in the natural health industry for more than 18 years. Karolyn is the publisher of the *Natural Medicine Journal* (www.naturalmedicinejournal.com) and has written hundreds of articles on the topic of natural health. She is also the managing editor of the *Better Nutrition Healthy Living Guide* series, which is a booklet and book publishing division that she created for AIM Media, publishers of *Yoga Journal*, *Vegetarian Times*, *Better Nutrition*, and other popular magazines. Karolyn's articles have appeared in numerous health publications and she has authored or coauthored several *Healthy Living Guides* on a variety of topics. Karolyn was named one of the top ten people of 2009 in integrative medicine and health care by John Weeks, who publishes an influential blog called The Integrator.

Karolyn is a cancer survivor and an avid horse enthusiast. She is an active volunteer with the Medicine Horse Program (www.medicinehorse .org) located in Boulder, Colorado, which is an innovative equine-assisted therapy program that helps high-risk youth.

Acknowledgments

We could not have written this book as comprehensively and accurately without the review, contributions, and corrections from our esteemed editorial advisory board, whose members are listed beginning on page xv. A special thanks to Donald Abrams, MD, who contributed the foreword to this edition. We are proud to have his valued input on this important topic.

Thanks to the staff of Ten Speed Press, especially our editor, Sara Golski, who with gentle persistence has helped us to make this edition so much better. Thanks to designer Chris Hall, copy editor Sheryl Rose, and proofreader Jennifer McClain. We also want to acknowledge the talented work of artist Ron Weed, whose illustrations debut in this edition. Thank you to Bill and Kathy Adams for letting us transform your wonderful home in Pagosa Springs into an incredible writing retreat. We would also like to thank the many cancer thrivers, loved ones, and experts who contributed their insights to this book. Their wisdom is invaluable.

Lise's Acknowledgments

My continuous delight in working with Karolyn Gazella has been amply renewed with the writing of this edition. Karolyn's incredible talent as a writer combined with her passion for truth-telling have indelibly marked her as my favorite author. Plus, I have the added benefit of her friendship, and as hard as it is keeping up with a princess, I am all in for trying.

I am incredibly blessed to have the most amazing friends. As I fought my way through my breast cancer treatments, every call, email, and visit from my friends reinforced the fact that love really is the mark of a life well lived. I would like to send a perpetual printed hug to my dear friends Jane Guiltinan, Cindy Breed, Wyler Hecht, Dan Rubin, Peggy Lean, Emily Payne, Karen Howard, Spencer Gunkle, Jake Birdsong, Zoe Allen, and Bethany Cook. You are all stunningly beautiful human beings.

My family is my bedrock. I don't know how I managed to land in such an incredible family, but I did. I am forever grateful for each of you—Ann Adams, Britt Ruhe, Alfie Alschuler, Elena Alschuler, Irene Nystrom, Colin Ruhe, Ericka Alschuler, Isaiah Ruhe, Aman Ruhe, Mason Alschuler, and Anika Alschuler. Britt, I would love you even without your cookies, although their deliciousness is an expression of who you are in this world. Thank you, Alfie, for your quiet, steady, and unflinching support, love, and admiration—it goes both ways! Elena, your bravery and compassion in the face of all that life has dealt you is an inspiration. A big thank you to my mom, Irene, for providing the finest example of the power of knowledge and information. Isaiah, Aman, Mason, and Anika—you each make me believe in the future. Colin, thank you for your generosity and kindness, and for always being on the other end of the phone. Ericka, the only reason we let you win in Scrabble is because of your big heart and sweetness. And, Ann, thank you, yet again, for so gracefully and unselfishly supporting me in this writing. I am grateful for every minute that I have had the good fortune to share with you in this life. You are exquisite.

Finally, I bow my head in heartfelt admiration to the many people diagnosed with cancer in whose journey I have had a part. You have each taught me more than you will ever know. Your bravery is unbelievable. You are my heroes.

Karolyn's Acknowledgments

I have wanted to write a book on cancer since my diagnosis in 1995. It is impossible to acknowledge everyone who has positively inspired my cancer journey since that time, but I appreciate each of you.

I would like to first thank my coauthor, Dr. Lise Alschuler. She is a healer in the truest sense: highly intelligent, yet acutely sensitive and caring. But what makes Lise really special is that she is a joy to be with. Her positive attitude is contagious and she demonstrated how deep her courage travels as she battled breast cancer. And although she drove me crazy with her early morning Tae Bo routine during our writing retreat, I can honestly say that I would not take on a project such as this with anyone else in the world. Words cannot describe how fortunate I feel to have spent time with Lise creating this new edition of our book. She has become one of my closest friends and for that I am truly blessed.

Much gratitude is extended to my friends for their love and support as they cheered me on throughout this project, especially Miriam Weidner, Veronica Smith, Kerrie Moreau, Deirdre Bell, Maria Dalebroux, Marian Hathorne, and Myra Eby. You all epitomize what true friendship is and I am proud to have you in my posse. To my four-legged best friends, Beau and Sundance—it's true, our horses are our best therapists!

To my large Midwest family who have encouraged me over the years, especially my four brothers, Mark, Dan, Rick, and Randy, and my sisters-in-law Patti and Linda. A special thanks to my father, Don Gazella, who taught me the value of hard work and persistence.

I recognize that I have something many people will never have: a sister and a best friend who are the same person. My sister, Kathi Magee, is a wonderful human being who continues to inspire me. She is the most amazing person I have ever met. It may sound clichéd, but words truly cannot describe the positive influence she has had on my life. Kathi and her two boys, Cody and Travis Magee, have given me a foundation upon which my life is built, and for that I am extremely grateful. My life is anchored by the love and support I receive from Susan Mesko. Susie, your kind heart, warm smile, and strong integrity continually remind me how lucky I am and make me want to be the best I can be. For that, I am truly grateful.

Finally, to my mom, Eunice Matzke Gazella, who represents all that is good and all that is spiritual. "You will be judged by how you treat others and what you give back," she told me as she waited to make her transition into heaven. She gave so much. Her radiance lives on in those of us who were blessed to have known her. Thanks, Mom.

Editorial Advisory Board

Shauna Birdsall, ND, Cancer Treatment Centers of America
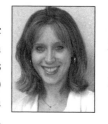
Shauna Birdsall graduated from National College of Naturopathic Medicine (Portland, Oregon) in 2000, and completed a residency in naturopathic medicine and oncology at Cancer Treatment Centers of America–Midwestern Regional Medical Center (Zion, Illinois) in 2002. Dr. Birdsall served as a staff naturopath at Midwestern Regional Medical Center, where she practiced in an innovative, integrative, team-based, holistic comprehensive cancer care center. Currently, Dr. Birdsall is the director of naturopathic medicine at Cancer Treatment Centers of America–Southwestern Regional Medical Center in Goodyear, Arizona. She is strongly committed to providing individualized, compassionate, scientifically based care to empower and provide hope to cancer patients.

Alexandria Concorde, MBBS, PhD, FRSM, Concorde Initiative (United Kingdom)
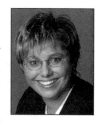
Alex Concorde is a U.K. specialist medical doctor with a primary degree in biochemistry and a multidisciplinary PhD in virology, pathology, immunology, and molecular genetics. She has developed a sophisticated new system of naturopathic medicine that takes a "mind-to-molecule" approach to preventing and treating complex stress, immune system, and hormone-related disorders.

Dr. Concorde is head of research and development for the Concorde Initiative and president of the International Association of Transformational Change (IATC). She tutors on master's programs for two U.K. universities and sits on a specialist section council of the United Kingdom's Royal Society of Medicine. She has received several prestigious research grants, is widely published, and is quoted in the U.K. national press.

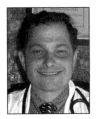
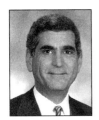
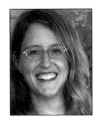

Mimi Guarneri, MD, FACC, Scripps Center for Integrative Medicine

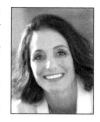

Erminia M. Guarneri earned her medical degree from SUNY Medical Center, graduating number one in her class. She served her internship and residency at Cornell Medical Center as chief medical resident. Dr. Guarneri is board certified in cardiology, internal medicine, nuclear medicine, and holistic medicine. She has been an attending interventional cardiologist at Scripps Clinic since 1995 and is the founding medical director of the Scripps Center for Integrative Medicine. An author and international lecturer, her articles have appeared in the *Journal of Echocardiography* and the *Annals of Internal Medicine*. Her book *The Heart Speaks* was featured on *Today*.

Tina Kaczor, ND, Private Clinical Practice

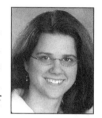

Tina Kaczor is currently in private practice in Eugene, Oregon, where she specializes in naturopathic oncology. Dr. Kaczor received her doctorate from the National College of Naturopathic Medicine in Portland, Oregon. Subsequent to graduation, she completed a residency in integrative oncology at Cancer Treatment Centers of America in Tulsa, Oklahoma. Prior to her naturopathic training, Dr. Kaczor received dual bachelor's degrees in English and biochemistry and conducted research in plant molecular biology, publishing her results in the peer-reviewed journal *Plant Physiology*. She is currently a member of the American Association of Naturopathic Physicians (AANP) and the Society for Integrative Oncology (SIO). She is also the president of the Oncology Association of Naturopathic Physicians (OncANP) and board certified in naturopathic oncology by the American Board of Naturopathic Oncology. She is the medical editor of the *Natural Medicine Journal* (www.naturalmedicinejournal.com).

Matthew Mumber, MD, Harbin Clinic

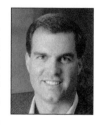

Matt Mumber is a practicing, board-certified radiation oncologist living in Rome, Georgia. He received his undergraduate and medical degrees from the University of Virginia and completed his radiation oncology residency at the Bowman Gray School of Medicine. He graduated from the 2002 associate fellowship program in integrative medicine at the University of Arizona. Dr. Mumber serves as the medical advisor for local and regional cancer initiatives through the Georgia Cancer Coalition, and is the president of the Georgia Society of Clinical Oncology. He founded Cancer Navigators

Inc. in 2002, a 501(c)3 corporation that provides nursing, education, and service navigation for those touched by cancer. He is the editor of *Integrative Oncology: Principles and Practice*, published by Taylor and Francis in 2006. Dr. Mumber facilitates residential retreats for cancer patients and is active in multi-institutional research trials.

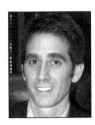

Dan Rubin, ND, FABNO, Rubin Medical Center

Daniel Rubin is a board-certified naturopathic oncologist in private practice in Scottsdale, Arizona. He received his BA in philosophy from the University of Iowa and his doctorate in naturopathic medicine from Southwest College of Naturopathic Medicine, in Tempe, Arizona, where he also completed his residency. Dr. Rubin is a member of the Naturopathic Physicians Board of Medical Examiners in the state of Arizona. He is assistant clinical professor of naturopathic medicine at Southwest College of Naturopathic Medicine, assistant editor of the peer-reviewed and indexed medical journal *Integrative Cancer Therapies*, the oncology editor of the peer-reviewed *International Journal of Naturopathic Medicine*, and serves on the editorial advisory board of *Hematology Oncology News and Issues*. He is the immediate past-president of the Oncology Association of Naturopathic Physicians and serves on the board of the American Board of Naturopathic Oncology Medical Examiners.

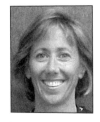

Susan Ryan, DO, Rose Emergency Medical Center

Susan Ryan received her medical degree from the College of Osteopathic Medicine of the Pacific in Pomona, California. She completed a residency in family medicine and a sports medicine fellowship and is board certified in both. She has served as a team physician for collegiate, Olympic, and professional athletes in many sports. Dr. Ryan actively teaches residents and medical students while practicing emergency medicine at Rose Medical Center in Denver, Colorado. She is a contributing author to *The Encyclopedia of Sports Medicine: Women in Sport*, and she has written numerous articles and given lectures about exercise and medicine.

Foreword

Receiving a diagnosis of cancer is a startling life event that often makes a person feel as if they have totally lost all sense of control. Suddenly they are at the mercy of their surgeon, radiation oncologist, medical oncologist, and chemotherapy nurse—and life as they knew it is, at best, put on hold. The emerging field of integrative oncology strives to return to the person living with or beyond cancer a sense that they can also participate actively in their journey back toward health. In the setting of a committed patient-practitioner partnership, the cancer patient is given a number of tools that they can integrate into their treatment program, empowering them to be an active member of the team and not a victim or bystander.

To date, however, there are few oncology professionals who are well-versed in the modalities patients seek to incorporate into their conventional cancer care. Most focus on targeting the tumor and ridding the body of malignant cells—certainly a noble venture. However, in doing so, the person living with the cancer is often overlooked. While cancer is the weed, integrative cancer care deals with the garden as well, making the soil as inhospitable as possible to growth and spread of the weed. Nutrition, supplements, physical activity, stress reduction, traditional Chinese medicine, mind-body interventions, spirituality—these are all incorporated as appropriate with the conventional cancer care regimen to optimize the patient's outcome, decrease symptoms associated with the cancer or its treatment, and maximize quality of life.

For the newly diagnosed individual, trying to sort through the vast amount of potential complementary interventions recommended by family or friends or encountered on the Internet can be a daunting experience.

There is so much information out there—how do you know whom to trust? A resource entitled *The Definitive Guide to Cancer* certainly inspires confidence, and rightly so! Now in its third edition, updated and authored by two renowned authorities who also happen to be cancer survivors themselves, this volume is an invaluable resource to cancer patients, their families, and their conventional care providers. Impeccably researched and thoroughly referenced, the authors have created a cancer guide that is both academic as well as totally accessible to those without formal medical training. The background chapters on cancer biology, treatment approaches, and supporting the key body functions are sound, up-to-date, and easy to absorb. The chapters summarizing each individual cancer type provide a concise summary of valuable information, both for the patient and cancer care provider.

As more people living with and beyond cancer seek to supplement their conventional therapies and even assist in reducing the risk of cancer in their family and friends, this text will remain an invaluable resource. With the latest information including targeted therapies, survivorship recommendations, and the ever-evolving soy controversy, this edition is completely current. The extensive tables on "Nutrient and Herb Interactions with Conventional Cancer Treatments" and the rated "Supplement Guide" are concise and meticulous and should be at the fingertips of every cancer patient and their care team. This evidence-based encyclopedic text, infused with experience and humanity, truly lives up to the promise of its name.

—Donald I. Abrams, **MD**, Chief, Hematology-Oncology, San Francisco General Hospital; Director of Integrative Oncology Research, UCSF Osher Center for Integrative Medicine; Professor of Clinical Medicine, University of California San Francisco; and President, Society for Integrative Oncology

Introduction

We wish there were no need for this book. We wish cancer were not so common—not so daunting. But the reality is that there is a desperate need for accurate, trustworthy information, and an even more urgent desire for a cure and, ultimately, an ironclad method to enhance quality of life.

If you're reading this book, chances are you or someone you love has been diagnosed with cancer. You are not alone. You have just gained access to a club that nobody wants to belong to—a club with an ever-increasing membership.

Cancer takes the life of one of every four people in the United States, second only to heart disease overall, but surpassing it in some age categories. More than 1,500 people die of cancer every single day. The future doesn't look any brighter. The next two decades will likely witness a 45 percent increase in the number of cancer diagnoses from 1.6 million in 2010 to 2.3 million by 2030. Although it is not yet the most common cause of disease-related death, surveys indicate it is certainly the most feared.

In addition to its physical and emotional toll, cancer has a devastating economic impact. Cancer is a very expensive illness. The National Institutes of Health estimates that overall costs associated with cancer were $228 billion in 2008.

Purpose of This Book

Our goal is to present information on integrative cancer prevention and treatment in a practical, useful manner so you will be able to make informed decisions based on your specific circumstances and comfort level. You have choices. We will present scientifically substantiated information that will help you make your decisions. We understand that the amount of information, the number of decisions, and the implications of those decisions can be overwhelming. This book is here to help.

Throughout this book, we adhere to the following guiding principles:

- Meeting our readers without judgment, wherever they are on their particular journey

- Scrutinizing the scientific literature and all information carefully and using only the highest-quality references and the most respected sources

- Being scientific yet compassionate while presenting the most accurate information as succinctly as possible

- Delivering informed hope, not false hope

In part I, you'll develop a better understanding of cancer: what it is, what causes it, and how to help prevent it. Part II explores treatment options: conventional treatments, complementary and alternative therapies, integrative treatment, and lifestyle choices that can help you most effectively fight cancer. You will learn about how to use complementary therapies to support conventional treatments and help offset some of the side effects of conventional treatments. You will also learn how to support your recovery after conventional treatment is over.

Part III discusses five important physiological systems and bodily processes—the immune system, inflammation, the endocrine system, blood sugar control, and digestion, detoxification, and elimination—and their relationship to cancer. You will learn how proper functioning of these systems will help you more effectively fight cancer.

Part IV contains separate chapters on 21 different cancers. Each chapter includes the causes, symptoms, diagnoses, conventional treatments, and complementary and alternative therapies for each cancer.

You'll also find valuable information beyond the end of the main text. There is a glossary of terms to help familiarize you with some of the technical terms that we use. There is also an appendix in which we've given dosage ranges for the herbs and supplements mentioned throughout the book.

Information Is Power

A study featured in *Annals of Oncology* regarding patient-doctor communication revealed a disturbing situation: nearly half of breast cancer patients interviewed said the information they received was "incomprehensible or incomplete." Most of the women rated social and psychological support as important, and yet only one-third had been referred to a support group. Nearly 60 percent said they wanted to speak to the medical staff more frequently.

"Patients who rated their communication as incomplete or incomprehensible had poorer quality of life even five years after their diagnosis," explains Jacqueline Kerr, author of the study. The researchers found that women who felt confused and inadequately informed experienced more depression, anxiety, irritability, and difficulty with relationships and were less able to participate in leisure activities. The project director, Dr. Jutta Engel, concludes, "Although these findings paint a bleak picture . . . information giving is a reasonably cheap intervention with much potential."

There is a lot to gain from accurate and trusted information. In a study featured in *Cancer Nursing*, researchers in Taiwan demonstrated that "informed patients reported significantly higher levels of hope than those who were not informed." Unfortunately, a great contradiction arises when you or a loved one is diagnosed with cancer: You want as much information as possible, and yet the sheer magnitude of what's available is overwhelming. To help you sift through all of this information and to make sense of it, this book will teach you how to evaluate sources and determine the quality of information.

About This Edition

This book is the third edition and follows our second edition from 2007. This edition updates all of the information based upon the most recent science. The information has been re-presented in concise, practical ways. Our hope is that you can use this edition to help you make key decisions in real time wherever you are in your experience of cancer. We have retained some of the explanatory information to support you in becoming an empowered individual with cancer. The basis of this book is an advocacy of integrative cancer care (oncology).

From our perspective, integrative medicine is the responsible blending of applicable traditional, supplemental, and complementary healing methods with appropriate conventional medical interventions. This should take place within the context of a safe, open, caring dialogue between the patient (and their loved ones) and their physician(s) and other health-care providers. Integrative medicine is a truly holistic approach that evaluates and considers all health-promoting approaches and then applies those that are most appropriate to prevention and treatment. The ultimate goal is enhanced quality of life and deep healing of the mind, body, and spirit. Integrative oncology takes advantage of the body's own capacity for self-healing. An integrative approach will bolster the patient's internal defense systems and help ease the side effects of conventional cancer treatments. The cornerstone of integrative oncology is combining evidence-based tools and approaches with an enhanced patient-doctor relationship. More patients are demanding this integrative approach.

Our hope is that in the future the term *integrative medicine* will no longer apply. It will no longer be integrative medicine; it will just be good medicine.

Scientific Credibility

Our most important goal has been to create a book that is not only trusted by readers but also respected by their physicians. To this end, we have cited solid original research, interviewed experts, and established a team of respected health-care practitioners for our editorial board. Utilizing the conventional medical standard for evaluating the evidence for therapies, we have developed our own rating system to help you make sense of the onslaught of data.

Some conventional doctors and researchers try to perpetuate the myth that there is no scientific substantiation, in the form of well-designed studies or otherwise, demonstrating that diet, lifestyle, nutrients, and herbs are safe and effective aspects of oncology. This is simply not true. You will notice that throughout this book we utilize the same journals as conventional medical practitioners use. Clearly, we have found an abundance of scientific information indicating the value of a wide variety of approaches presently available. Scientifically substantiated treatment options go far beyond the three ways conventional medicine deals with cancer—drugs, surgery, and radiation.

In regard to those doctors (or patients) who say there is no scientific information on the safety and effectiveness of diet, lifestyle, nutrients, and herbs for use in cancer prevention and treatment, they obviously have not done a literature search recently! We are impressed with the research we have gathered for this book, and we are confident that you and your doctor will be as well. Because of the sheer volume of information available, we have primarily chosen to feature the most recent scientific studies, though we do occasionally refer to older studies because they are so significant in this area of integrative oncology.

We encourage you to share this text with your doctor. Even more importantly, we encourage you to work with health-care professionals, clinics, and hospitals that are receptive to an integrative approach to cancer prevention and treatment.

Treatment Success

We have also looked closely at how we define cancer treatment success. Our focus is on healing from cancer, which refers to an internal process of becoming whole and feeling harmonious with yourself and your environment. Healing pertains to all levels of being, bringing a person's true character into focus and healthy expression. Here's how we define cancer treatment success:

- Accepting and embracing positive and negative emotions with love and nonjudgment so we can enjoy the journey no matter where we are on the path

- Enhancing quality of life—physically, mentally, and spiritually—by connecting the mind, body, and spirit in order to grow and gain peace

Success relies on internal awareness just as much as external factors. You cannot force success; you just need to make room for it. Those who transition from this life should not be judged unsuccessful. Perhaps cancer was meant to be a vehicle for them—a stepping-stone.

It has been said that the true measure of a life is not reflected in the number of years lived, but in how one lived those years on this earth. This is particularly true for people with cancer. The measure of a life is calculated by how we spend our days and how we treat others. These are outcomes not dictated by chemotherapy, radiation, surgery, or supplements. Cancer success comes in the form of realization, personalization, connection, contentment, and grace, which can't be measured in a test tube, diagnostic lab, or doctor's office. Regardless of the physical outcome, these measures of success are embedded in one's heart and soul. Not even cancer can steal the true measure of a life well lived.

Our Connection to Cancer

Cancer patients and their loved ones are fighting a multidimensional battle against a mammoth opponent. We understand the overwhelming feelings that accompany a cancer diagnosis. Our personal experiences with cancer have helped us bring a unique perspective to this complex and frightening topic. Cancer has profoundly touched our lives, and it has motivated us to join forces to write this book.

We take great pride in the scientific detail that has informed the creation of this book. However, for us cancer is more than facts and figures, outcomes and data. To us, cancer also represents a personal, emotional, and intimate exploration beyond the statistics. We would like to share our personal stories with you to help illustrate the close connection we have to this topic and to you.

Lise's Story

I know the disease of cancer well—all too well. Since the last edition of this book, I was diagnosed with it myself. My story begins, however, much earlier than that, and it begins with my father when I was in third grade. I burst into the study, breathless with excitement. "Dad! Dad! I know what I want to be when I grow up!" My father looked up from his work with a broad smile and a twinkle in his eyes. "Really," he said. "Well, you had better come here and tell me." I climbed onto his lap and solemnly told him that I had decided to become a nurse. He paused for a moment. "You know, that is a wonderful idea. Have you considered the idea of becoming a doctor?" I considered this for a long moment and then replied, "I like that idea; I will become a doctor." I never let go of that goal. Thirty-five years later, now a doctor, I can vividly recollect that memory of sitting on my father's lap and, at his gentle prodding, determining what would ultimately become my life's work.

As can be the case with career aspirations, my path has not been linear; rather, I've weaved through different landscapes collecting experiences and knowledge along the way. After completing an undergraduate degree in medical anthropology from Brown University, I was headed toward conventional medical school. However, despite my lifelong ambition to become an allopathic medical doctor, I realized that my heart was not in that path. I withdrew my applications to conventional medical school. Fortunately, I was able to keep my dreams of becoming the kind of doctor that I envisioned alive in my discovery of naturopathic medicine.

My work as a naturopathic physician has been immensely gratifying. The medicine I practice respects the wisdom of every individual and supports their inherent healing capacities. I am able to employ the healing powers of nature in a scientifically robust manner to help people rediscover health and wellness. I spent the first ten years of my professional career practicing general naturopathic medicine. Then, in 2002, I left my job as clinic medical director at Bastyr University Natural Health Clinic for the opportunity to work as a naturopathic physician and administrator in a midwestern hospital north of Chicago. This hospital, part of Cancer Treatment Centers of America, embraces an integrative model of cancer care. This work gave me an intense appreciation for the complexity of cancer and for the scientific rigor required when applying natural therapies. I have been continually awed, amazed, touched, angered, broken, and healed by the very brave people I encountered—both patients and their loved ones—who were coping with cancer. My work in this area transformed me and continues to remind me daily about what is important.

My work experience alone would have been enough motivation to join Karolyn in writing this book. However, in February 2005, my father called me from a hospital in California to tell me that he had just been diagnosed with pancreatic cancer. The tumor in his pancreas was large and cancer cells had already spread to regional lymph nodes. His prognosis was grim. My father was a man who embodied the very essence of robustness. He had a career of dizzying accomplishment as a professor of education and psychology. He raised four children with fierce love and unsuppressed pride and joy. Despite severe knee injuries, at the age of 64 he rode a hand-powered tricycle from North Carolina to Massachusetts. His appetite for life was voracious. My father has been a mentor, friend, and inspiration to me. His call brought me to my knees. How could this happen to my dad? Why pancreatic cancer of all cancers? Why now? All unanswerable questions, all questions I continue to ask.

As Karolyn and I wrote the previous edition of this book, I was living the world we were describing through my father's experience with cancer. Seventeen months of a heart-wrenching, painful, and also wonderful odyssey accompanied my writing. My siblings and our partners banded together around my father. We fumbled our way through the maze of decision making, emotional ups and downs, and continued uncertainties that cancer creates. My father subjected his body to surgery, chemotherapy, radiation, and experimental drugs and steadfastly ingested a daily regimen of supplements that could constitute a meal in and of themselves. My father far outlived his statistical prognosis and enjoyed 17 months of good health. Despite "failing" conventional treatment, with the disease having slowly spread into his lungs, liver, and more lymph nodes, he felt, as he put it, "better now than I did before I was diagnosed!" While he attributed his wellness to his supplement and lifestyle program, his own grace and determination in fighting this illness, along with the deep love many people felt for him, also sustained him. He became alternately scared, panicked, and angry, but somehow he always continued to resurface into, as he puts it, "living life exuberantly." On August 3, 2006, my father passed away from pancreatic cancer, surrounded by his children. (His story is featured on page 342.) His brave fight inspires me to this day to live my own life exuberantly, mindfully, and respectfully.

Inspiration was just what I needed when, in October of 2008, at the age of 42, I learned that I had breast cancer. The unreality and shock of this diagnosis was as real for me, in spite of my extensive professional and family experience with cancer, as it is for anyone. While my relatively healthy and prevention-oriented lifestyle did not prevent cancer, it certainly did promote my health. I didn't feel ill after my diagnosis, but rather found myself feeling like a healthy person with cancer. The subsequent treatments of surgery, chemotherapy, and radiation put my health to the test. Despite the rigors of treatment, I continued to feel like a healthy person who had cancer and manifested some pretty vigorous reactions to the strong therapies of chemotherapy and radiation. I have also learned firsthand the power of natural therapies in managing side effects of surgery, chemotherapy, and radiation. I experienced the power of natural supplements, exercise, stress management, and diet in maintaining and strengthening my wellness both during my conventional treatment and after. Now, just over a year from my diagnosis, I feel better than ever, truly transformed by my experience.

Living in the world as a person with cancer has been a deeply meaningful experience. I continued my professional life throughout my treatment, which included giving several talks at conferences on the topic of cancer, integrated treatment, and prevention. Standing up on stage without any hair, being a visible bearer of cancer and disclosing that I had just received a chemotherapy treatment or a radiation treatment infused my words with authenticity. Cancer both humbled and emboldened me. My sister once remarked on my apparent optimistic and positive attitude. I explained that despite the challenges of this disease and its treatments, I was receiving many gifts—that having cancer opened a door into a room, a door that only cancer can open. The room is filled with gifts. Some gifts look scary or feel very heavy, and there are so many that it can feel bewildering and confusing. But everything in this room in some way teaches me how to experience life more fully, more gratefully, and with more love.

What if someone were to offer you a magic button that you could pin onto your clothing and whenever anyone looked upon this button, they would automatically express unrestrained compassion and loving kindness toward you. Would you take this button? Of course! Well, cancer is that button. I have been incredibly honored by the love, care, and concern expressed to me by friends and strangers alike upon learning of my diagnosis. More love, care, and concern in the world sounds like a beautiful thing to me—another gift of cancer. It is my hope that my experiences infuse the knowledge contained within these pages with loving kindness and that the final product is a gift and a trusted tool for those who must also walk this path.

Karolyn's Story

In 1993, I experienced a professional dream come true as I started my own small publishing company. My mom was my first employee and my sister, Kathi, was my second. The three of us were incredibly close. Not only did we work together each day, we socialized and were best friends. People would comment on how they admired the three of us for being able to work so closely and still maintain strong friendships with one another. I felt truly blessed to have such a close relationship with the two of them.

My parents have six children: me, Kathi, and our four brothers. Kathi is my older sister and she is protective of me. Our mom showed us by example the positive impact of hard work, integrity, and spirituality. She was a caring individual that people were drawn to.

Just two years into the business, we were pleased it was doing so well. But we were soon blindsided as cancer paid its first visit to our immediate family. Previously, we had seen aunts and cousins stricken with this horrible disease.

When Kathi walked into my office after her routine annual physical, she was crying. Her doctor had found a lump in her breast and it would require a biopsy. We were scared. We had just attended the funeral of an aunt who died a painful death due to metastatic breast cancer. Other aunts had died of cancer, as well as our maternal grandmother. To us, cancer equaled death.

"Let's not panic," I thought. But it was hard not to. My mom took the news especially hard. The thought of losing a child was more than she could manage.

At the young age of 35, in July 1994, Kathi entered the operating room not knowing what to expect. The surgeon came out to deliver the news to us. He said the word *cancer* and my mom's knees buckled. I quickly stretched my arm around her to keep her standing. I'm not sure what was worse, hearing that word, or seeing my mom's reaction to it.

Nearly every day after the diagnosis, while my sister recovered at home, my mom would come into my office each morning, sit in the chair across my desk, and cry. She was so afraid. It was heartbreaking to witness how devastated this strong, spiritual, selfless woman was. She could not bear the thought of possibly losing one of her children to the same illness that took her mom, sisters, and sister-in-law (who was also a dear friend). Her morning tears seemed to purge her system for a short time, allowing her to make it through the day. She never cried in front of Kathi because she didn't want to negatively affect Kathi's recovery.

Kathi had a lumpectomy followed by radiation. She was so strong. I think that having two young sons motivated her to fight hard. She was determined to win this battle. And she did.

A few months after Kathi's surgery, Mom developed flulike symptoms and her back pain worsened. We attributed the back pain to a serious horseback riding accident she had had several years prior. But the flulike symptoms were oddly persistent. I remember her being ill at Thanksgiving, and then a few weeks later at our company holiday party she still wasn't feeling well. She was not the type to see a doctor without a lot of prodding. But when she developed jaundice, she could no longer avoid our persistence. We hoped it was something simple, maybe gallstones. I wish that had been the case.

She was admitted to the hospital immediately. They found a huge tumor in her bile duct and five different tumors in her liver. A liver biopsy confirmed that the cancer originated in her pancreas. My brother Dan and I were in her hospital room when the oncologist delivered the news. Advanced pancreatic cancer. He told us there was no hope. Without a tear in her eye, my mother calmly asked how long she had. When he said three months at the most, the shock and disbelief welled up inside me like hot lava. I wanted to scream. I saw the color run from my brother's face. I began to quietly cry at her bedside and she comforted me. This would be her way as she transitioned from this life.

Just five days before Christmas Day, I eased my mom into my car and took her home to die. Mom's health deteriorated quickly, and my sister and I took turns staying with her. Wonderful hospice nurses helped us care for her so she could die at home. Three weeks from the date of her diagnosis, on January 6, 1995, at the age of 58, my mom died at home with my sister at her side. Mom left this life as she lived it—with grace, dignity, and unconditional kindness and love. She was an incredible role model for me and she continues to influence my life.

The physical toll Mom's death took on us was overwhelming. We were tired and emotionally devastated by our loss. Soon after Mom died, I began experiencing severe pain in my lower abdomen. Fueled by fear and denial, I would ignore the pain until it caused me to double over. I finally went to see the doctor.

Less than three months after my mom's death and two days after my thirty-third birthday, I was operated on for ovarian cancer. In less than eight months, my immediate family experienced three cancers, one taking the life of our mom.

My tumor was large—two inches. It had completely enveloped my left ovary and was growing down my uterus. I had a complete hysterectomy—removal of both ovaries and the uterus. Because it was on the outside of the ovary, my local doctors recommended a potent chemotherapy regimen. I went to the University of Wisconsin–Madison to get some advice and finally decided to delay chemotherapy and simply continue to monitor my blood work. I would start chemotherapy if I couldn't get my blood work in the normal range.

I changed my diet, began exercising, used a variety of antistress techniques, focused on my mind as well as my body, and took lots of dietary supplements. Within a year, my blood work was in the normal range. I had avoided chemotherapy entirely. On March 28, 2010, I celebrated the fact that I have been cancer free for 15 years.

Shortly after the previous edition of this book was released, I received a call from my sister. She had cancer again. This time would prove to be more challenging—a more virulent cancer meant that chemotherapy would be required. I was with her when she interviewed her first oncologist. She had the second edition of this book in her hand and told the oncologist that she was receptive to chemotherapy, but she wanted to use an integrative approach that included dietary supplements. The doctor dismissed her quickly and looked at me and said, "So you had ovarian cancer?" I said, "Yes." "And you still have your breasts?" I said, "Yes, I have healthy breasts and I don't care to remove them out of fear of 'possibly' getting breast cancer." She shook her head and looked back at my sister who said, "We'll let you know what we decide," and we walked out of the office knowing that she would not choose that doctor. The second oncologist was completely different. She said, "I don't know much about integrative oncology and dietary supplements, but I appreciate this book and we will work together on this." That's the doctor my sister chose. Today, my sister is thriving. She has shown me once again why she is my mentor and an inspiration. I feel truly honored and blessed to have her as my best friend.

The pall of cancer that hangs over our family tree has piqued the curiosity of university researchers. Our extended family of cousins on my mom's side chose to do genetic testing with Creighton University. Not surprisingly, they discovered that some of our family members have the "cancer gene." Kathi has been tested and, not surprisingly, has the gene. I have chosen not to get tested because I already live my life as if I had the gene. I would not change my course.

Although conventional medicine would say that Mom lost her battle with cancer, I think differently. She gave us significant emotional and spiritual tools we could use to fight our own cancers. She created a living template for us to use and pass on for generations to come. The gifts she gave us are far more powerful than any cancer gene imaginable.

I live my life differently thanks to cancer. I am humbled to join my sister and the millions of other cancer "thrivers" who are alive and well today.

Part I
Understanding Cancer

one

The Cancer Experience

Cancer results from the uncontrolled growth of abnormal cells. As these cells continue to divide, they form into cancerous tumors. With destructive precision, a cancerous tumor redirects blood flow to itself as it leaches off its healthy cellular neighbors. Cancer cells can invade other tissues within the body and produce additional tumors. The frenzied development of a cancerous tumor can overwhelm the organ or tissue where it is located. Left unchecked, many cancers can eventually destroy enough tissue that the body loses its ability to sustain life.

This monstrous demolition can be mirrored emotionally in the person with cancer. The physical chaos and damage is only a part of the story. Cancer brings with it thundering amounts of anger, anxiety, or fear, which can render someone less able to cope emotionally. Even for the most stoic of souls, three simple words—"you have cancer"—can create a simmering internal panic. This panic can be both reflected and magnified in loved ones. A cancer diagnosis goes well beyond the patient, and takes its toll on loving family and friends as well. Sometimes it can be even more difficult being a caregiver or support person and watching a loved one struggle.

Although a cancer diagnosis can bring on a fear of dying, cancer is not a death sentence. That may be difficult to believe if you are in the throes of a recent diagnosis or struggling with treatment. However, not all people diagnosed with cancer physically succumb to the disease. And even among those who do die from cancer-related causes, there are some who experience tremendous wellness and healing in the process. Cancer offers an opportunity for deep reflection and introspection, no matter what the outcome of the disease. It helps us consider the whole of life rather than the sum of its material parts.

Coping with cancer requires us to first embrace it. After it shakes us to our very core, we concede the emotional storm it has created. During a conversation with mind-body-spirit pioneer Rachel Naomi Remen, MD, who has worked with thousands of cancer patients, she explained that ignoring fear can prevent us from healing. She recommends that people with cancer invite it in. "Although it is expressed in a very constricting way, fear is the will to live. What's under the fear is a desire for life, and we need to somehow get to that. That means going through the fear, not denying it." Discovering our inner strength enables us to face the unknowns associated with a cancer diagnosis. Over the years, Dr. Remen has found that "the experience [of having cancer] can be transformative."

For both patients and their loving supporters, this will be a highly individualized and personal process. There is no right way to cope with cancer. Whether you are the one with the diagnosis or a loved one is, you will want to patiently take one step at a time. The first step is to understand what cancer is.

Cancer Defined

Technically, cancer is not one disease. It is a complex illness with more than 200 variations. A cancer malignancy is characterized as a locally invasive and destructive growth pattern caused by the development of genetically altered cells. The cancer is typically designated based on the organ it originates in. There are five major types of cancer:

- *Carcinomas*, the most common type of cancerous growth, are solid tumors that may affect almost any organ or part of the body. They can spread to other parts of the body via the lymphatic fluid or the bloodstream. Carcinomas may occur in the skin, mouth, nose, throat, lungs, genitourinary and gastrointestinal tracts, and glands, such as the breasts or thyroid.

- *Leukemias* form in the blood and bone marrow and are not solid tumors. The abnormal white blood cells associated with leukemias replace healthy white blood cells and circulate throughout the bloodstream.

- *Myelomas* are tumors that originate in bone marrow plasma cells, the antibody-producing white blood cells. Myelomas were formerly considered rare, but their incidence is increasing.

- *Lymphomas* are cancers found in the glands and nodes of the lymphatic system. Lymph nodes are the body's filtering system, helping to remove toxins and impurities. These small, round masses of tissue are concentrated in the neck, groin, armpits, spleen, center of the chest, and around the intestines. Lymphomas are solid tumors usually made up of abnormal white blood cells. Hodgkin's and non-Hodgkin's lymphoma are the most common forms of lymphatic cancer in the United States.

- *Sarcomas* are the rarest of the five types. Sarcomas are solid tumors that arise from connective tissue, such as bone and muscle. Sarcomas can also form in the surrounding connective tissues of major organs, including the bladder, kidneys, liver, lungs, and spleen.

The process of developing cancer is known as carcinogenesis, which literally means "the birth of cancer." The cancer process begins with damage to a cell. Specifically, one or more genes in cellular DNA (deoxyribonucleic acid) become damaged, which is referred to as genetic mutation. This is significant because DNA is the critical information-carrying part of the cell. When the DNA is repeatedly damaged, the cell loses its ability to repair the damage, begins to behave abnormally, and divides uncontrollably. Scientists have confirmed that genetic mutations activate the process of carcinogenesis. This becomes important when considering ways to prevent cellular damage to ward off cancer, something we'll discuss in subsequent chapters.

As damaged or malignant cells divide, more mutations occur, a process known as promotion. Malignant cells eventually become numerous enough to join together to form a solid tumor, or they simply circulate throughout the body, wreaking havoc on other healthy cellular systems. Most anticancer therapies attempt to halt the growth of cancerous cells. Radiation therapy and some chemotherapy agents damage DNA so much that the malignant cells can no longer divide; instead, they undergo a process either of cellular rupture and destruction or of apoptosis, which may be thought of as cellular suicide. Other chemotherapy agents interrupt the process of cell division, effectively halting cellular replication and eventually sending the cell down the path of apoptosis.

How Does Cancer Grow?

Rapidly growing cancer cells are not only hearty, they are demanding. Their appetite for nutrients, oxygen, and blood far exceeds that of healthy cells. At the same time, they can also survive under a variety of internal conditions. According to a recent issue of *Cancer Research*, Japanese researchers discovered that, despite their voracious needs, cancer cells also have an amazing ability to tolerate extreme conditions, including a low supply of nutrients and oxygen. They discovered that cancer cells have the ability to modify their energy metabolism to sustain growth while simultaneously minimizing their need for nutrients and energy. Cancer cells can also develop resistance to specific chemotherapy drugs. It is this adaptability and resilience that makes cancer such a daunting and dangerous opponent.

Like a biochemical vampire, the cancer cell's nectar of choice is blood. The human body is fertile ground for these bloodthirsty cells. As long as the cancer cell has access to blood, it is less likely to die. In fact, cancer cells go to great lengths to ensure they have a sufficient blood supply. The body's process for developing blood vessels is known as angiogenesis. Cancer cells hijack this mechanism by sending signals to existing blood vessels, redirecting their growth and creating their own blood supply. Finding ways to shut down the blood supply to a cancerous tumor, known as antiangiogenesis, is critical to stopping its growth. Tumor cells produce vascular endothelial growth factor (VEGF) to help create new networks of blood vessels that will grow toward the tumor. Drugs and natural substances that block the action of VEGF will prevent the formation of new blood vessels and in so doing deprive the tumor of the nutrients it needs to grow, thrive, and spread.

Cancer cells aren't bound by the same rules of internal cellular control as are normal cells. Self-preserving cancer cells produce telomerase, an enzyme that allows the cancer cell to override the process that normally limits the life span of the cell. The presence of telomerase contributes to the abnormally long life of a cancer cell. Another critical internal control mechanism that has gone awry in cancer cells has to do with repairing cellular damage. Healthy cells contain tumor suppressor genes, which suppress cell division to allow a damaged cell to repair itself or, if the damage is too great, to self-destruct (as mentioned previously, this is known as apoptosis). Tumor suppressor genes are often underactive in cancer cells. The most recognized tumor suppressor gene is p53. Unfortunately, this key gene is one of the genes most susceptible to damage. In fact, p53 is damaged in over 50 percent of all cancers. This can be caused by a variety of toxic and inflammatory insults that cause oxidative damage to the gene. Some people also inherit a susceptibility to sustaining damage to this tumor suppressor gene. If the p53 tumor suppressor gene can't do its job, cancer cells are free to break the rules and continue dividing despite being damaged. Finding effective ways to stimulate apoptosis in cancer cells before they become too resistant and overpowering is a critical component in any integrative treatment approach. At present, a great deal of cancer research is focused on compounds that can activate tumor suppressor genes or can stimulate apoptosis.

Unfortunately, cancer is adaptable and those cancer cells that are best adapted will survive, with their survival characteristics becoming stronger

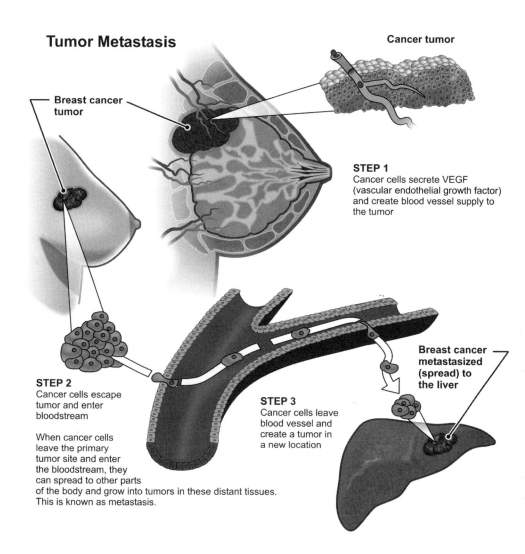

Tumor Metastasis

Cancer tumor

Breast cancer tumor

STEP 1
Cancer cells secrete VEGF (vascular endothelial growth factor) and create blood vessel supply to the tumor

STEP 2
Cancer cells escape tumor and enter bloodstream

When cancer cells leave the primary tumor site and enter the bloodstream, they can spread to other parts of the body and grow into tumors in these distant tissues. This is known as metastasis.

STEP 3
Cancer cells leave blood vessel and create a tumor in a new location

Breast cancer metastasized (spread) to the liver

with each new generation of cells. Basically, cancer will do everything it can to survive and grow. Unlike healthy cells, cancer cells that metastasize (move from one part of the body to another) exhibit little or no cell-to-cell adhesion. Most cells in the body—other than circulating blood cells—bond with one another to form well-defined tissues. Cancer cells, on the other hand, are free agents thoroughly adapted to foster their own growth and movement. Once metastasis has occurred, cancer becomes more powerful and much more difficult to treat. This is when cancer can be most life-threatening.

While it is clearly a complicated disease process, carcinogenesis and tumorigenesis are examples of basic biology gone awry. What should be a simple biological procedure of cell division and growth can quickly turn into a chaotic and complex illness. A seemingly innocent mutation multiplies exponentially with no boundaries or limitations, following its own rules. The aggressive intruder then steals oxygen, nutrients, and blood from unassuming healthy cells in order to survive and thrive. A bountiful blood supply, growth factors, circulating hormones, and many other contributors encourage its growth and sustainability. From this process, the life-changing diagnosis of cancer emerges.

Cancer Diagnosis

Treatment success is dependent upon accurate information. It is important to determine exactly where the cancer exists and the type of cancer cells present.

The primary cancer site is the part of the body where the cancer first develops. Even if the cancer spreads to other parts of the body, it is always described in terms of the primary site. For example, if pancreatic cancer spreads to the liver, it is still referred to as pancreatic cancer; specifically pancreatic cancer metastatic to the liver. According to the National Cancer Institute's Surveillance, Epidemiology, and End Results (SEER) training module, knowing the primary site is critical in diagnosis and treatment because it may help determine how the tumor will behave. The most common primary cancer sites are the skin, lungs, breasts, prostate, and colon.

The main techniques used to determine if cancer is likely to be present are as follows:

- Direct observation, including signs and symptoms
- Advanced imaging technologies
- Lab tests

Ultimately, diagnosis depends upon looking at the suspicious tissue under a microscope. Tissue must be removed for this microscopic evaluation. This procedure is called a biopsy. The National Cancer Institute textbook *Informed Decisions* states that "biopsy is preferred to establish, or rule out, a diagnosis of cancer." This confirmation provides conclusive evidence needed to avoid misdiagnosis. Testing of cancerous tissue samples can also provide valuable information regarding type, grade, and stage, which will help determine the most effective treatment plan.

Cancer Terminology

Tumor size and aggressiveness become critical when determining treatment and prognosis. One measure of aggressiveness is cellular differentiation. Cellular differentiation refers to the process whereby cells progressively acquire

Can Animal Intuition Diagnose Cancer?

For years, dogs have been trained to assist people who are impaired physically or visually. They can sniff out bombs, drugs, and victims of disaster. Is it possible then that your faithful pooch can detect cancer?

According to researchers at the Pine Street Foundation in San Anselmo, California, the answer is a resounding yes. Their pilot study, featured in the journal *Integrative Cancer Therapies*, demonstrated that five ordinary household dogs could be trained to detect cancer by smelling exhaled breath samples. The dogs were trained in a matter of weeks. If they detected cancer, they were to stay in front of the sample. If they did not detect cancer, they were to ignore the sample.

The researchers found that overall sensitivity of dog detection compared to biopsy-confirmed conventional diagnosis was an amazing 99 percent for lung cancer and 88 percent for breast cancer. These diagnostic results are comparable to chest X-ray for lung cancer and mammography for breast cancer. The researchers speculate that the dogs could have been responding to odors caused by cancer symptoms such as inflammation, infection, or necrosis (tissue death) rather than the cancer itself.

This was a blind study, meaning that the dog handlers and experimental observers did not know which breath samples were from diagnosed cancer patients and which were from the control group, people who did not have cancer. In addition, the dogs did not have any previous encounters with the participants who gave the samples.

Previous studies have confirmed that there are distinguishable biochemical patterns in exhaled breath. Unfortunately, we have yet to develop a technology that can use these patterns for accurate diagnosis. In the meanwhile, perhaps our canine companions can be trained to provide an effective and low-cost method of early cancer detection.

the individual characteristics of their fully mature cell type. Cancer cells are typically poorly differentiated, or immature, cells. At birth, a human infant has about five trillion cells differentiated into about 100 different cell types. For example, red blood cells have the designated duty of transporting oxygen and carbon dioxide. White blood cells, on the other hand, are charged with the task of destroying foreign organisms or scavenging and cleaning up damaged cells. All of the body's differentiated cells are programmed to live, die, and be replaced on a specific schedule. Without this differentiation, cancer cells do not function as normal cells.

A pathology report from biopsied tissue determines how closely the cancer cells resemble normal, healthy cells. In a poorly differentiated cancer, the tumor cells bear almost no resemblance to normal cells of that particular tissue. Cancer cells that do not resemble the healthy cells associated with that tissue are referred to as undifferentiated. This system of cell differentiation is used to help "grade" the cancer. The higher the grade, the more undifferentiated, aggressive, and difficult to treat the cancer is. This means that the prognosis is usually much more positive with grade 1 cancers than grade 4 cancers.

The Major Players of Your Immune System

The immune system guards the body against foreign and disease-producing substances. It is a complex system that relies on many different players and a variety of feedback mechanisms. Its workers are various white blood cells, including 1 trillion lymphocytes and 100 million trillion antibodies produced and secreted by the lymphocytes. Because of the importance of the immune system in preventing and treating cancer, it's important to understand the key players in this team effort.

Lymphatic system: This system encompassing capillaries and blood vessels, lymph nodes, the spleen, and the thymus collectively absorbs tissue (lymph) fluid and circulates it toward the major veins in the torso of the body. Bacteria and other disease-causing organisms in the fluid are destroyed as it moves through the lymphatic system, before it is returned to the blood.

Lymph fluid: Lymph fluid flows throughout the body in the lymphatic vessels, helping to maintain the fluid level of cells. It delivers nutrients to cells and carries waste products to the bloodstream for elimination. The human body has one to two quarts of lymph fluid, accounting for 1.5 to 3 percent of body weight.

Lymph nodes: These clusters of immune tissue work as filters or "inspection stations" for detecting foreign and potentially harmful substances in the lymph fluid. Cells inside the lymph nodes examine the lymph fluid, collected from body tissues, for foreign matter. While the body has many dozens of lymph nodes, they are mostly clustered in the neck, armpits, chest, groin, and abdomen.

Leukocytes: This is another name for white blood cells. Leukocytes are divided into two types—granulocytes (neutrophils, basophils, eosinophils) and agranulocytes (monocytes and lymphocytes)—according to the shape of the nucleus and the presence or absence of granules within the cells. Leukocytes, formed in the bone marrow, spleen, and thymus, destroy infectious organisms, clean up damaged cells, and begin the cellular repair process. Leukocytes travel within the lymphatic system and penetrate into tissues in response to chemical alarm signals sent by injured tissues.

Neutrophils: These white blood cells are formed in the bone marrow and released into the blood, where they comprise 54 to 65 percent of the total number of leukocytes. The principal activity of the neutrophil is to ingest foreign particles, especially virulent bacteria and fungi.

Lymphocytes: A type of white blood cell, lymphocytes usually constitute 25 to 33 percent of the total count, but their numbers increase during infection. Produced in the bone marrow and found in lymph nodes, lymphocytes come in two forms: T cells, which are matured in the thymus gland and have many functions in the body's immune response; and B cells, which produce antibodies to neutralize antigens (molecules on the surfaces of damaged cells or bacteria). Lymphocytes are found in high numbers in the lymph nodes, bone marrow, spleen, and thymus gland.

T cells: T cells specialize their immune function to become helper T cells, suppressor T cells, or natural killer cells. Helper T cells facilitate the production of antibodies by the B cells. Suppressor T cells suppress B cell activity.

Antibodies: These protein molecules are made from amino acids by B lymphocyte cells in the lymph tissue. They are set in motion by the immune system against a specific antigen (a molecule that damaged cells or bacteria display, which acts as a signal for immune activity). Also referred to as immunoglobulins, antibodies may be found in the blood, lymph, colostrum, and saliva and in the gastrointestinal and urinary tracts, usually within three days after the first encounter with an antigen. The antibody binds tightly with the antigen as a first step in removing the cell or organism from the system or destroying it.

Immunoglobulins: Another name for antibodies. Each lymphocyte produces a specific antibody, or immunoglobulin. There are five main types of immunoglobulins, grouped according to their concentration in the blood: IgG, IgA, IgM. IgD, and IgE.

Natural killer cells: Natural killer cells (NK cells) are a type of nonspecific, free-ranging immune cell produced in the bone marrow and matured in the thymus gland. NK cells can recognize and quickly destroy virus and cancer cells on first contact. Armed with an estimated 100 different biochemical poisons for killing foreign proteins, they can kill target cells without having encountered them previously. As with antibodies, their role is surveillance, to rid the body of foreign or aberrant cells. NK cells can destroy cancerous cells before they multiply and cause disease. Decreased numbers of NK cells have been linked to the development and progression of cancer, as well as chronic and acute viral infections and other deficiencies of the immune system.

Phagocytes: White blood cells that ingest and destroy microorganisms, cell debris, and other particulate.

Macrophages: Macrophages are the mature form of the white blood cells known as monocytes, which are produced in the bone marrow, then circulate in the bloodstream for a few days before entering tissues, where they develop into macrophages. Macrophages can "swallow" germs and foreign proteins, then release an enzyme that chemically damages, kills, or neutralizes whatever is ingested. The name means "big" (*macro*) "swallower" or "eater" (*phage*). Macrophages are the filter feeders of the immune system, ingesting everything that is not normal, healthy tissue, even old body cells or cancer cells.

Cytokines: A grouping of distinct proteins produced primarily by white blood cells, cytokines act as signals to other immune cells to regulate inflammation or other immune responses. Cytokines include monokines, lymphokines, interleukins, interferons, tumor necrosis factor, erythropeitin, and colony-stimulating factors.

Interferon: Familiar to many as a cancer treatment, interferon is a natural protein produced by white blood cells in response to a virus or other foreign substance. Interferon enables virally infected cells to be recognized and killed by T lymphocytes and also stimulates macrophages.

Interleukins: A type of cytokine that enables communication among leukocytes and other cells active in an inflammatory or immune response.

Thymus: Located behind the breastbone, the thymus is a lymphoid organ that secretes thymosin, a hormone that strengthens immune response. The thymus is also where T cells mature into fully functioning cells. Once mature, the T cells migrate to other lymphoid tissue such as the spleen and lymph nodes, where they control immune responses. The thymus gland grows until puberty and begins to shrink during adulthood, once it has produced the majority of T cells needed for a fully functional immune system.

Spleen: Located near the stomach, the spleen is like a large, spongy lymph node except that it filters blood rather than lymph fluid. Blood enters the spleen and travels through progressively smaller vessels and through the inner pulp of the spleen. Bacteria, foreign particles (antigens), and damaged and old red cells are trapped in the spleen and eliminated.

The National Cancer Institute's grading system is as follows:

- Grade 1 = well differentiated
- Grade 2 = moderately differentiated
- Grade 3 = poorly differentiated
- Grade 4 = undifferentiated

In addition to receiving a grade, some cancers are also referred to as having stages. Cancer develops over time, sometimes quietly with little or no warning, and sometimes very rapidly. In the continuum of cancer progression rates, quick metastasis (spreading) lies at the most dangerous end of the spectrum. Some cancers are aggressive and fast moving, while others are more indolent, demonstrating far less activity than their dangerous counterparts. Cancer can be detected at any stage along its growth and development continuum.

The system of stages is conventional medicine's method of describing the extent of the disease at the time of diagnosis. Staging allows the doctor to determine a prognosis and recommend a regimen of treatment. The stage of a particular cancer is based on the tumor's size and location and whether it has spread. The primary stages are as follows:

- Stage I is the earliest, most curable stage, with only local tissue involvement.

- Stage II cancer has spread to some surrounding tissues and perhaps to nearby lymph nodes.

- Stage III cancer has metastasized to distant lymph nodes.

- Stage IV cancer has spread to distant organs or other parts of the body; this stage is the most advanced and difficult to treat.

Other systems and terminology are also used to describe cancers. For example, in the TNM system (tumor, nodes, and metastases), T indicates the size and extent of the primary tumor, N indicates involvement of nearby lymph nodes (if any), and M indicates distant metastases. An example for breast cancer would be T2 N1 M0, which indicates that the tumor is of a moderate size and has spread to nearby lymph nodes but not to more distant parts of the body. The term *in situ* describes cancer that hasn't spread beyond the localized layer of cells where it developed. An invasive cancer, on the other hand, has spread beyond the layer of tissue in which it originated.

For a tumor located in a part of the body where it can be felt, imaging is still required in order to determine its accurate size. Imaging is also an important way to detect tumors at an earlier stage in their growth. A tumor that is detected by touch is larger than a tumor that can only be detected by ultrasound. For example, the average size of a breast tumor when first detected by mammography is about 800 million cells, or about ⅛ of an inch in diameter. However, the average size of a breast tumor found manually is about 1 inch in diameter, which represents about 2.5 billion cells. You can see that there is a big difference.

The Body's Ability to Heal

Is cancer overwhelming? Yes. Is it insurmountable? Absolutely not. Just ask the more than ten million people in the United States who have a history of cancer. The human body is designed to win this battle. In fact, most all of us have circulating cancer cells—the only reason we don't have a diagnosis of cancer is because we have been successful in destroying and eliminating these cancerous cells. We each have body systems, cells, and pathways set up to help prevent and defeat cancer. Diet, lifestyle, the external environment, and genetic makeup all influence the body's ability to fight cancer. Altering these influences where possible and supporting the body's anticancer processes are critical components of any cancer prevention and treatment plan.

The cornerstone of integrative cancer prevention and treatment is supporting the body's natural ability to protect and heal itself. Conventional oncology severely underestimates the body's potential for self-healing. The body has an innate cellular system of checks and balances that works to keep us well. This internal system normally prevents cells from duplicating too many times. Every time a normal cell divides, it loses a part of itself. Eventually, it cannot duplicate, and finally it dies, sometimes to be replaced. Aging is associated with more cells dying than are being replaced.

Although cancer is cunning and adaptable, don't underestimate the immune system, the body's first line of defense against invaders. A sophisticated and intelligent network of cells focused on communicating with one another, the immune system has its own army of cancer killers that circulate throughout the entire body. The body contains a legion of immune system cells— 1 trillion white blood cells alone—which join forces with trillions of antibodies, lymphocytes, T cells, natural killer cells, macrophages, and others to create a formidable anticancer team (for more about these cells, see the sidebar "The Major Players of Your Immune System" on pages 10 to 11). It is a massive effort of more than 20 trillion immune system cells working tirelessly on your behalf. (The role of the immune system in the prevention and control of cancer will be discussed more thoroughly in chapter 8.)

The immune system isn't alone in playing a significant role in preventing and treating cancer. Researchers have discovered that other key body functions are just as critical. Your body's status in regard to the following factors can have a major impact:

- Inflammation

- Hormonal influences

- Insulin resistance

- Digestion and detoxification

Understanding the connection between these body systems and cancer prevention and treatment is absolutely critical, so we've included an entire chapter on each. But first, we need to look at potential causes. In order to effectively prevent and treat cancer, we need to understand its causes as best we can. There are a number of known and speculated causes of cancer, and the next chapter is devoted to this complex and important topic.

two

Causes and Diagnosis of Cancer

Every one of the more than 200 different types of cancer starts the same: After a cell mutates, instead of destroying itself it multiplies uncontrollably. Nature has designed our cells to divide a finite number of times. While we are still in the womb, we automatically stop producing the cell-dividing enzyme telomerase. Researchers from the Swiss Cancer Research Institute have speculated that the shutting down of this enzyme is a mechanism designed to protect us from cancer. They describe normal cells as tightly packaged coils and go on to explain that cancer cells unravel the coil and flip the telomerase enzyme switch back on. This enables the cancer cells to divide infinitely and spread.

Cancer is caused by many contributing factors collaborating over a long period of time. The causes of cancer are difficult to identify because it takes years for these interdependent precipitating elements to culminate into a cancer diagnosis. But why do some people get cancer while others remain cancer free?

The American Cancer Society's book *Informed Decisions* offers this perspective: "The very fact that only some of the people exposed to most cancer-causing agents develop the disease proves its multi-step nature. If there were a single, or simple, cause, then everyone, or nearly everyone, would fall ill."

Although in general we cannot pinpoint a single cause of cancer, we can identify cancer-causing agents (carcinogens) and cancer-promoting activities that work together to encourage the development and spread of cancer. Cancer causes, which are as varied and individualized as cancer itself, can be

Do Parasites Cause Cancer?

In some parts of the world, people are exposed to parasites; if left untreated, they can remain in the body for extended periods of time. During this time, significant inflammatory damage can be done to the digestive tract, liver, and in some cases distant organs. Is cancer part of this damage? While some people believe that parasites can cause cancer, there is no scientific evidence to support this direct link. At best, a parasitic infection could contribute to inflammation and additionally deplete certain nutrients, which in turn could increase the possibility of other cancer-causing agents stimulating carcinogenesis. However, this is theoretical. It can be dangerous to assume that an undiagnosed parasitic infection is the cause of someone's cancer and then launch into an antiparasite supplement program as a sole cancer treatment. The antiparasite program will not stop the cancer. More appropriate treatment should not be delayed in favor of an antiparasite program.

controllable, uncontrollable, external, or internal. Although the potential causes of cancer are numerous, they can be placed into these basic categories:

- Genetics and family history (5 to 10 percent)
- Obesity and dietary habits (35 percent)
- Environmental influences (25 percent)
- Lifestyle factors (30 percent)

Even in the case of genetic cancers, the activation of the gene may depend on a variety of factors. There is also a distinct difference between genetically caused cancers and cancers that arise from family history.

Genetics and Family History

The same system that created us is what cancer uses to overtake us: cell division. We begin as a single cell that divides after fertilization. The division continues: Two cells become four, then eight, and so on. By the time we reach adulthood, we are made up of about 75 trillion cells.

In the center of each cell (the nucleus) there are DNA molecules that contain our genetic information, passed down from our parents. DNA directs whether we will be tall or short or have brown or blue eyes. Heredity is the transmission of these genetic characteristics to the child.

We know that damage to DNA can cause cancer to develop. Genetically influenced cancers develop when a specific mutation is passed on from one generation to the next. Although the mutation is transferred, the inevitability of cancer is not. In some cases, the chance of developing cancer due to a genetic mutation is very high. But in most cases, genetics determine a propensity toward the development of cancer but don't predict it conclusively. We are not indelibly tattooed with the same destiny as our parents. If that were the case, there would be no individuality or uniqueness. And while we inherit a specific genetic code, we are also influenced by our surroundings, diet, lifestyle, and emotions.

In fact, genetic cancers are considered uncommon. Overall, genetic cancers only make up about 5 percent of all cancers. With breast and ovarian cancer, the percentage increases to about 10 percent. That means 90 to 95 percent of all cancers have nothing to do with inheriting a deformed gene.

A variety of studies involving identical twins have demonstrated that while both twins have the same DNA, often only one develops cancer. In the case of breast cancer, if you have inherited the BRCA1 or BRCA2 gene, you have a 40 to 80 percent lifetime risk of developing breast or ovarian cancer before age 70. Considering that the average woman has a 12.7 percent risk of developing cancer over her lifetime, the contribution of the BRCA gene is significant and women with BRCA mutations need to be especially diligent regarding cancer prevention and early diagnosis.

The important descriptive word regarding genetic cancer is *predisposition*. While your genes may predispose you to getting cancer, you can utilize the prevention methods outlined in the next chapter to reduce the chances of any cancer genes becoming activated. Preventing cancer does not mean that you won't get cancer—it means that your chance of developing cancer is less.

Family history is quite different from genetic predisposition. While genetic cancers are always caused by inherited gene mutations, family history refers to a clustering of cancer cases in a family unit that may have causes other than a mutated gene. We've probably all heard the statement "cancer runs in my family." A family history of cancer is said to exist when a person has a first-degree relative (mother, father, sister, brother, or grandparent) with a certain type of cancer. Breast, ovarian, prostate, and colon cancers are most closely associated with a family history.

People with a family history of cancer may not have a specific mutated gene; rather, they may have "inherited" cancer-promoting activities. For instance, children of smokers are more likely to become smokers themselves. Thus, it is important to consider whether it is the cancer-promoting lifestyle that is passed on to the next generation, rather than a genetic mutation. Regardless, people with a family history need to be even more diligent about reducing or eliminating cancer risk factors. "Even with a family history," explain the authors of *How to Prevent and Treat Cancer with Natural Medicine*, "in most cases lifestyle and dietary factors have been found to have a greater impact than genetics on cancer risk."

Obesity and Dietary Habits

While a lower percentage of cancers can be attributed to a genetic mutation, a high percentage are directly related to obesity. In fact, recent studies have confirmed that being overweight or obese is responsible for one in six cancer

Body Mass Index Calculator

BMI	19	20	21	22	23	24	25	26
Height (feet, inches)				Body weight (pounds)				
4'10"	91	96	100	105	110	115	119	124
4'11"	94	99	104	109	114	119	124	128
5'0"	97	102	107	112	118	123	128	133
5'1"	100	106	111	116	122	127	132	137
5'2"	104	109	115	120	126	131	136	142
5'3"	107	113	118	124	130	135	141	146
5'4"	110	116	122	128	134	140	145	151
5'5"	114	120	126	132	138	144	150	156
5'6"	118	124	130	136	142	148	155	161
5'7"	121	127	134	140	146	153	159	166
5'8"	125	131	138	144	151	158	164	171
5'9"	128	135	142	149	155	162	169	176
5'10"	132	139	146	153	160	167	174	181
5'11"	136	143	150	157	165	172	179	186
6'0"	140	147	154	162	169	177	184	191
6'2"	144	151	159	166	174	182	189	197
6'3"	148	155	163	171	179	186	194	202
6'4"	152	160	168	176	184	192	200	208
	Healthy weight						Overweight	

deaths in the United States, second only to smoking. Overall, excess weight accounts for about 17 percent of cancer deaths. For men, being overweight increases the chances of dying of prostate cancer by 34 percent. For women, being heavy more than doubles the risk of dying of breast cancer.

Currently, the typical Western diet promotes obesity and thereby contributes to the development of cancer. In addition to adding pounds without purpose, a poor diet fails to nourish the important anticancer systems of our body. Remember, the body is designed to beat cancer, but it can only do the work when it is fueled properly. Asking your body to defend you against cancer without the proper nutrition would be like expecting your car to run after you have filled up the tank with water.

27	28	29	30	31	32	33	34	35
Body weight (pounds)								
129	134	138	143	148	153	158	162	167
133	138	143	148	153	158	163	168	173
138	143	148	153	158	163	168	174	179
143	148	153	158	164	169	174	180	185
147	153	158	164	169	175	180	186	191
152	158	163	169	175	180	186	191	197
157	163	169	174	180	186	192	197	204
162	168	174	180	186	192	198	204	210
167	173	179	186	192	198	204	210	216
172	178	185	191	198	204	211	217	223
177	184	190	197	203	210	216	223	230
182	189	196	203	209	216	223	230	236
188	195	202	209	216	222	229	236	243
193	200	208	215	222	229	236	243	250
199	206	213	221	228	235	242	250	258
204	212	219	227	235	242	250	257	265
210	218	225	233	241	249	256	264	272
216	224	232	240	248	256	264	272	279
Overweight			Obese					

Source: Adapted from *Clinical Guidelines on the Identification, Evaluation, and Treatment of Overweight and Obesity in Adults: The Evidence Report*. 1998. NIH/National Heart, Lung, and Blood Institute (NHLBI).

As a whole, people in the United States don't consume the anticancer nutrients we need; instead, we fill up on cancer-promoting foods like refined sugar, excess carbohydrates, fat, and meat. These foods weaken immunity, promote an inflammatory response, disrupt sugar metabolism, and stimulate the release of cancer-promoting hormones. (The complex interactions between foods, cancer, and these important body systems will be explained in much more detail in chapter 4.)

Recent research directly links excess weight to increased risk of death from cancer. That should provide good motivation to maintain a healthy, normal weight. Avoiding excess pounds, eating a healthful diet, and exercising is a direct and controllable way to help prevent cancer—and it's something you can start doing today. We will go into much more detail about diet and exercise later in the book.

Environmental Influences

An important factor in remaining disease free is maintaining or creating a healthy environment for optimal cellular functioning. Unfortunately, aspects of our environment are directly damaging to cells. The air you breathe, the water you drink, the food you eat, the chemicals you touch, and the devices you use (cell phones, microwaves, X-rays) can, to varying degrees, create cellular damage.

When this damage is to the DNA of our cells and is severe enough, the development of cancer can begin. Many environmental factors can make a person more vulnerable to cancer. These environmental factors are called carcinogens. To gauge your risk, see the chart "Evaluating Your Exposure to Environmental Toxins" beginning on page 24. Here are some of the most common environmental carcinogens:

● Agricultural use of pesticides and herbicides (see the sidebar "Organic: The Healthier Choice" on page 23)

● Genetically modified crops

● Hormones, such as estrogen, in the food supply

● Smoking and secondhand smoke

● Toxic chemicals released into the air, soil, and water such as asbestos, lead, and radon

● Occupational exposure to toxins such as benzene

● Ionizing and nonionizing radiation

● Home exposures, such as polybrominated diphenyl ethers (PBDEs), which are flame retardants used to treat upholstered chairs, sofas, foam mattresses, and cushions

● Cleaning products that contain chlorinated hydrocarbons, chloroform, and trihalomethanes

● Gardening pesticides and herbicides

● Paraphenylenediamine, parabens, phthalates, talc, and propylene glycol, found in hair products, cosmetics, deodorants, powders, skin creams, and nail polish

Exposure to carcinogens can increase the chances of developing cancer. The body has natural mechanisms in place to detoxify, repair, and rejuvenate, and it continually goes through a process of detoxification and repair in response to exposure to these substances. However, increasing external toxins can overwhelm these systems. The undetoxified carcinogens then damage cellular DNA and cause mutations.

The most troubling aspect of increasing environmental toxins is the negative health impacts these foreign compounds are having on our children. A recent study featured in the journal *Occupational and Environmental Medicine* confirmed a link between childhood leukemia and exposure to toxic pesticides in common household products.

Perhaps the most pervasive and offensive environmental carcinogen is secondhand smoke, which is especially harmful to children. Active smoking produces 50 different known carcinogens. Comparatively speaking, secondhand smoke is a toxic cocktail, containing 4,000 chemicals in a complex mixture in the smoke emitted from smoldering tobacco between puffs and exhaled smoke. The American Cancer Society estimates that secondhand smoke is responsible for about 3,000 lung cancer deaths among nonsmokers every year, further stating that "numerous studies have documented increased risk of lung cancer among nonsmokers exposed to secondhand smoke at work and at home." There is also thirdhand smoke, which is the residue from smoke that collects on smokers' hair, clothing, and furniture. This residue contains heavy metals, carcinogens, and trace radioactivity. Thirdhand smoke exposure is particularly dangerous to children who are more likely to touch these areas and then ingest these compounds. Lead is another major environmental culprit. This toxic metal is present in the air, soil, and water. Because of lead pipes and lead-based paints, older homes generally present a greater risk of lead exposure. Even low levels of this all-too-common metal have been linked to an increased risk of cancer.

Unfortunately, our drinking water—which should be a foundation of good health—is often burdened not just with lead, but with a wide variety of toxic substances. While chlorine does kill disease-causing microbes in the water, studies have demonstrated that it also creates toxic chemicals called trihalomethanes (THMs). THMs have been shown to cause cancer in animals and have been linked to miscarriage and other pregnancy risks in women. According to a Reuters Health report, there is a connection between THMs and human bladder cancer. Depending on the source of your drinking water, it may also contain toxic metals, radioactive minerals or radon, and a wide variety of synthetic and possibly toxic chemicals, including some that are added as part of the treatment process. Municipal drinking water may even contain prescription medications. According to a

2008 Associated Press investigation, there were numerous pharmaceuticals including estrogen, antibiotics, and mood stabilizers found in the drinking water of millions of homes.

Tap water isn't the only beverage to watch out for. The Environmental Working Group (EWG), a nonprofit environmental investigation team providing information about ways we can protect ourselves from environmental pollutants, issued a report warning that popular children's juices and sodas sold at major national retail outlets contain two ingredients that can form the toxic carcinogen benzene. "Benzene is a potent carcinogen that has no place in foods and drinks targeted to children," says Richard Wiles, senior vice president of EWG. In February 2006, the Food and Drug Administration (FDA) revealed that some soft drinks were found to contain benzene at levels up to 10 to 20 parts per billion, which is four times the acceptable limit in drinking water. Benzene has been linked to leukemia and other cancers.

According to a recent report in the *Journal of Midwifery and Women's Health*, contaminants that threaten children not only show up in soda pop and our water supply, they have also made their way into breast milk. The group of chemicals known as persistent organic pollutants (POPs) are chemicals that are either manufactured for a specific purpose or produced as a by-product of incinerated waste. These dangerous chemicals include dioxins, PCBs (polychlorinated biphenyls), and DDT, among others. Levels of PCBs in the breast milk of European and North American mothers are higher than those of women in nonindustrialized nations. PCBs are also found in meat and fish. As the report explains, "POPs are very stable compounds that are not readily degraded in the environment nor completely metabolized or excreted by organisms. As they are consumed and stored by one organism after another, these substances bioaccumulate in the food chain."

EWG, in collaboration with Commonweal, a nonprofit health and environmental research institute in Northern California, and Mount Sinai School of Medicine in New York, found an average of 91 industrial compounds, pollutants, and other chemicals in the blood and urine of nine volunteers. Altogether, a total of 167 different chemicals were found in these people, who do not work or live near an industrial facility.

Genetically modified crops are also problematic. Even though genetically modified foods have helped reduce hunger in famine-stricken regions around the world, the long-term risks are unknown. Impacts on human DNA (and that of other species) and potential cellular damage that may contribute to illness should be carefully evaluated. Until then, it becomes even more critical to eat organic foods whenever possible (see the sidebar "Organic: The Healthier Choice" on the opposite page).

Organic foods are produced without pesticides, synthetic fertilizers, antibiotics, supplemental hormones, or genetic engineering. They don't contain artificial ingredients and they aren't irradiated. Organic farmers often emphasize use of renewable resources as well as land and water conservation. Organic standards in the United States are currently regulated by the U.S. Department of Agriculture. These standards and the regulation of these standards continue to be hotly debated; however, we highly recommend choosing organic foods whenever possible.

Lifestyle Factors

Making healthful lifestyle choices will help reduce your chances of getting cancer. Conversely, some choices may increase your chances of getting cancer. For example, lack of exercise and increased consumption of alcohol are both linked to cancer. And smoking has been conclusively shown to cause cancer. Lack of exercise or physical activity influences cancer development and growth by encouraging excess weight and obesity. Sufficient exercise has a positive impact on metabolism, immunity, and elimination, so it only makes sense that exercise reduces the risk of cancer. Alcohol is often overlooked as a cause of cancer. A report on alcohol and cancer in the journal *Lancet Oncology* concluded that the more alcohol consumed, the higher the risk of developing cancer, especially cancers of the mouth, larynx, esophagus, liver, colon, and breast. There is some evidence that alcohol consumption may be linked to pancreatic and lung cancer as well.

Researchers at the National Institutes of Public Health in Denmark found that men who consume more than two drinks per day are more than three times more likely to develop rectal cancer as compared to nondrinkers. The study monitored nearly 30,000 Danish men. A study presented at the 41st Annual Meeting of the American Society of Clinical Oncology, in 2005, found that women who drank the equivalent of a half glass of wine a day were 6 percent more likely to develop breast cancer. Women who drank up to two glasses a day faced a 21 percent increased risk of breast cancer.

Organic: The Healthier Choice

Organic foods are gaining in popularity and availability throughout the world. This is good news not only for consumers, but also for our environment. Conventional farming not only contaminates the food that is grown, but also contributes to the pollution of our air, water, and soil. In addition, conventional farming practices strip our soil of health-promoting minerals and other nutrients. A Native American proverb states, "We do not inherit the earth from our ancestors, we borrow it from our children." Organic farming techniques help us take care of what we are borrowing. Organic foods are also better for our health in the long run.

Organic foods are free of added hormones, pesticides, synthetic preservatives, and other toxic compounds. It is especially important to choose meat and dairy from organically fed animals in order to avoid exposure to added hormones and antibiotics, which can damage our health when consumed frequently. Organic foods are better for our health, our environment, and frequently have higher nutrient content than the processed alternatives. According to a presentation by Charles Benbrook, PhD, at the Ecofarm 2009 conference, an evaluation of 236 studies demonstrated that organic foods were nutritionally superior in 61 percent of the cases.

Evaluating Your Exposure to Environmental Toxins

Cancer type	Substances that increase risk	People at special risk
Bladder	Cigarette smoke Artificial sweeteners Alcohol Arylamines Chlorinated drinking water Arsenic Coffee	• Those exposed to cigarette smoke • People working in the following industries: plumbing, heating, and air conditioning; rubber and plastic production; automotive parts and supplies; transportation and material moving; aluminum; leather; and dry cleaning • Teachers, records clerks, and housekeepers
Brain	Radiation and electromagnetic fields Chemicals such as polymers, iron, chromium compounds, lead, cadmium, aromatic hydrocarbon compounds, arsenic, mercury, and petroleum products	• Oil refinery and petroleum workers • Chemical, pulp, and paper workers • Cell phone users • Radiologists, medical workers, firefighters, butchers, computer workers, electricians and electrical equipment operators, farmers, janitors, painters, and those who work in food processing
Breast	Hormonal factors (hormone replacement therapy, oral contraceptives) Toxic chemicals, especially pesticides, heavy metals, organochlorines (DDT, hexachlorobenzene, dioxins), and air poluution Alcohol use and poor diet Smoking and secondhand smoke	• Individuals experiencing increased lifetime exposure to estrogen—those with earlier- or longer-duration menses, later menopause, or later-age pregnancy • Agricultural communities and others exposed to pesticides; those exposed to by-products of plastic production or plastic incineration • Those with a family history of breast cancer

Cancer type	Substances that increase risk	People at special risk
Kidney	Organic solvents such as trichloroethylene; pesticides and herbicides	• Agricultural communities and others exposed to pesticides • People working in the following industries: dry cleaning; railway; mining; and metallurgy
	Chemicals such as copper sulfates, benzene, benzidine, Creosol (present in asphalt) coal tar, soot and pitch	
	Mustard gas, vinyl chloride, and DNT (dinitrotoluene)	
	Cutting or lubricating oil	
Leukemias	Chemicals such as dioxins, benzene, and DDT	• Workers in industrial facilities—chemical manufacturing, gasoline storage, petroleum refineries, and coke ovens—as well as the automobile, dry-cleaning, and color printing industries • Dental and radiological technicians and radiation therapists • Agricultural workers
	Diagnostic radiation, such as X-rays	
	Air pollution: carbon monoxide, hydrocarbons, particulate matter, sulfur dioxide	
	Asbestos	
	Nitrous oxide gas (and other anesthetic gases used in surgery)	
	Industrial solvents	
	Aromatic hydrocarbons	
	Benzene and trichloroethylene	
	Cigarette smoke	
	Radon	
Lung	Chemicals such as dioxins, benzene, and DDT	• Those exposed to motor vehicle exhaust and petroleum products • Smokers and those exposed to secondhand smoke • Industrial workers exposed to asbestos: miners, mill workers, mariners
	Air pollution: carbon monoxide, hydrocarbons, particulate matter, sulfur dioxide	
	Asbestos	
	Cigarette smoke	
	Radon	

Evaluating Your Exposure to Environmental Toxins *(continued)*

Cancer type	Substances that increase risk	People at special risk
Lymphomas	POPs (persistent organic pollutants)	• Those experiencing breakdown of the immune system • Those exposed to environmental toxins, agricultural pesticides and herbicides, emissions from solid waste incinerators, dry-cleaning chemicals, household maintenance supplies
	Phenoxy herbicides (such as Agent Orange)	
	Chlorophenols	
	Dioxins, organic solvents, chlordane, PCBs (polychlorinated biphenyls)	
Myeloma (blood cancer)	Ionizing radiation	• Those with repeated infections or lowered immune functioning • Those exposed to cigarette smoke • Agricultural workers, as well as those exposed to benzene and other pesticides • Workers with higher exposure rates to chemicals
	Dark-colored hair dye	
	Agricultural and industrial chemicals: paints, petroleum, industrial solvents, pesticides	
	POPs (persistent organic pollutants)	
Prostate	Synthetic estrogens or estrogen-like compounds	• Those consuming food from cans lined with varnish • Users of plastic products (food wrap, test tubes, drinking water bottles) • Workers employed in agriculture, electrical utilities, coal-burning power plants, or hazardous waste incinerators or exposed to cement kilns • Those who work at or live near coal-burning power plants
	Alkylphenols	
	Pesticides, insecticides, and herbicides	
	PCBs (polychlorinated biphenyls)	
	Electromagnetic fields	
	Lead and cadmium	
	Bisphenol-A (BPA)	
Skin (Melanoma)	Sun exposure (harmful UV rays)	• Users of tanning equipment • People using pressure-treated wood • Agricultural workers and those exposed to weed killers, insecticides, and fertilizers • Those who work at or live near coal-burning power plants and those working with or exposed to high-voltage power lines or capacitor manufacturing • Workers in the electronics industry
	CFCs (chlorofluorocarbons) and PAHs (polycyclic aromatic hydrocarbons)	
	Solvents and other hazardous organic compounds such as benzene	
	Electromagnetic fields	
	Phenoxy herbicides (such as Agent Orange)	

Cancer type	Substances that increase risk	People at special risk
Testicular	Hormone-disrupting chemicals present in paints, pesticides, detergents, hair spray, perfume, car seats, vinyl flooring, wallpaper, and elsewhere	• Men whose water supply is contaminated with estrogen from birth control pill residues • Agricultural workers and those exposed to pesticides and herbicides • Plastics industry workers
	Xenestrogen chemicals: organochlorines, PCBs (polychlorinated biphenyls)	
	Phthalates	

Those who drank more than two drinks a day were 37 percent more likely to develop breast cancer. In menopausal women, the risk was even greater with a half glass of wine daily increasing their chance of breast cancer by 18 percent. Other studies have found similar results with other types of alcoholic drinks, thus the risk is due to the alcohol, not to the type of drink. It is now generally well established that one daily alcoholic drink increases the risk of breast cancer by approximately 10 percent.

Is There a Cancer Personality?

We've identified the major causes of cancer, but some people say there is a "cancer personality"—traits that may actually determine your risk of developing cancer. While it is interesting to explore such theories, this type of designation can be dangerous. The simple fact is, not every person with cancer is negative, mean, or unhappy; happy, nice, peaceful people get cancer too.

Does a person's attitude cause cancer? We believe not. Can a person's attitude contribute to successful prevention or treatment? We definitely say yes. Cancer development and growth has multidimensional influences. So, it makes sense that your attitude or your personality may play some role.

Some of the most interesting studies regarding cancer prevention and treatment involve humor. A literature review featured in the *Clinical Journal of Oncology Nursing* demonstrated the following benefits of humor:

● Assists with pain management and increases comfort levels

● Lessens anxiety and discomfort, helping cancer patients relax

● Positively affects immunity by increasing natural killer cell activity

● Improves physical stress responses and influences stress hormones to increase overall feelings of well-being

While we do not believe personality can cause cancer, we do feel that a positive attitude that includes laughter, love, and kindness will help strengthen any cancer treatment plan. Finding ways to appreciate and nurture the positive aspects of your life is an important part of cancer prevention and treatment. Early detection and diagnosis are equally as important as cancer prevention strategies.

Early Detection and Diagnosis

Without a doubt, treatment success and remission rates increase dramatically when the cancer is detected early—and the earlier, the better.

Prevention is the most important and reliable cancer-fighting tool that exists today. But because we cannot prevent cancer entirely, it is critical to detect it early. One of the hallmarks of an integrative treatment approach is to detect signs of cancer as early as possible, obtain appropriate treatment, and then take practical, proactive steps to prevent its recurrence.

Screening tests are different from diagnostic tests. Early detection occurs through screening, which is appropriate for people who do not have symptoms but are interested in uncovering illness at the earliest and most treatable stage (see the screening guidelines from the American Cancer Society beginning on the opposite page). Diagnostic tests, on the other hand, are for people who have symptoms and want to find the cause.

Screening and Early Detection

Early detection entails being diligent and taking responsibility. Part of this responsibility lies in becoming familiar with your body so that you can detect changes that might signify the development of cancer. (See the sidebar "Getting to Know Your Body" on page 37 for early detection tips.) In addition to self-examination, there are certain screening examinations and tests that may detect cancer early in its development. Sometimes, however, the mere thought of having a test that could uncover cancer can be paralyzing. Fear about the test outcome may cause people to avoid screening tests. But if they are ultimately diagnosed with cancer, these people have lost valuable time when their cancer might have been caught earlier and treated more effectively. The opposite is also true: People can obsess about early detection to the point where their fear disrupts their quality of life. Neither avoidance or overuse of screening tests is appropriate, but being vigilant and mindful about screening is of the utmost importance.

There are several types of screening tests. For a list of common screening tests, refer to the chart "Common Cancer Screening Tests" on page 33.

American Cancer Society Screening Guidelines for the Early Detection of Cancer in Average-risk Asymptomatic People

Cancer Site: Breast   Population: Women, age 20+

Test or Procedure	Frequency
Clinical breast examination (CBE)	For women in their 20s and 30s, it is recommended that clinical breast examination (CBE) be part of a periodic health examination, preferably at least every three years. Asymptomatic women aged 40 and over should continue to receive a clinical breast examination as part of a periodic health examination, preferably annually.
Mammography	Begin annual mammography at age 40.[1]

Cancer Site: Colorectal   Population: Men and women, age 50+

Test or Procedure	Frequency
Stool DNA test	Interval uncertain, starting at age 50
Flexible sigmoidoscopy, or	Every five years, starting at age 50
Fecal occult blood test (FOBT)[2] and flexible sigmoidoscopy,[3] or	Annual FOBT (or or fecal immunochemical test (FIT) and flexible sigmoidoscopy every five years, starting at age 50
Double-contrast barium enema (DCBE), or	Every five years, starting at age 50
Colonoscopy	Every 10 years, starting at age 50
CT colonography[4]	Every five years, starting at age 50

Cancer Site: Prostate   Population: Men, age 50+

Test or Procedure	Frequency
Digital rectal examination (DRE) and prostate-specific antigen test (PSA)	Health care providers should discuss the potential benefits and limitations of prostate cancer early detection testing with men and offer the PSA blood test and the digital rectal examination annually, beginning at age 50, to men who are at average risk of prostate cancer, and who have a life expectancy of at least 10 years.[5]

American Cancer Society Recommendations *(continued)*

Cancer Site: Cervix   Population: Women, age 18+

Test or Procedure	Frequency
Pap test	Cervical cancer screening should begin approximately three years after a woman begins having vaginal intercourse, but no later than 21 years of age. Screening should be done every year with conventional Pap tests or every two years using liquid-based Pap tests. At or after age 30, women who have had three normal test results in a row may get screened every two to three years with cervical cytology (either conventional or liquid-based Pap test) alone, or every three years with an HPV DNA test plus cervical cytology. Women 70 years of age and older who have had three or more normal Pap tests and no abnormal Pap tests in the past 10 years and women who have had a total hysterectomy may choose to stop cervical cancer screening.

Cancer Site: Endometrial   Population: Women, at menopause

Test or Procedure	Frequency
Women, at menopause	At the time of menopause, women at average risk should be informed about risks and symptoms of endometrial cancer andstrongly encouraged to report any unexpected bleeding or spotting to their physicians.

Cancer-related check-up   Population: Men and women, age 20+

On the occasion of a periodic health examination, the cancer-related checkup should include examination for cancers of the thyroid, testicles, ovaries, lymph nodes, oral cavity, and skin, as well as health counseling about tobacco, sun exposure, diet and nutrition, risk factors, sexual practices, and environmental and occupational exposures.

[1] Beginning at age 40, annual clinical breast examination should be performed prior to mammography.

[2] FOBT as it is sometimes done in physicians' offices, with the single stool sample collected on a fingertip during a digital rectal examination, is not an adequate substitute for the recommended at-home procedure of collecting two samples from three consecutive specimens. Toilet bowl FOBT tests also are not recommended. In comparison with guaiac-based tests for the detection of occult blood, immunochemical tests are more patient-friendly, and are likely to be equal or better in sensitivity and specificity. There is no justification for repeating FOBT in response to an initial positive finding.

[3] Flexible sigmoidoscopy, together with FOBT, is preferred, compared to FOBT or flexible sigmoidoscopy alone.

[4] Individuals with a personal or family history of colorectal cancer or adenomas, inflammatory bowel disease, or high-risk genetic syndromes should continue to follow the most recent recommendations for individuals at increased or high risk.

[5] Information should be provided to men about the benefits and limitations of testing so that an informed decision about testing can be made with the clinician's assistance.

Source: American Cancer Society. *Cancer Prevention & Early Detection: Cancer Facts and Figures 2009.* Atlanta: American Cancer Society, Inc.

Sometimes tests are done to screen for risk factors associated with cancer and not cancer specifically. For example, along with a Pap test, women can also be tested for human papillomavirus (HPV). HPV has a strong association with cervical cancer, so that is why many gynecological screenings include testing for HPV.

The majority of screening tests are used to survey the body or certain tissues for the presence of abnormal cancerous cells and tumors. These screening tests can uncover the presence of cancer at an early stage in its growth, allowing for more treatment options, including, in many cases, surgical removal of the cancerous tissue. However, some tests presently being used are not as sensitive as would be ideal. For example, a chest X-ray can be used to detect the presence of lung cancer, but by the time the cancer can be detected via a chest X-ray, it has already advanced to a stage that may make complete remission extremely difficult. For this reason, some lung cancer screening experts recommend annual ultrafast chest CAT scans for smokers over the age of 50.

Some screening tests can also yield false results—either negatives or positives. Either scenario is laden with its share of problems. A false negative can give a false sense of relief and delay treatment until a time when the cancer has grown to a stage that makes it much less treatable. A false positive, on the other hand, may cause the person to undergo treatment that is actually unnecessary and could be costly to their well-being. Fortunately, commonly recommended screening tests have very low rates of both false negatives and false positives. Additionally, most initial screening tests that yield a positive result are confirmed by follow-up tests to reveal any false positives and confirm true positives.

Two common statistical measures of the usefulness of a screening test are sensitivity and specificity. Sensitivity refers to the probability that a test will show a positive result when cancer exists; specificity is the probability that a negative test result occurs when cancer is absent. A test that has high sensitivity and high specificity is much less likely to cause false positives or false negatives. These values reflect the effectiveness of screening methods and help medical practitioners know how much they can rely upon the results of these screening tests. Common screening tests are continually evaluated for their sensitivity and specificity so that practitioners and the public can make informed decisions and be aware of the most advantageous times to obtain certain screening tests. This is why, for instance, it is not generally recommended that women under the age of 40 obtain annual mammograms. The natural density of breast tissue in women under 40 makes mammograms less accurate for this group, with low specificity and sensitivity resulting in false positives and false negatives.

Breast Thermography: Advances in Breast Imaging

Mammography has long been considered the gold standard of breast cancer screening. When combined with a physical exam, mammography can help detect cancer early. Unfortunately, mammography has the following limitations:

- It exposes the breast tissue to harmful radiation.

- It isn't sensitive to fast-growing tumors in the preinvasive stage.

- It's less sensitive for women using hormone replacement therapy.

- It's difficult to interpret findings in large, dense, or fibrocystic breasts.

- It cannot show areas near the chest wall in most women.

In addition, mammography does not detect ductal carcinoma in situ (DCIS), which is the most common precancerous abnormality (although it can detect abnormal calcification that may indicate DCIS).

Breast thermography is a new technology that provides women and doctors with an alternative or additional screening method. Using infrared sensors to detect heat and increased blood flow, it yields a computerized image that indicates suspicious areas in red. Research has demonstrated that cancerous tissue is hotter than noncancerous tissue. While some studies have deemed the temperature variance to be coincidental, Japanese researchers featured in *Surgery Today* confirmed a direct correlation between the results of thermography when compared to confirmed invasive ductal carcinoma.

Researchers featured in the *American Journal of Roentgenology* recommend using thermography along with mammography to determine if a tumor is benign or malignant. This could help avoid a large percentage of unnecessary biopsies performed as a result of false positives from mammograms. This would be extremely valuable, as approximately 85 percent of mammogram-initiated biopsies are found to be benign. Preliminary research indicates that thermography produces about 10 percent false positives. The study featured in the *American Journal of Roentgenology* included 875 biopsied lesions and demonstrated 97 percent sensitivity in predicting malignancies. A concern regarding breast thermography is that there is no certification available as of yet for thermographers. Until this certification exists, the quality of thermography can vary significantly from one center to the next.

While the research on breast thermography is still preliminary, the technique is safe and noninvasive and is likely to become an excellent adjunct to mammography. Thermography should not be used as a sole diagnostic measure. Many insurance companies will not cover this screening method because the technology is too new, but centers offering thermography are now available in most major cities.

When done at the right time, most screening tests have incredible value and can contribute positively to the fight against cancer. Beyond helping to find cancer when it is most treatable, test results from early detection techniques can also provide information that contributes to the success of the treatment plan. An ultrasound, for example, can help pinpoint location and size of a tumor prior to surgery, allowing for a more efficient and successful surgical removal.

Physical Exam

Physical examination is another important component of cancer screening. A physician performs a physical exam during an annual check-up to check for

Common Cancer Screening Tests

Test name	Description	Who benefits	Type of cancer detected	Comments
Pap	Gentle scrapings of cervical and vaginal tissue	Sexually active females and adult women	Cervical and vaginal	Noninvasive test; occurs as part of annual gynecological examination.
Mammogram	Radiographic imaging of breast tissue	Women	Breast	Routine mammograms every two years are recommended beginning at the age of 50, unless you have a high risk. This test results in some radiation exposure and discomfort due to breast compression during the examination.
Fecal occult blood test	Tests sample of feces for blood	Men and women	Colon	Positive results are not diagnostic, but require additional testing.
Colonoscopy	A flexible viewing tube allows visualization of the entire colon	Men and women	Colon	Inserted into the colon under light anesthesia.
Sigmoidoscopy	A flexible viewing tube allows visualization of the last part of the colon	Men and women	Colon	Requires no anesthesia.
Breast MRI	Magnetic resonance imaging of tissue	Women	Breast	Used as a screening test in high-risk women, especially with dense breast tissue.
Prostate-specific antigen (PSA)	Measures a specific protein in the blood released by prostate cells	Men	Prostate	Elevations in PSA are not necessarily diagnostic but do require further evaluation and ongoing monitoring.
Ultrasound (sonography)	High-frequency sound waves detect structural differences in examined tissue	Men and women	Breast, ovarian, heart, liver, bladder, testes	Noninvasive test with no known risks.

cancerous lumps, cancerous skin lesions, and other signs of organ distress that can be associated with cancer. An annual physical exam is especially important for women who are concerned about developing breast cancer. You should also do some self-screening by paying special attention to certain areas. Men can do a self-exam of the testicles, and women can do breast self-exams. It is a good idea to get to know your body. This will help you be aware of changes. For more information on what to look for, refer to the sidebar "Getting to Know Your Body" on page 37.

Proper Diagnosis

Different from screening, diagnostic testing is used to identify the cause of symptoms. The goal of diagnostic testing is to confirm the presence or absence of a disease. Undergoing diagnostic testing for cancer, while essential, is a process wrought with anxiety. Fear is opportunistic and often preys upon those beset by unknowns. For a person awaiting definitive test results, the cancer nightmare strengthens with each passing day. Knowledge is a gift that comes with a cancer diagnosis. The diagnosis is a life-changing shock, but power comes with the knowing.

Accurate diagnosis needs to happen in order to successfully treat cancer with an integrative approach—or any other approach. Results of diagnostic testing not only confirm or rule out cancer, they also help guide future decisions about treatment. Diagnostic testing clarifies the cause and location of symptoms and establishes the extent of the disease.

Remember, many symptoms that can be linked to cancer can also be tied to other, non-life-threatening illnesses. The presence of blood in fecal material, for example, can be the result of a variety of intestinal problems. Stomach pain can turn out to be an ulcer rather than stomach cancer. And a benign ovarian cyst can be the cause of menstrual irregularities. Diagnostic tests will help to determine the cause of these symptoms. The results of diagnostic testing may rule cancer out, or identify it as the likely cause of symptoms.

Before you agree to any diagnostic tests, the American Cancer Society recommends that you ask these key questions:

- What will we learn from this test?

- What are the alternatives to the test?

- What are the possible side effects, complications, or risks of the test?

- What happens during the test?

- Is any part of the test painful or uncomfortable?

- What further tests may be needed if the results are positive?

- Will this test be covered by my insurance?

Following are some of the most common methods used in conventional medicine to confirm or rule out a cancer diagnosis (listed in alphabetical order).

Biopsy: According to the American Cancer Society, "The most definitive diagnostic test is a biopsy, the removal of a piece of tissue for microscopic evaluation." A biopsy can be done via a needle aspiration, an endoscopy, or surgical removal. The type of biopsy performed depends on the location and size of the suspected tumor and the amount of tissue needed for an accurate diagnosis. Depending on what's required, this procedure can be done in a physician's office, an outpatient surgical facility using local anesthesia, or a hospital using general anesthesia. Depending on the location and the amount of tissue taken, a biopsy can have few complications or can be associated with discomfort, pain, bleeding, infection, or scarring.

Blood tests: There are two categories of blood tests: specific and nonspecific. Although blood tests are not used to determine a definitive cancer diagnosis, they do provide valuable information regarding overall health and organ function. Specific blood tests measure substances in the blood known as tumor markers. (For more information about tumor markers, see the sidebar on page 36.) Tumor markers may come directly from a tumor or may be a result of the body's response to a tumor. Tumor markers are not routinely used as general screening tests because some noncancerous lesions can elevate certain tumor markers. Plus, not all cancers shed tumor markers into the blood. However, in the context of a suspicious lesion or mass, tumor markers can help to confirm the need for further diagnosis and also can be used later to monitor the success of treatment interventions. Nonspecific blood tests include a complete blood count and blood chemistry test. These tests are used to detect the presence of anemia and immune system irregularities, and to look for chemicals in the blood that indicate organ dysfunction.

Computed tomography (CT) scan: A CT scan can be considered a hybrid X-ray combining radiography with computer technology. The scanner rotates to create a front-to-back, two-dimensional image of internal structures. No hospitalization is required. It offers more detail than a conventional X-ray, but involves higher exposure to radiation. According to the American Nuclear Society, a CT scan of the head and body delivers 110 millirems (mrem; the unit of measurement with radiation), while a film X-ray of the chest delivers 6 mrem. Nonetheless, CT scans are a critical part of most diagnostic (and staging) workups and help establish the presence, size, and location of tumor tissue.

Magnetic resonance imaging (MRI): MRI is an imaging technique that uses radio waves and magnetic fields to view the body from all directions. It produces a high-quality, two-dimensional image and is especially useful when dealing with areas that are difficult to view with a typical X-ray or CT scan, such as the brain or joints. It does not detect calcifications, which limits its ability to detect some precancerous and cancerous growths (for example, certain types of breast tumors).

Positron emission tomography (PET): A PET scan is a type of noninvasive nuclear medicine imaging. A PET scan measures important blood flow, oxygen use, and glucose (sugar) metabolism. Highly active (metabolic)

Tumor Markers in the Blood

"Since cancer is actually a hundred different diseases, it's unlikely that one test will screen all types of malignancies," explain the authors of *Informed Decisions*. "However, tests can now detect certain molecules, often a type of protein, produced by specific types of cancer."

These molecules, referred to as tumor markers, can be identified in the blood. While the idea of detecting cancer through a simple blood test is exciting, tumor markers are typically used to monitor treatment success after cancer is diagnosed. This is because other noncancerous conditions can also elevate tumor markers. The tumor marker tests are only useful once cancer has been diagnosed and once the cancer has been determined to cause elevations in its associated tumor markers. In this instance, the tumor markers can serve as reliable indicators of increased or decreased cancer growth. Some of the most established tumor markers include the following:

- Carcinoembryonic antigen (CEA) is elevated in colorectal, gastrointestinal, kidney, stomach, breast, pancreatic, liver, and lung cancers.

- Carbohydrate antigen 125 (CA 125) is primarily elevated in ovarian cancer but can be elevated in cancers of the endome-trium, pancreas, stomach, and colon, and especially with invasive cancers.

- Carbohydrate antigen 15-3 (CA 15-3) is elevated in breast cancer, especially if it has spread (metastasized) to other parts of the body.

- Prostate-specific antigen (PSA) is elevated in prostate cancer.

- Carbohydrate antigen 19-9 (CA 19-9) is elevated in pancreatic cancer and other cancers of the digestive tract.

Once again, elevated levels of these tests do not conclusively indicate cancer. For example, high levels of CA 125 can indicate endometriosis, pelvic inflammatory disease, benign ovarian cysts, or other gynecologic issues. CA 125 levels can even be elevated during menstruation or pregnancy. Elevated PSA can occur with prostatitis and enlarged prostate, which are both noncancerous conditions.

These tumor marker blood tests also miss cancers, and even when a low number is present cancer may still be found. Tumor markers can provide information, especially in the context of diagnosed cancer; however, this technology needs more research and fine-tuning before it can be a reliable diagnostic tool.

tissues including cancerous tumors utilize more glucose. Radioactive glucose is injected into the patient prior to the examination. The tissues with high glucose uptake are easily visualized in the PET scan. PET scans are often combined with CT scans to provide more complete information about suspicious areas.

Surgery: Exploratory surgery is performed when a physician wants to get a firsthand view of internal tissues and organs. Depending on what is found, tissue samples can be taken, or lymph nodes, tumors, or organ tissue may be removed. Diagnosis by surgery is not without risk. Exploratory surgery usually requires a hospital stay and a recovery time. Because visual inspection of the tissue does not suffice to confirm cancer, the removed tissue is usually analyzed microscopically afterward. One significant advantage of surgical diagnosis is the ability to do surgical staging, which uses the surgeon's visual and other findings to determine the overall stage of the cancer.

Getting to Know Your Body

The message of prevention is that cancer is most treatable in the earliest points of its development. The key is to detect the presence of cancer early enough that you can treat it with an immune-enhancing, body-supportive, nontoxic approach. This works best when the body's tumor burden is relatively small—in the earliest phases of the cancer's development.

Here are signs that may indicate the presence of cancer.

1. **A lump or thickening in the breast or testicles.** Self-examination of the breast and testicles offers the best protection against breast and testicular cancer. A lump or thickening in the breast, or any noticeable change in the testicles, is an early warning sign. Such signs are grounds for an immediate medical examination.

2. **A change in a wart or mole.** Changes in warts or moles may be indicative of melanoma or squamous cell carcinoma. Skin cancers may appear as dry, scaly patches, as pimples that never go away, or as inflamed or ulcerated areas. Warts or moles that grow or bleed and persistent mouth sores should be checked.

3. **A skin sore or a persistent sore throat that does not heal.** Sores that do not heal may also be indicative of melanoma. A persistent sore throat or hoarseness, a persistent lump in the throat, or difficulty swallowing may indicate cancer of the pharynx, larynx, or esophagus. These cancers are readily treated when caught early.

4. **A change in bowel or bladder habits.** Do not ignore ongoing urinary difficulty, constipation, chronic diarrhea, abdominal pains, rectal or urinary bleeding, or dark tarlike stools; these symptoms should be regarded as signs to seek professional help.

5. **A persistent cough or coughing up blood.** Coughs that become chronic, especially in smokers, should be checked. If there is a tumor in the air passages that lead into the lungs, they may be partially obstructed or irritated or even bleed. Coughing may be a sign of this obstruction or irritation.

6. **Constant indigestion or trouble swallowing.** Difficulties in swallowing or continued indigestion, nausea, heartburn, bloating, loss of appetite, or bowel changes may be symptoms of colon cancer or cancer of the stomach or esophagus. Unexplained weight loss is also an indicator that something may be wrong.

7. **Unusual bleeding or vaginal discharge.** The early stages of uterine endometrial cancer, later stages of cervical cancer, and some ovarian cancers can cause unusual bleeding or vaginal discharge. Prompt attention to these symptoms means a better chance of catching cancer at its most treatable stage. In the case of cervical cancer, Pap tests can detect problems before the later stages cause bleeding.

8. **Chronic fatigue.** General feelings of chronic fatigue accompany any type of cancer that is rapidly progressing. Fatigue along with decreased appetite and night sweats is particularly concerning and necessitates prompt evaluation.

If you are experiencing any of these signs or symptoms, contact your physician immediately.

Ultrasound: Because no radiation is used, ultrasound is considered one of the safest diagnostic methods for many cancers. It's also one of the most effective. Ultrasound involves using the echoes of high-frequency sound waves to create an image of the inside of the body. It is not effective in detecting brain, lung, or intestinal tumors because the sound wave cannot break through gas-filled spaces. It also cannot penetrate bone; however, it is effective at differentiating cysts from solid masses and can provide access to soft tissues that don't show up clearly with a conventional X-ray.

X-ray: This common diagnostic procedure involves sending high-energy beams of radiation through the body to create shadows on film. Bone and dense tissue are easily viewed on an X-ray because they show up white. X-rays are widely used because the technique is painless, easy, and fairly inexpensive. However, because of the dangers of radiation exposure, this evaluation should be used only when necessary. Because radiation exposure can be a cause of cancer, an effective prevention program involves reducing exposure to all sources, including excessive X-rays. If you feel uncomfortable receiving X-rays, discuss other options with your doctor.

Information Is Power

There can be false comfort in not knowing. Sometimes a potential answer is so frightening that we avoid asking important questions. We need to try to resist the temptation that allows fear to befriend our denial. Getting the answers we need helps us make informed decisions on how to move forward each step of the way. Early detection and accurate diagnosis of cancer segue into effective treatment and an improved prognosis. You can gain strength from the information you receive, no matter where you are in the process.

three

Prevention Is Paramount

Whether you are trying to prevent an initial diagnosis of cancer, or focusing on preventing a recurrence, the rules are the same. There are proactive steps you can take through diet and lifestyle. Surprisingly, however, there is actually still some debate about the topic of cancer prevention. Some authorities assert that cancer is one of the most preventable serious illnesses of our time. Other experts believe the basis for cancer is so entrenched in our genetic makeup that any effort to manipulate this genetic destiny is futile. The truth is likely someplace in the middle. While cancer is a disease of the genes, genetic expression is not static. Factors in our lives such as how we feel, what we are exposed to, what we eat, and how much weight we carry can influence and guide expression of our genes. These lifestyle factors can stimulate the repair of damaged genes and silence the expression of mutated genes. Conversely, lifestyle factors can also contribute to more genetic damage and promote the expression of already damaged genes.

Learning to Live Well

The ultimate demonstration of self-love and respect is to proactively nurture your body, mind, and spirit. The marriage of physical, emotional, and spiritual health is not only the foundation of cancer prevention, but also the key to achieving optimal wellness and vitality. Unfortunately, life can sometimes get in the way of living—especially healthy living.

Choosing Safe Skin Care Products and Cosmetics

By Myra Eby and Susan Mesko

The skin can be considered the largest organ of the human body. It provides an important protective barrier against hazardous materials and pathogens. And yet many of us choose to expose our skin to even more toxins. Every day researchers are learning more about the health risks of certain ingredients found in many skin care products and cosmetics. These ingredients have been found to be the culprit in health problems ranging from allergic reactions to birth defects to cancer.

Many of us are not fully informed about the ingredients listed (or not listed!) on the lotions and potions we so liberally apply to our skin. What do you really know about parabens, propylene glycol, quaternium-15, imidazolidinyl urea, diazolidinyl urea, and fragrances, just to name a few? One of the most interesting discoveries of skin care research is that up to 60 percent of your favorite skin care or cosmetic products may be absorbed through the skin, and that percentage continues to increase. This means that chemical preservatives, fragrances, fragrance maskers, coloring agents, and stabilizers in your body care products are being introduced into your bloodstream every time you apply a cream, lotion, deodorant, or anything else to your skin. These toxic ingredients are stored and can accumulate in the human fatty tissues, systemically affecting health and vitality.

The Environmental Protection Agency (EPA) has identified 5,000 different chemicals found in cosmetics alone. Let's take a look at some of the most common, and most toxic.

Parabens, such as ethyl-, butyl-, propyl-, and methylparaben, are generally used as preservatives. It is not uncommon to find at least two types in any given product. These chemical preservatives are found in almost all body care products and can easily accumulate inside various body tissues. One reason parabens are dangerous is because they mimic estrogen. Recent evidence indicates that topical parabens have been detected in human breast tumors. Women are especially at risk when using underarm deodorants containing parabens after shaving because shaving makes it very easy for these chemicals to enter the skin. This is also a vulnerable spot because of the concentration of lymph nodes located there, which are connected to breast tissue. Since parabens mimic estrogen, they can act as cell proliferators on estrogen-dependent breast cells.

Demands, commitments, pressures, and the fast-paced world we live in can make it difficult to cultivate and sustain healthy habits. Exercise is often bumped to next week's to-do list. We are continually tugged in different directions, yanked from the salad bar, and dropped in the fast-food drive-through line. Morning meditation is hijacked and replaced with coffee, muffins, and a meeting. Not to mention the fact that our world is full of dangerous and harmful chemicals—including the styrene in that disposable coffee cup, the plastic wrapper around that microwaved muffin, and the new carpet in the meeting room.

But for those of us trying to prevent a cancer recurrence, enhancing our overall health will help add quantity and quality to the years we have left. The first step in making changes and setting goals is to assess where you are right now. So to that end, and without judgment, take some time to evaluate your life. On a piece of paper, write down your answers to these questions:

Allergic hypersensitivity to parabens is also quite common.

Other preservatives, such as DMDM hydantoin, imidazolidinyl urea, and quaternium-15, create a chemical reaction that can release trace amounts of formaldehyde into the skin, causing a toxic effect at the cellular level. Formaldehyde can cause joint discomfort and many other health problems. Imidazolidinyl urea and diazolidinyl urea, the most commonly used preservatives after parabens, are also a primary cause of contact dermatitis, or skin inflammation.

Beware of personal care products containing phthalates (pronounced THA-lates), as these chemicals soak into the skin and accumulate over time. According to a study conducted by the Centers for Disease Control in 2000, more than 75 percent of Americans tested had traces of phthalates in their urine. Virtually all fragrances contain phthalates, and they're also commonly found in hair sprays and nail polish. Phthalates have been linked to liver toxicity and genital malformation and are suspected to contribute to cancer.

Synthetic colors are equally bad, as they can be carcinogenic. Avoid anything listing "FD&C" or "D&C" followed by a number as an ingredient.

Look for products containing natural coloring agents instead.

While vegetable oils may seem like a benign, or even healthful, ingredient, they can be problematic. Unless they are cold-pressed, they have a tendency to turn rancid relatively quickly. Free radicals are then created, setting up a carcinogenic environment in the skin. Avoid any products that contain oils not described as cold-pressed.

By making healthy choices for your skin, you are safeguarding your health. Take the extra moment to read labels carefully. Try to avoid products containing the previously mentioned toxins, and choose "all-natural" products whenever possible. However, be aware that just because a product is labeled "all-natural," that doesn't mean it is truly safe. If you are unsure about an ingredient, err on the side of caution and choose another product.

Myra Eby is the founder of MyChelle Dermaceuticals and Susan Mesko is an industry consultant. MyChelle Dermaceuticals is devoted to providing active and effective skin care products that are safe for consumers and the environment. It is one of only a few skin care lines completely free of parabens and other toxic ingredients.

1. How many hours a week do you spend working?

2. How many hours a week do you spend playing?

3. How many hours a week do you spend doing some type of spiritual practice (praying, meditating, volunteering, connecting with nature)?

Next, make a list of activities, things, and people that make you feel happy, at peace, and fulfilled. How many hours a week do you spend with those people or doing those things? At the end of your life, no matter when that occurs, what will you cherish more: money or moments; power or peace; chaos or caring? A life well lived is a life well loved, and that begins with self-love. Don't let everyday obstacles get in the way of such devoted self-love.

Be gentle with yourself. Consider following the 80/20 rule: If you make healthy choices 80 percent of the time, it is fine to bend the rules the other

20 percent. The idea is to make the effort and move in the right direction. You may not be able to achieve 80/20 right away, but you'll be surprised at how quickly you can get there. Who knows, there may be days, even weeks, when you make healthy choices 90 percent or even 100 percent of the time!

To prevent a cancer recurrence it is important to focus on diet, dietary supplements, the mind-body connection, and physical activity. Let's start by looking at diet.

The Power of Food

As a nation, we are obsessed with food. Fast-food restaurants and their billboards clutter our city streets. Volumes have been written on the topic of food. Newsstands are littered with magazines about it, and there is even an entire television network devoted just to food. We savor it, discuss it, and even plan our lives around it. And we consume a lot of it. In the process, we've also managed to supersize our health risks dramatically over the past few decades.

The kind of food eaten has nearly as big an impact on health as the amount—and sometimes more. In fact, much of the malnutrition in the world can be attributed to unhealthy food or consumption of "empty calories" (highly processed foods lacking important vitamins, minerals, and other essential nutrients). Though it may seem surprising, many obese individuals are actually significantly malnourished.

But foods have both the power to harm and the power to heal. Understanding both sides of the equation is important. Rather than allowing food to have power over you, you can create a winning partnership with it. Proactive cancer prevention shifts the energy, placing emphasis on healthful, fresh, and whole foods packed with essential nutrients, turning calories into cancer-fighting fuel.

Sometimes what we ingest has clear ramifications. If you drink coffee daily, think back to a time when you tried to give it up or had to do without. Remember the headache? Have you ever experienced heartburn after too many pieces of pepperoni pizza or constipation after eating too much cheese? The good news is that this dynamic works both ways. You can prevent ill effects by avoiding certain foods, and even better, you can enhance your health by making certain food choices.

Some foods contain significant nutrients that help keep your body healthy and operating at peak capacity. While it is true that different people have different dietary needs and that what is healthy for one person may not work as well for another, there are some common denominators. Here are just a few examples of cancer-fighting foods and spices:

- Tomatoes contain the powerful antioxidant lycopene, which supports a strong immune system.

- Whole grains contain lignans that positively influence hormonal activity.

- Citrus fruits contain flavonoids that enhance immunity.

- Soy contains certain sterols that can reduce the development of some cancer cells.

- Broccoli contains sulforaphane and other compounds that help stimulate detoxification and immunity.

- Cruciferous vegetables, such as cabbage, cauliflower, and brussels sprouts, contain indole-3-carbinol, which has been shown to have anticancer properties.

- The peel of an apple contains phenolic compounds that help prevent unhealthy cells from dividing and spreading.

- Kale is high in vitamins A and C, as well as fiber, which are all perfect nutrients to help prevent cancer.

- Garlic contains several key compounds that inhibit the activity of cancer cells and help with detoxification.

- Turmeric contains curcumin, a powerful anti-inflammatory substance, shown to help prevent and treat some cancers.

- Rosemary contains carnisol and other active compounds that can help prevent and treat cancer.

Many of these foods and spices share a common characteristic: They are colorful. At mealtime, look closely at your plate. If it is primarily white or beige, you need to add some color. Fruits and vegetables will add that color, as well as a healthy dose of potent anticancer nutrients. (For more information on specific nutrients to prevent cancer, refer to the chart "Healing Foods" on pages 46 and 47. Also, chapter 4 goes into more detail about how to build a strong anticancer foundation with foods.)

There is no question that diet plays a huge role in cancer prevention. According to a report by Dr. Edward Giovannucci, professor of nutrition and epidemiology at Harvard, at least 70 percent of colon cancers may be prevented with moderate changes in diet and lifestyle. He states that "many of the diet and lifestyle risk factors for colon cancer are the same for cardiovascular disease and for some other cancers, so focusing on the modifiable risk factors for colon cancer is likely to have many additional benefits beyond this cancer."

The ultimate cancer prevention diet should follow the simple guidelines outlined below.

Consume more	Consume less
Colorful fruits and vegetables	Added sugar
Organic foods	Preservatives, additives, artificial colors/ flavors
Whole grains	Alcohol and soft drinks
Nuts, seeds, and oils rich in omega-3 and monounsaturated fats (fish oils, flax oil, and olive oil)	Refined carbs (processed sugars, white rice, breads and pastas made with processed flours)
Purified drinking water	Saturated/trans fats (red meat/fried foods)
Green tea	Smoked and processed meats

We've all heard the term *empty calories*. These are foods with no redeeming nutritional qualities and nothing to offer us other than taste. These foods should be avoided. According to the authors of *The Encyclopedia of Healing Foods*, these foods contain lots of sugar and fat, which "fill you up so you don't have room for the good stuff—the foods that give your body a fighting chance to prevent cancer and other diseases." Foods in the empty calories category include soft drinks, candy, fried foods, chips, pastries, and crackers (unless they're made with whole grains).

Sticking with a strong cancer prevention diet may require that you become a label reader. Eating on the run, while not desirable, is occasionally necessary. When purchasing prepared food items, be especially wary of added sugar in its many guises. It may appear on the ingredient label in many different forms, including glucose, sucrose, fructose, maltose, lactose, dextrose, corn syrup, evaporated cane juice, and white grape juice concentrate. These added sugars contribute to inflammation, temporarily cripple the immune system, and over time contribute to the development of insulin resistance—all of which can promote cancer. Also avoid products with partially hydrogenated ingredients and trans-fatty acids. Thanks to new federal legislation, there is a separate listing for trans fats in the fat section of all food labels. Partially hydrogenated oils and trans fats contribute to inflammation, hamper immune system activity, and even directly damage genes, which can ultimately lead to the development of cancer.

Choosing the most healthful water source is also significant. More than two-thirds of our body is water, and our cells and tissues are literally bathed in a water environment. Drinking an adequate amount of water is critical to support optimal cellular and tissue function. Tap water, especially from municipal sources, may contain carcinogenic compounds. Filtered or purified water and water-rich fruits and vegetables are the best sources of water.

Food plays a significant role in any cancer prevention plan, and almost any diet, no matter how healthy, can be improved in this regard. Be receptive to new foods and new ways of eating. Elevate your awareness of what you eat, when, and why, and be more conscious about what you put into your body. (See below for the 2005 revised guidelines from the USDA.) Knowing how important this is to your health should provide any needed motivation.

Supplemental Insurance

When it comes to cancer prevention, there is a special type of supplemental insurance available—dietary supplements, that is. Nutritional supplements may consist of just one ingredient or a combination, and they may contain vitamins, minerals, amino acids, herbs, glandular extracts, and more. Dietary supplements are just that, *supplements* to the diet. It is always best to get as many nutrients as you can from food, not pills. But when diet falls short, supplements may help fill in the gaps. In addition, supplements can be used to stimulate certain processes in the body for a specific outcome.

Anatomy of MyPyramid

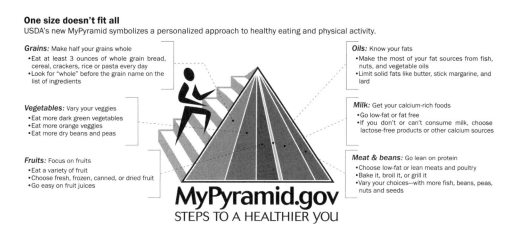

One size doesn't fit all
USDA's new MyPyramid symbolizes a personalized approach to healthy eating and physical activity.

Grains: Make half your grains whole
- Eat at least 3 ounces of whole grain bread, cereal, crackers, rice or pasta every day
- Look for "whole" before the grain name on the list of ingredients

Vegetables: Vary your veggies
- Eat more dark green vegetables
- Eat more orange veggies
- Eat more dry beans and peas

Fruits: Focus on fruits
- Eat a variety of fruit
- Choose fresh, frozen, canned, or dried fruit
- Go easy on fruit juices

Oils: Know your fats
- Make the most of your fat sources from fish, nuts, and vegetable oils
- Limit solid fats like butter, stick margarine, and lard

Milk: Get your calcium-rich foods
- Go low-fat or fat free
- If you don't or can't consume milk, choose lactose-free products or other calcium sources

Meat & beans: Go lean on protein
- Choose low-fat or lean meats and poultry
- Bake it, broil it, or grill it
- Vary your choices—with more fish, beans, peas, nuts and seeds

MyPyramid.gov
STEPS TO A HEALTHIER YOU

Healing Foods

Foods	Key nutrients	Benefits
Broccoli, brussels sprouts, cabbage, cauliflower, radishes, turnips, watercress	Indole-3-carbinol, glucosinolates, vitamin C	Enhancing detoxification
		Protecting DNA
		Inhibiting tumor formation
Carrots, peppers, green vegetables	Vitamins A and C, carotenoids, lutein, fiber, calcium, magnesium	Antioxidant function
		Immune enhancement
Citrus fruits (lemon, grapefruit, orange)	Vitamin C, fiber, potassium, flavonoids (limonoids, hesperidin, rutin), ellagic acid	Antioxidant function
		Preventing tumor invasion
		Enhancing detoxification
		Immune enhancement
Dark berries and grapes	Bioflavonoids (anthocyanidins), resveratrol	Immune enhancement
		Antioxidant function
		Cell protection
		Enhancing detoxification
Whole wheat and other whole grains	Vitamin E, zinc, selenium, fiber, lignans	Elimination and detoxification
		Immune enhancement
Green tea	Polyphenols (including epigallocatechin-3-gallate, abbreviated EGCG)	Antioxidant function
		Inhibiting tumor formation
		Interfering with signaling for tumor growth
		Preventing genetic damage and cancer formation

Foods	Key nutrients	Benefits
Garlic and onions	Allicin, S-allyl cysteine, selenium, flavonoids (quercetin)	Blocking formation of cancer-causing agents
		Preventing tumor growth
		Antioxidant function
		Immune enhancement
Spices (especially ginger, rosemary, and turmeric)	Carnosol, curcumin, flavones	Antioxidant function
		Enhancing detoxification
		Inhibiting tumor formation
		Immune enhancement
		Antinausea (ginger)
		Anti-inflammatory (curcumin and ginger)
Tomatoes	Lycopene	Inhibiting tumor formation and carcinogenic activity
Legumes and beans (soybeans, garbanzo, kidney)	Phytic acid, genistein, fiber, isoflavones, phytoestrogens, protease inhibitors	Blocking estrogen receptors
		Inhibiting tumor formation
		Interfering with carcinogenic activity
		Modulating hormones
Nuts and seeds	Vitamin E, essential fatty acids, calcium, magnesium, zinc, fiber, protease inhibitors, sterols	Antioxidant function
		Modulating hormone receptors
Mushrooms	Polysaccharides, beta-glucan, fiber	Immune enhancement
Cold-water fish (salmon, cod, halibut)	Vitamin D, essential fatty acids (eicosapentaenoic acid, epa; docosahexaenoic acid, dha)	Immune enhancement
		Inhibiting tumor formation

Supplements are an important part of an integrative cancer treatment program in order to help repair physiological processes that contribute to cancer development. Impaired immunity, inflammation, endocrine disturbances, insulin resistance, and insufficient detoxification are each linked to cancer formation and can be corrected with lifestyle and supplemental interventions. This is discussed in further detail in chapters 8 to 12. Nutritional supplements are also important in the active treatment of established cancer. Many supplements have powerful anticancer effects. The chapters on specific cancers (chapters 13 to 34) highlight supplements that are an important part of an integrative treatment plan.

The supplements you take should be chosen to meet your individual needs, deficiencies, or activity level. A woman trying to prevent breast cancer may take different supplements than a man trying to manage prostate cancer. A young competitive athlete will have a different supplement regimen than a middle-aged weekend warrior. Dietary supplements can help you fill in the gaps based on your specific health goals. Qualified health-care providers such as integrative physicians and naturopathic physicians can guide the most appropriate use of supplements in the context of cancer.

If your diet is lacking in the foods listed in the chart "Healing Foods" on pages 46 and 47, you may want to consider taking one or more dietary supplements to provide you with additional insurance. If you are uncertain whether the quality and variety of the foods in your diet are able to meet your nutritional needs, consult a qualified dietician, naturopathic doctor, or integrative physician to determine whether you would benefit from supplementation.

The Mind Matters

The human body has billions of nerve cells and countless chemical messengers that connect the brain to the heart, immune system, digestive tract, reproductive system, and every other system of the body. Every cell is either directly or indirectly connected to the others via the central nervous system. There is no question that there is a complex and efficient connection between mind and body.

Researchers are also confirming that there is a direct link between emotions and health. "We can understand through the language of science that emotions and disease are connected," explains Esther Sternberg, MD, from American University, "and disturbances of emotions can change your physical health and physical disease can change your emotional health." Additionally, "Every single person should be informed that the mind has a huge impact on the body and there are ways you can take advantage of that," says Tracy Gaudet, MD, with the Duke Center for Integrative Medicine.

Research in this area is on the rise and the concept is beginning to gain mainstream acceptance. Science is confirming that we have a much better chance of being healthy if we nurture positive thoughts and emotions and try to reduce stress and anxiety. Conversely, negative emotions such as anger and depression can impair our health. This is not to suggest that any one individual should take on the entire responsibility for developing cancer. Cancer growth is influenced by a multitude of factors, many of which are not within our control. Taking the blame for having cancer causes unnecessary suffering and does not encourage the attitude that will help us make different choices to improve our health and recovery. Instead of focusing on blame and guilt, it is far more healing to use cancer, or cancer prevention, as an opportunity to learn self-forgiveness, gratitude, and hope. Being aware without judgment is the first step. From there you can begin to incorporate more health-enhancing thoughts and emotions into your daily life.

The most powerful health-promoting emotion of all is love—giving it, receiving it, and even participating in activities you love. Love goes far beyond romantic love. It comes from inside and outside of us. It is cultivated in our social interactions and connections with family and friends. Love can come from oneself, a pet, a supportive or welcoming environment, or an activity. Whether you love hiking in the mountains or curling up with a good book, do what you love and do it often.

"The healing power of love and relationships has been documented in an increasing number of well-designed scientific studies involving hundreds of thousands of people throughout the world," writes Dean Ornish, MD, in his groundbreaking book *Love and Survival: The Scientific Basis for the Healing Power of Intimacy*. One of the greatest benefits of allowing more love into your life is that it fosters forgiveness—of yourself and of others. Life can be hard, and people sometimes make mistakes and do things that are hurtful to themselves or others.

A diagnosis of cancer forces a person to recognize her or his mortality. This perspective is a powerful refocusing lens that gives people the opportunity to let go of emotions that may hinder wellness and their ability to enjoy whatever time life grants them. When asked what they would do differently if they had the opportunity, most people with cancer say things like "Spend more time with the people I love," "Argue less and forgive more," or "Trust and let go of fear, anger, and pain." Using this wisdom from people diagnosed with cancer, we can all improve our wellness now. We can let go of anger and hurt and move into the state of grace granted by forgiveness and compassion for others and ourselves. With love and forgiveness, a sense of wellness can infuse your entire being in spite of any physical impediments. From that space, everything else—including making healthy choices in regard to diet, supplements, and exercise—becomes so much easier.

Health-Enhancing Activities

Physical activity has many health-promoting benefits. Exercise can stimulate the immune system, reduce inflammation, improve self-esteem, enhance mood, increase oxygenation, and help maintain a healthy weight. It's amazing that something as simple as moving will provide that much benefit.

"There are ways that you can exercise without really 'exercising,'" according to Mark Hyman, MD, in his book *UltraMetabolism*. "You don't have to go to the gym, run on a treadmill, and pump iron to stay in shape. Just start moving around more." One of Dr. Hyman's specific suggestions is wearing a step counter as you move throughout the day. He sets a goal of 10,000 steps per day.

The most important aspects of exercise are to choose an activity or activities that you will stick with and then be consistent. The best way to be successful at this is to make exercise fun and enjoyable. If you find walking boring, but enjoy reading, listen to books on tape while you walk. If you find it hard to motivate yourself to ride your bicycle but you miss spending time with your friends, make regular biking dates. If your routine becomes boring, change it from time to time to keep your enthusiasm up. Increase your physical activity as you get in better shape. Try not to fall into the weekend warrior trap; it's much better to be active every day than it is to do something strenuous for a few hours on the weekend. For more information on exercise and cancer prevention, refer to the sidebar "Exercise Is Medicine" on page 52.

Not all health-enhancing activities involve movement. In fact, research has demonstrated that the act of just sitting can be an amazing cancer prevention tool—it's called meditation. Many clinical studies have shown that meditation improves quality of life, reduces pain, decreases anxiety and depression, and enhances energy levels. More recent research indicates that meditation can also increase positive immune activity. According to a 2003 report in *Psychosomatic Medicine*, "A randomized study of relaxation, meditation, and hypnosis training in asymptomatic HIV-positive men found improved T cell counts in the treatment group which were maintained at one-month follow-up."

Stress reduction is critical in any effort to promote health (and this is probably one reason meditation has such beneficial effects). For example, stress has observable impacts on the rate of healing, as demonstrated by Ohio State University husband and wife research team Drs. Ronald and Janice Glaser. They made a small circular incision, smaller than an eraser on the end of a pencil, on the arms of two groups. One group consisted of caregivers of people with Alzheimer's disease. The other group was matched for age and financial circumstances but had considerably less stress in their lives. The unstressed group healed a full nine days sooner than the stressed group. The photos from the study were remarkable, as they visually conveyed the noticeable difference between the two groups.

The Center for Integrative Medicine at Jefferson Medical College chose to study medical students because these students face significant academic and psychosocial stress. Researchers taught one group of medical students mindfulness-based stress reduction techniques that included meditation and then compared them to a control group of students who didn't use these techniques. The students practicing stress reduction techniques had significantly less tension, anxiety, confusion, and fatigue than the control group.

In her book *My Grandfather's Blessings*, Rachel Naomi Remen, MD, has a somewhat different perspective on stress. "After 20 years of working with people with cancer, I have come to realize how much stress is caused by the sad fact that many of us believe in one way and live in quite another. Stress may be more a matter of personal integrity than time pressure, determined by the distance between our authentic values and how we live our lives."

Stress reduction comes from awareness, from quietly yet confidently embracing who you really are. You'll feel less stress if you focus on being in the moment and truly relishing the nuances of any given experience. Meditation is one way to get closer to your true self and reinforce the idea of being present in the moment.

Beyond exercise and meditation, there are many other ways to enhance your health. The key is finding activities that are meaningful or rewarding for you. That may mean getting in touch with your creative side by writing or other artistic endeavors. Journaling can be particularly effective, as it allows you to express your emotions and process your thoughts. Or you may find that playing or listening to music can reduce feelings of stress and increase your sense of contentment and joy. As with exercise, the key is to find health-enhancing activities that you enjoy and are comfortable with and then make them part of your routine. Like a seamstress making a quilt, take each piece of healthful living and sew it into the fabric of your life, creating a blanket of protection and wellness.

Be Proactive

Before we can even think of cancer treatment, we must first review the core principles of proactive prevention. As much as possible, these prevention principles should become a way of life. As mentioned previously, each of us has cancer cells circulating in our body at this very moment. If your body is healthy and functioning properly, its ability to detect, target, kill, and eliminate these errant cells is strengthened. If your body is overwhelmed and unhealthy, it may not be able to perform this ongoing search-and-destroy

Exercise Is Medicine

By Susan Ryan, DO

Sports medicine is often thought to deal only with the prevention and treatment of injuries. Many believe the pinnacle of sports medicine is the care of elite athletes. Sports performance can be enhanced by the advances within this specialty; however, the contributions of exercise medicine to overall health and disease prevention are often underestimated.

We all experience the gentle—and sometimes not so gentle—tug of aging. Every physiologic system undergoes a gradual decline in its operational efficiencies. Although exercise does not prevent these changes in their entirety, it can certainly slow down the process.

The scientific evidence involving exercise medicine is gathering momentum. Study after study shows that our bodies respond favorably to a variety of exercise loads as we age. Increased strength and flexibility and improvements in neuromuscular function and balance can be expected from an exercise program. As we age, this translates into the preservation of our independence.

Exercise has long been touted to help in the prevention of a variety of diseases. Much of this data has been gathered through epidemiologic studies, the largest of which is the Framingham Study, which has followed more than 5,000 people over three generations. This study has provided critical data that increases our understanding of disease prevention.

For so many years, the cornerstone for cancer prevention in conventional medical practice has been early detection. Early detection can find precancerous changes or early cancer at a stage when prompt treatment can prevent long-term illness and extended treatment. However, even before early detection, there is vast opportunity to engage in preventive behaviors and choices that may avert the formation of cancer altogether. These modifiable risk factors, that is to say, the things that each of us can do to decrease risk, have gained increasing attention in the scientific community, and we now have a much better understanding of these factors and what we can do to minimize them. One of the most commonly studied modifiable risk factors is exercise.

More than 20 large studies have investigated the relationship between exercise and cancer prevention. And while there are confounding variables that are difficult to isolate, such as diet or alcohol use, these studies have revealed some very clear relationships between exercise and the prevention of many cancers.

In three separate studies, published in the *Journal of the National Cancer Institute*, the *New England Journal of Medicine*, and the *Journal of the American Medical Association,* breast cancer risk on average was decreased by 30 to 40 percent for women exercising moderately and even more for those who exercised three to four hours a week. This risk reduction was evident at every level of risk for women with breast cancer. Obesity and adult weight gain have clearly been linked to the risk of breast cancer in more than 100 studies. As little as 5 to 10 pounds of excess weight can increase risk by 20 percent, and 40 to 50 pounds doubles the risk of breast cancer. There is credible evidence that exercise can significantly decrease risks of many other cancers, including colorectal, endometrial, and prostate cancers. The scientific data confirming the connection between exercise and cancer prevention is becoming stronger with each passing year.

You may be concerned about your genetics or hopeful that a cancer "cure" will be discovered, but these factors are beyond your control. In the meanwhile, there is something simple you can do to help prevent cancer. So, get out of your chair and do something—anything—because exercise is medicine.

Susan Ryan, DO, is board certified in both sports medicine and family medicine. She has been a team physician for Olympic, professional, and collegiate athletes in multiple sports. She is also on this book's editorial advisory board.

mission. You can support your body in this crucial task by focusing on creating and maintaining a healthy body, mind, and spirit.

Cancer is a complex and tenacious illness, and a multidimensional, integrative approach is needed to help defuse its energy. Diet and other aspects of lifestyle, as well as an understanding of the significant connection between body and mind, can have a huge impact on whether or not a person develops cancer. In addition to understanding the basics of proactive prevention, we can go deeper by building a strong foundation with diet, nutrition, and stress reduction. Sometimes doing all the right things may not prevent cancer, however, in our personal experiences and from the experiences of many cancer patients, a prevention-based lifestyle supports overall health. As a result of prevention, you can be a healthy person with cancer and that can make a world of difference in how you experience cancer treatment and recovery.

Part II
Treatment Approaches

Building a Strong Foundation with Diet, Nutrition, and Stress Reduction

After a cancer diagnosis, you are faced with many decisions, but one decision should be clear: to support your body by building a strong foundation featuring a health-promoting diet and lifestyle. This may mean drastic changes for some or just fine-tuning for others. Whether you choose a conventional approach to treatment, an integrative approach, or no treatment at all, making appropriate diet and lifestyle changes is paramount.

When it comes to making dietary adjustments, you may just need to alter your perspective. Food provides much more than comfort or fuel—it is a critical component of any cancer treatment plan. A healthy diet needs to become a way of life. The anticancer nutrition plan focuses on making choices that will stimulate your body's innate ability to fight cancer.

Food as Medicine

More than 2,000 years ago, Hippocrates advised, "Let your food be your medicine and let your medicine be your food." We need to reclaim this wisdom. Nutrition is powerful in its own right, and on the cancer battlefield it has a role alongside chemotherapy drugs, the surgeon's knife, and radiation therapy. In fact, because poor food choices can play a role in the development of many cancers, a healthy diet should be viewed as a critical part of the first line of defense. In most cases, however, diet alone will not cure cancer.

Foods that heal contain so much more than just calories, carbohydrates, proteins, and fats. They also contain vitamins, minerals, and other essential nutrients that are critical for good health. Many of these essential nutrients also play an important role in bolstering the body's ability to kill cancer.

Here are just a few critical cancer-fighting vitamins, minerals, and other nutrients and some of the tasty foods they're found in:

- **Vitamin A and carotenes**: Carrots, peppers, apricots, spinach, and mangoes

- **Vitamin C**: Peppers, broccoli, guavas, cauliflower, strawberries, and papaya

- **Vitamin D**: Cold-water fish and dark green leafy vegetables

- **Vitamin E**: Whole grains, seeds, and nuts

- **Folic acid**: Beans, asparagus, lentils, walnuts, and spinach

- **Calcium**: Kelp, cheese, almonds, and watercress

- **Magnesium**: Wheat bran, brown rice, cashews, peanuts, tofu, and figs

- **Potassium**: Bananas, oranges, lima beans, and avocados

- **Selenium**: Brazil nuts, whole wheat bread, and orange juice

- **Zinc**: Fresh oysters, pumpkin seeds, ginger root, and pecans

- **Flavonoids**: Colored fruits such as cherries, grapes, blueberries, and strawberries

- **Essential fatty acids**: Fish, shellfish, flaxseeds, and sea vegetables

Vitamins and essential minerals are, by their very definition, essential for good health. But science is discovering a whole new world of healing compounds in plant foods. Most whole grains, fruits, vegetables, herbs, and spices contain specific active compounds called phytochemicals (*phyto* meaning "plant") that can make a positive contribution to health. These compounds can actually stimulate specific body functions on the cellular level.

Researchers at the M. D. Anderson Cancer Center reviewed a variety of phytochemicals found in fruits, vegetables, and herbs to determine how they can help treat cancer by influencing cell-signaling pathways. By disrupting important cellular signals, these agents can potentially stop cancer growth, prevent angiogenesis, and even cause cancer cell death (apoptosis). They studied a long list of agents, including the following:

- 6-gingerol (found in ginger)

- Anethole (found in anise, camphor, and fennel)

- Beta-carotene (found in carrots)

- Capsaicin (found in red chiles)

- Catechins (found in green tea)

- Curcumin (found in turmeric)

- Diallyl sulfide, S-allyl cysteine, and allicin (found in garlic and onions)

- Diosgenin (found in fenugreek)

- Ellagic acid (found in pomegranates)

- Eugenol (found in cloves)

- Genistein (found in soybeans)

- Indole-3-carbinol (found in cruciferous vegetables)

- Limonene (found in citrus fruits)

- Lycopene (found in tomatoes)

- Resveratrol (found in red grapes, peanuts, and berries)

- Silymarin (found in milk thistle)

- Ursolic acid (found in apples, pears, and prunes)

The researchers conclude that "extensive research during the last half century has identified various molecular targets [that are influenced by these phytochemicals] that can potentially be used not only for the prevention of cancer but also for treatment."

While that list is quite impressive, there are scores of other nutrients, herbs, and foods being studied for cancer prevention and treatment. Nutrients receiving a great deal of research attention include vitamin D, folic acid, selenium, coenzyme Q10, glutathione, and essential fatty acids (specifically, EPA and DHA from cold-water fish). Herbs of interest include rosemary (which contains the phytochemical carnosol), turmeric (which contains the phytochemical curcumin), and green tea (notably, EGCG). Certain whole foods or components of them also show particular promise, including olive oil, flax oil, active compounds in various mushrooms, active compounds in rice bran, and lignans found in flaxseed, whole grain cereals, and other foods.

Getting Back to Basics

It's tempting to jump on the bandwagon of dietary fads. We all want to believe that our answers lie in some new miracle food or easy-to-follow diet doctrine. However, simply adopting the latest diet fad isn't the answer. Rather, we must look to the past—before the era of fast-food restaurants, before preservatives and hydrogenation became the mainstays of mass-produced food, and before white flour became an unfortunate symbol of refinement. We need to look way back to those simple times when most of the foods we ate were whole, fresh, and seasonal, when we ate what came out of the ground and dessert was a bowl of berries.

We can take advantage of the amazing power of simple foods to support essential body functions. To construct the perfect anticancer diet, we need to get back to these basics. The foundation is to eat plenty of colorful vegetables and fresh fruits (organic whenever possible). We recommend seven to ten servings of fruits and vegetables a day. (For more information, refer to the sidebar "How Many Servings Do We Need?" at right.) If that's a daunting prospect, vegetable juices and protein-enriched fruit smoothies are great ways to more easily get all of those servings and the beneficial nutrients they provide. Whole grains, beans, seeds, and nuts provide fiber and important vitamins and minerals and should also be abundant in your diet. Fresh cold-water fish is a great source of protein as well as beneficial omega-3 fatty acids. Because of the fat content, limit dairy to one to two servings of organic dairy products daily. And don't forget to drink plenty of water. Proper hydration is essential for everyone, but especially those with cancer.

Eat More Vegetables and Fruits

The scientific evidence linking vegetable intake to cancer prevention and treatment is impressive and continues to grow. There are long-term and large epidemiological studies consistently showing that the people who eat the most vegetables have the lowest incidence of all types of cancer. Studies have shown that vegetables in the diet improve immune function and strengthen liver detoxification. Scientists are also discovering how compounds in vegetables help protect DNA from damage that would otherwise lead to cancer.

Of special interest are the cruciferous vegetables such as brussels sprouts, kale, broccoli, and cabbage. Many studies have shown these vegetables can help prevent cancer. Newer research involving components of these important vegetables, such as sulforaphane, actually show they may have the ability to destroy established cancer. Fruits are also very important to any cancer-fighting plan. Fruits contain active compounds called flavonoids. Flavonoids protect fruits from being damaged by the ultraviolet rays of the sun. Scientific research is confirming that some of those flavonoids have similar effects in us. Specifically, flavonoids exert cancer-preventive effects and also stimulate a variety of anticancer actions within our bodies. Here are just a few flavonoids from fruits to focus on:

● Phenolic compounds (in apples)

● Resveratrol (from red grapes)

- Anthocyanidins (from berries)

- Limonoids (from citrus fruits)

(For more information about the active compounds in foods, refer to the "Healing Foods" chart on page 46.) Increasing your consumption of organic fresh vegetables and fruits is the first and most important step toward building an anticancer foundation of health. In addition, there are several other dietary aspects to consider.

Whole Grains for Health

Some researchers argue that whole grain intake is even more important than eating fruits and vegetables. Many people don't realize that, in addition to being great sources of fiber, whole grains provide important vitamins and minerals. According to a review featured in the *Journal of the American Dietetic Association*, "Whole grain foods are valuable sources of nutrients that are lacking in the American diet, including dietary fiber, B-vitamins, vitamin E, selenium, zinc, copper, and magnesium."

Unfortunately, most Americans are not getting enough whole grains to receive the immense health benefits these foods can provide. In 2004, researchers from the University of Minnesota reported that the average American was eating less than one serving of whole grains daily instead of the recommended three servings. Other dietary intake studies have confirmed that Americans are not eating enough whole grains.

Dietary fiber has been shown in several clinical studies to prevent some cancers—most notably, cancers of the

How Many Servings Do We Need?

According to the Optimum Health Food Pyramid, your daily diet should, on average, consist of the following:

Vegetables = 5 to 7 servings

Seeds, nuts, and healthy oils = 4 servings

Whole grains = 3 to 6 servings

Beans (legumes) = 2 to 3 servings

Fruit = 2 to 3 servings

Protein = 2 to 3 servings

Dairy (organic, if possible) = 1 to 2 servings

If you'd rather avoid dairy, you can substitute calcium supplements or calcium-rich foods, such as almonds and sea vegetables.
What's in a serving? Here'a guideline:

Vegetables = 1 cup of raw leafy vegetables, ½ cup of raw nonleafy, ½ cup cooked vegetables, or ½ cup fresh vegetable juice

Seeds or nuts = ¼ cup

Healthy oils = 1 tablespoon

Whole grains = 1 slice whole wheat, rye, or other whole grain bread, ½ cup whole grain cereal, ½ cup cooked whole kernel corn, 1 small ear of corn, or ½ cup cooked whole grain pasta

Beans (legumes) = ½ cup cooked

Fruit = 1 medium fruit; ½ cup cut-up fruit; 1 cup berries; 4 ounces of 100 percent juice; or ¼ cup dried fruit

Protein = 3 to 4 ounces (the size of a deck of cards)

Dairy = 1 cup milk, yogurt, or cottage cheese, or 1 ounce cheese

colon. However, the value of whole grains as an anticancer food goes beyond fiber. Whole grains have been shown to help rid the body of excess circulating hormones, stabilize blood sugar levels, maintain healthy weight, and stimulate immunity. Whole grains include foods such as whole wheat, oats, and brown rice. An emphasis on whole grains is important because they contain more nutrients and complex carbohydrates than refined grains. For more information about carbohydrate metabolism and the downside of eating refined carbohydrates, see chapter 11, "Insulin Resistance."

The Lowdown on Fats

Until recently, fats in general received a very bad rap. Many people tried to avoid dietary fats as much as possible, thinking this made for a healthy diet. As it turns out, the situation is much more complicated. Excessive dietary fats, especially saturated fats, have been implicated in increased risk of cancer, along with other serious diseases. But certain fats are good for you, and in fact, some are so important as to be termed essential fatty acids (EFAs)—essential because they can't be created within the body, but are required for various metabolic functions. And when you realize that fats are present in every cell membrane and every organ and tissue in the body, you can see that it's important to include some fat in the diet. The question is, which fats are best? To answer this question, we need to take a closer look at the chemistry of fats.

Saturation refers to the number of hydrogen atoms that are linked to the carbon atom backbone of a fatty acid. When all of the carbon molecules in the chain are linked by single bonds, this allows for the greatest number of hydrogen atoms to be attached to the carbon backbone; such fats are referred to as saturated fats (i.e., they are saturated with hydrogen). Monounsaturated fats have one double bond between carbon atoms, with the result that the overall molecule contains one less hydrogen atom than possible. Polyunsaturated fats contain multiple double-bond linkages between carbon atoms and thus even fewer hydrogen atoms. Most vegetable oils contain a combination of monounsaturated and polyunsaturated fats.

Health Risks Associated with Saturated Fats

Saturated fats are found in animal products like butter, cheese, whole milk, cream, and fatty meats. Coconut, palm, and palm kernel oils also contain saturated fats, although the saturated fats in coconuts are medium-chained triglycerides that are readily utilized for the production of energy and do not carry the same risks as do other saturated fats. This makes coconut fat an exception to the rule. While saturated fats are more closely linked to increased risk of heart disease than other types of fat, the link between this "bad" fat and cancer is becoming stronger. According to an MSN report provided by the American Institute for Cancer Research, a reason saturated fats can contribute to cancer is because they cause insulin problems. New studies show that too much saturated fat can decrease insulin production, which leads to a rebound effect of overproduction of insulin. Insulin is a growth factor for many cancers.

Several studies have linked a diet high in animal fats to an increased risk of developing some cancers. To reduce saturated fat consumption, we need to reduce our consumption of animal products. As a point of reference, a 4-ounce T-bone steak (broiled or grilled) delivers a whopping 26.5 grams of fat. The goal is for fat to comprise no more than 30 percent of the diet and to try to significantly reduce consumption of saturated fat. Recommended daily fat intake for a 2,000-calorie diet is 65 grams. If you eat a 10-ounce T-bone steak, you've already exceeded your limit for the entire day. Excessive consumption of saturated fats from animal sources contributes to insulin resistance and obesity, and introduces bioaccumulated toxins and hormones into your body. All of these factors contribute to cancer formation and development and can also inhibit treatment and recovery.

Trans Fats

Another category of fats to avoid is trans fats. Although they occur in minute quantities in certain foods, the vast majority of the trans fats we consume are created synthetically by heating liquid (unsaturated) fats in the presence of hydrogen. This is done to make them more solid (for example, to make margarine) and to make them more stable, thus increasing the shelf life of foods made with trans fats—a boon to the big business of prepackaged foods. In addition to increasing the amount of saturation, this process also alters the very structure of the molecule, converting it into a straighter, more linear molecule—a form the body isn't accustomed to metabolizing. When these trans fats are incorporated into cell membranes, they impede energy metabolism and also interfere with the function of certain anti-inflammatory substances. For more information on the link between inflammation and cancer, refer to chapter 9.

In fact, these fats are so bad for the body that effective January 1, 2006, food manufacturers were required to list both saturated and trans fat amounts on package labels. According to the Harvard School of Public Health, "Now that trans fat must be listed on food labels, some companies are scrambling to remove them from their products." This is remarkable, considering that the FDA once estimated that 100 percent of crackers and 95 percent of prepackaged cookies contained harmful trans fats. Many cities and states including New York City, Philadelphia, and California have now banned trans fats from restaurants. We hope other states will follow this lead. Until trans fats are banned more widely, read labels carefully and avoid consumption of trans fats whenever possible.

Essential Fatty Acids

Now that we've discussed the bad fats, let's take a look at the good ones. Essential fatty acids (EFAs) are divided into two primary categories: omega-3 and omega-6 fatty acids. The average American gets more than enough omega-6s from diet, so for most of us, obtaining enough omega-3s is the problem.

In reality, there's just one essential omega-3 fatty acid (alpha-linolenic acid, or ALA) and one essential omega-6 (linoleic acid, or LA). From these basic building blocks the body can manufacture all of the other omega-3s such as eicosapentaenoic acid (EPA) and docosahexaenoic acid (DHA), as well as omega-6s, which include gamma-linolenic acid (GLA). However, there's a metabolic cost to doing so. For people whose systems are compromised by cancer, it's preferable to avoid that metabolic expenditure by directly consuming the important omega-3s, such as EPA and DHA, in the form of dietary supplements. Although omega-3s are available from both plant sources (particularly flaxseeds, but also pumpkin seeds, sunflower seeds, walnuts, and leafy green vegetables) and animal sources (especially fish and shellfish), plant sources mostly contain omega-3 fatty acid as ALA with only minimal EPA and no DHA. So for therapeutic purposes, eating cold-water fish or supplementing with fish oil capsules is your best bet.

Recent research shows a direct link between omega-3s and effective cancer treatment. Here are just a few examples from this exciting area of investigation:

- Women with diagnosed breast cancers were randomized to eat either a 25-gram flaxseed muffin or a placebo muffin from the time of their initial biopsy until surgical removal of the breast tumor (approximately one month). The removed tumors were analyzed and those from women consuming flaxseeds showed increased apoptosis (cell death) and decreased proliferation.

- An Australian study of untreated pancreatic cancer patients showed improvement in quality of life and weight gain in patients who drank a protein energy drink and took an oral nutritional supplement with omega-3 fatty acids.

- Some studies have demonstrated that diets rich in omega-3 fatty acids are associated with a lower risk of breast and colon cancers.

- Preliminary animal studies indicate that omega-3 fatty acids can help make tumors of various types more sensitive to chemotherapy drugs.

The Bottom Line on Fats

Saturated fats, most commonly found in animal foods, are associated with numerous health risks, and reducing your consumption of these is a good idea. It's worth repeating that trans fats should be avoided. Healthier oils include monounsaturated and polyunsaturated fats such as olive, avocado, macadamia, and flax. Of these, olive oil is monounsaturated, making this a better choice for high-heat applications than polyunsaturated fats, which are more readily damaged by high heat. Because it contains monounsaturated fat, olive oil is less susceptible to damage than many other vegetable oils, so it is good to use in cooked dishes. Because of its very high percentage of polyunsaturated fats and especially omega-3 fatty acids, flax oil should never be heated. As healthy as it is when uncooked, when damaged by heat it can form dangerous compounds.

The Importance of Protein

One of the most undervalued components of a strong anticancer diet is protein. Protein helps maintain and build muscle mass. It can also help boost white blood cell counts and overall immunity. "Undergoing conventional cancer therapy may require as much as 50 percent more protein than usual," according to Michael Murray, ND, Tim Birdsall, ND, Joseph Pizzorno, ND, and Paul Reilly, ND, the authors of *How to Prevent and Treat Cancer with Natural Medicine*. The authors go on to state that "smoothies are an ideal—and delicious—way for people with cancer to consume lots of high-quality protein." People fighting cancer typically require between 60 and 100 grams of protein daily.

Although red meat may seem like the ideal way to obtain protein, it's actually not always the best choice. Red meat contains saturated fats that contribute to insulin resistance and increased cancer risk, and if it is not hormone free or all natural it also contains residues from pesticides, antibiotics, and hormones given to the animal. Red meat can also be difficult to digest, contributing to inflammation in the digestive tract. If red meat is your preferred protein source, you can minimize some of the associated health risks by choosing lean meat from organically raised and grass-fed cows. Meats such as elk, bison, and buffalo also have a healthier fatty acid profile and are healthier choices.

Good sources of protein include hormone- and antibiotic-free eggs, yogurt, seafood, and organically fed, free-range chicken; nuts, seeds, and legumes; and whey protein powder. You can create unique and yummy protein-rich smoothies by blending a variety of fruits (frozen or fresh), yogurt, and nonfat milk (organic, if possible), rice milk, or soy milk and adding about an ounce of high-quality whey protein powder per smoothie. Flavored whey protein powders can provide an extra flavor boost. We recommend whey protein powder because it contains a good balance of essential and nonessential amino acids, which are the building blocks of protein.

Among the essential amino acids, glutamine is especially important. Not only is it the most abundant amino acid in the body, it's also involved in more metabolic tasks than other amino acids. "Glutamine is especially important as a source of fuel for white blood cells, and for cells that divide rapidly, such as those that line the intestine," explain the authors of *How to Prevent and Treat Cancer with Natural Medicine*. "It has become an important component of intravenous feeding mixes in hospitals since double-blind studies have shown that it dramatically increases survival in critically ill patients."

Avoiding Unhealthy Foods

Food can be good medicine if you make the right choices. The foods mentioned previously can positively influence your health. Equally important is to avoid those foods that can cause harm. Here are some of the worst offenders:

- Simple sugars should be avoided or limited to avoid creating immune deficiencies and insulin resistance (discussed in chapters 8 and 11).

- Refined carbohydrates (such as white bread, pasta, white rice, and anything made with white flour), should be consumed only in moderation. Refined carbohydrates are rapidly broken down into simple sugars, so they also contribute to insulin resistance.

- Sodium from excess salt can disrupt electrolyte balance and contribute to fluid retention (edema).

- Additives and preservatives can overwhelm the body's detoxification process.

- Hydrogenated fats can directly damage DNA; these fats are the main ingredient in many margarines and are commonly used in convenience foods and other prepared foods.

- Alcohol should be consumed only in moderation, if at all, as it contributes to inflammation and insulin resistance.

Every day, make a conscious effort to eat more healthful foods and avoid those that are harmful. Step by step, you will get closer to the perfect anti-cancer diet.

What about the Macrobiotic Diet?

Macrobiotics was introduced to Western society from Japan in the 1920s. Macrobiotics—macro meaning "large" and bios meaning "life"—was originally thought of as a spiritual way of life featuring a simple diet of brown rice, miso soup, sea vegetables, and foods with no preservatives, additives, and other toxins. The initial philosophy of macrobiotics combined living simply with a spiritual, physical, and communal discipline oriented toward respecting the planet while searching for inner peace. Considered more than a diet, it was a way of life.

While many people still embrace the macrobiotic way of life, others primarily follow the dietary fundamentals. In his book *Comprehensive Cancer Care*, mind-body cancer expert James Gordon, MD, defines the basic macrobiotic diet as follows:

- 50 percent whole grains

- 25 to 30 percent seasonal vegetables

- 5 to 10 percent beans, bean products, and sea vegetables

- 5 to 10 percent soups and broths made with miso, a fermented soy product, and vegetables and beans

- Fruits in moderation and sometimes fish

- Organic food

According to Dr. Gordon, while the percentages may have shifted over the years, the premise of the macrobiotic diet is similar to recommendations of the American Cancer Society: choose foods from plant sources while limiting intake of high-fat foods, particularly from animal sources. In its most basic form, macrobiotics is a mostly vegetarian, whole foods diet. It is generally low in calories, composed of highly nutritious foods, and devoid of detrimental foods. It is hard to argue with such a solid dietary strategy. However, caution is strongly advised in cases of advanced or aggressive and fast-growing cancers.

In general, scientific data regarding macrobiotics as a cancer treatment is limited. In a paper featured in the *Journal of Nutrition* in 2001, researchers from Columbia University explained that "macrobiotics is one of the most popular alternative or complementary comprehensive lifestyle approaches to cancer" because of "remarkable case reports of individuals who attributed recoveries from cancer . . . to macrobiotics."

It is true that women consuming a macrobiotic diet have lower circulating estrogen levels, implying a potential reduction in breast cancer risk. This type of diet may also be helpful in delaying progression of cancers diagnosed at early stages or preventing their recurrence. And certainly, there are a wide variety of health benefits associated with such a diet. However, the Columbia researchers concluded that the "empirical scientific basis for or against recommendations for use of macrobiotics for cancer therapy is limited."

Macrobiotics, as well as other diets promoted as cancer cures, is likely more effective for prevention than treatment, especially in cases of advanced cancers. Mounting an effective immune response against advanced or aggressive cancer requires tremendous amounts of protein and calories, and a macrobiotic diet may be insufficient to meet these needs. A macrobiotic diet could do more harm than good if it causes a person with advanced cancer to lose additional lean body mass. Before committing to a macrobiotic diet or a similar regimen, cancer patients should consult with a dietician and have their percentage of body fat and lean body mass calculated. These measurements should be monitored to ensure that diet isn't contributing to a decrease in lean body mass, which can aggravate cachexia or malnutrition—potentially fatal complications of cancer or cancer therapy.

When Getting Adequate Nutrition Is a Challenge

The dietary concepts discussed thus far are appropriate for those who are interested in preventing cancer or for cancer patients with intact digestive systems who can control their nutritional intake. In certain situations of more advanced cancers, people may not be able to eat or digest sufficient quantities of food to get all of the nutrients they need from their diet. However, obtaining adequate calories with balanced protein, fat, carbohydrates, and healing micronutrients is just as important for these individuals, if not more so.

People having difficulty eating or maintaining weight may want to invest in a juicer. The nutrients in fresh vegetables and fruits are more easily absorbed when they are juiced because the fiber is removed. What remains is water and sugars from the vegetable or fruit, along with the majority of its vitamins, minerals, and other healthful nutrients. In this form, the nutrients can more readily saturate the system to produce energy and provide health benefits more rapidly. If one consumes freshly juiced fruits and vegetables regularly over a long period of time, it is important to add additional fiber to the diet to compensate for the fiber lost in the juices. Whole grains, legumes, nuts, and seeds are good sources of fiber.

In addition, it is important to note that fresh vegetable and fruit juices are high in natural sugars and can elevate your blood sugar level. This triggers the release of insulin, which clears excess sugar from the blood, but can also result in hypoglycemia, or low blood sugar. Hypoglycemia can make you feel shaky, nervous, sleepy, confused, or weak, and it can also cause you to crave more sugar to bring your blood sugar level back up again, creating a vicious cycle that can ultimately lead to insulin resistance (chapter 11 will cover this in detail). In addition to creating unpleasant symptoms, these sorts of blood sugar fluctuations are hard on the pancreas. To avoid this, you can add protein powder to fresh juices, dilute them with water, or take longer to drink them.

Medical intervention may be necessary to ensure adequate nutrition in certain situations, such as blockage of the digestive tract; severe digestive side effects from conventional treatments; issues that keep the person from eating, such as anorexia, severe depression, or confusion; pain that makes it difficult to swallow or chew; or surgery that has removed part of the gastrointestinal tract. Additionally, some cancer patients have difficulty maintaining adequate body weight and muscle mass. Known as cachexia, this is a serious muscle wasting condition associated with cancer. It has been estimated that 40 percent of cancer patients do not die from cancer, but from malnutrition. Many nutrients, specifically essential fatty acids, can help prevent and reverse cachexia.

In all of these situations, enteral or parenteral nutrition can be critical to the person's survival and quality of life. In enteral nutrition, nutrients are delivered in a liquid form by using a tube to deliver nutrients directly into the stomach or the beginning part of the intestines (the jejunum). Liquefied food is the most basic and natural form of enteral nutrition. In parenteral nutrition, specially formulated nutrients are infused through a venous IV.

Start Today

A growing body of evidence shows that nutrition can play an important role in preventing and treating cancer. While the idea of food as medicine may not sound appetizing, healthy food choices are not only good for you, they can be very tasty, too. There are so many wonderful cookbooks packed with healthy recipes. Find one or two that appeal to you and start exploring the delicious world of healthy eating. You may soon find yourself to be quite the connoisseur.

Within a short period of time, you will feel the benefits of eating healing foods. By making some simple dietary changes you can increase your energy, sleep better, think more clearly, and feel stronger. Making conscientious nutrition choices can also help strengthen your immune system; reduce inflammation; balance hormones; stabilize blood sugar levels; and improve digestion, elimination, and detoxification. Supporting these physiological systems will have enormous health benefits, not the least of which is helping you heal from cancer. When it comes to cancer treatment, healing foods are not just the fuel that makes the body run, they are the sparks that ignite each critical cancer-fighting body system. When combined with significant lifestyle factors, this becomes the strong foundation that integrative cancer care is built upon.

Lifestyle Factors That Make a Difference

"I've spent many years learning how to fix life, only to discover at the end of the day that life is not broken. There is a hidden seed of greater wholeness in everyone and everything. We serve life best when we water it and befriend it," Rachel Naomi Remen, MD, eloquently explains in her wonderful book *My Grandfather's Blessings.* She goes on to remind us that "in befriending life, we do not make things happen according to our own design. We uncover something that is already happening in us and around us and create conditions that enable it."

Dr. Remen has pinpointed the vital essence of lifestyle factors that positively influence cancer prevention and treatment, creating conditions that enable the healing power that is ever present within us. We need to establish an internal and external healing environment that influences mind, body, and spirit. This environment begins with healthy lifestyle choices that support our innate healing abilities, improve the body's response to cancer treatment, and improve quality of life.

Used alone or in combination, the activities discussed in this chapter are healing. While they will not, in and of themselves, cure cancer, they will certainly contribute to a successful cancer treatment program. Scientific interest in and validation of these lifestyle factors is on the rise. Their positive physical and emotional benefits have piqued the curiosity of many prestigious universities and research facilities. Respected medical journals such as the *Journal of Clinical Oncology*, *Journal of the American Geriatrics Society*, *Journal of the American Medical Association*, and *Annals of Internal Medicine*, to name a few, are publishing new and exciting research making the connection between a healthy lifestyle and cancer treatment.

Following publication of Dr. Dean Ornish's study of prostate cancer patients in 2005, a representative from the American Cancer Society commented that "the take-home message is that an active lifestyle combined with a healthy diet definitely decreases the risk of many types of cancer and in the case of early non-aggressive prostate cancer, it may slow disease progression." A representative from the National Cancer Institute said, "There's a building body of evidence that lifestyle may affect cancer progression. This is a very important area, and this is one more important lead that indicates a crucial direction for more research."

Yes, scientists and the medical community are taking note. What has caught their attention? In addition to dietary modifications, they are looking at how stress, exercise, and meditation affect a person's experience of cancer. Lifestyle factors that can positively influence cancer healing are as diverse as the people who practice them. And as with diet, these interventions are most successful when they move beyond being goals or occasional efforts; they're most effective when they become a way of life—a way of thinking, believing, and being. Here are some of the many options available to you:

- *Exercise and movement*: Strength training, yoga, walking, dance, qigong, and swimming are just a few of the possibilities. There's something for everyone, which is a good thing, as exercise or movement is so important.

- *Bodywork*: Choose from a wide variety of massage techniques, or consider chiropractic or osteopathic manipulation (it is important to inform your oncologist about your intention to receive chiropractic or osteopathic manipulation, so that you can be sure this treatment will be safe for your condition).

- *Meditation*: There are a variety of ways to meditate. The key is to find a meditation style that fits your lifestyle and personality. For some people, just being outside in nature is meditative and restorative. Others may experience the calming effects from a meditation practice based upon focused awareness on breathing.

- *Creativity*: Consider art, music, or journaling.

- *Experiencing positive emotions*: Anything that increases your daily experience of emotions such as love, happiness, and fulfillment will be good for you.

- *Spirituality*: Though most commonly associated with religious practice, prayer, or spiritual meditation, spirituality can be experienced in many ways. Anything that brings a sense of purpose and connectedness to your life can be considered a spiritual practice.

As diverse as this list is, most of the options mentioned have something in common: they can positively influence mood, enhance immunity, and reduce stress. And although all of these effects promote healing, stress reduction is leading the charge when it comes to lifestyle factors that can have a positive impact on an overall cancer prevention and treatment plan.

Reducing Stress Is Essential

Stress can come in a variety of forms. Although negative events like divorce or being fired are obviously stressful, you may be surprised to learn that some positive events, such as a wedding or a promotion, can be stressful too. Stress may be as minor as a buzzing fly or as monumental as a cancer diagnosis. Between all of those extremes lies an expansive spectrum of stress. We all have our favorite methods of stress management, whether it's a long, hot bath, playing with pets, a visit to the spa, or squeezing a small ball while sitting through a stressful meeting. Why do we so desperately want to shake off the stress that hangs on us? Because we know it (or our attitude toward it) negatively affects our health. But does stress cause cancer or cause it to spread? There is no conclusive evidence demonstrating that stress, in and of itself, causes cancer. However, many studies have confirmed that ongoing stress can contribute to the development and progression of cancer. While it's probably impossible to eliminate stress altogether, it does make sense to try to find ways to minimize the various stressors in our lives and shore up our ability to cope with those stressors.

Stressors are agents or conditions that can lead to a stress response. They can disrupt your internal balance. When this balance is disrupted, various physiological systems kick into action to try to reestablish balance. This is automatic and somewhat inexplicable, like a cat always landing on its feet. If the body detects imbalance, countless actions instantaneously occur to shift the body back into its comfort zone. All systems work together—cardiovascular, neurological, nervous, endocrine, immune, digestive—to maintain that balanced internal state known as homeostasis.

A certain amount of stress is normal, and the body is designed to manage it. In fact, stress is essential to life. Stress causes us to adapt and change, and over time, this contributes to our physical, mental, spiritual, and emotional development. The stress response can also help us cope more effectively in acute situations. We have all felt that nervous feeling prior to a big event, a difficult conversation, or a deadline. In those cases, the stress response helps us focus and tackle the issue head-on. However, according to Harvard medical professor and stress expert Herbert Benson, MD, prolonged stress or repeated acute stress can overload us, compromising our performance and eventually our health.

Stress can be physically damaging when the body gets accustomed to being out of balance. When being on high alert becomes the norm, homeostasis becomes foreign and unrecognizable. In this high-alert state, the body releases stress-induced chemicals causing organs and tissues to function differently in response. The normal functioning of the immune system is also affected. Immune cells behave differently, amplifying certain alarm reactions while neglecting their normal housekeeping tasks. And if the body's systems are constantly vigilant and focused on perceived stressors, they cannot do their job of killing cancer (this is discussed in detail in chapter 8).

Researchers at Ohio State University published a paper analyzing the association between age, stress, and immune function. They found that the immune system is affected by both aging and psychological stress. Each can disrupt immune function and have a potentially negative impact on health. Even worse, the effects of stress and age interact. Older adults can have more immune system impairment due to stress than younger adults because physiological stress both mimics and exacerbates the effects of aging. Life can be hard and unpredictable, and it isn't possible to avoid major life stressors. Divorce, death of a loved one, losing a job, and serious illness can rear its ugly head. But we can support our bodies through these difficulties with a healthful diet, healing lifestyle, and activities that quiet the mind and encourage internal peace.

Choosing stress-reducing activities is an individualized process. Putting on boxing gloves to work out frustrations may be perfect for some, while meditation may be the answer for others. Yoga, walking, golf, horseback riding, or tennis can all be great stress-reducing activities—if they're right for you. Or you may find that reading, journaling, praying, or listening to music helps you relax. Experiment and try different things. When you find a few enjoyable activities that help you relieve stress, stick with them and incorporate them into your regular routine.

One technique is so effective and yet so quick and easy to use that we encourage everyone to use it: deep breathing. Many of us fall into a habit of breathing shallowly—only into the chest. A few deep, diaphragmatic breaths can be enormously healing and help wash away stress and its biochemical debris. The diaphragm is the muscle that separates your chest and abdominal cavities, and a truly deep, diaphragmatic breath involves breathing so that this muscle expands downward. To check how you're breathing, place one hand on your chest and the other on your stomach. In diaphragmatic breathing, the hand on your stomach should move more than the hand on your chest. Next time you're overwhelmed by stress or overtaken by a strong negative emotion, give diaphragmatic breathing a try and see how it affects you.

Be aware of your emotions and how you are feeling. The more that you are aware of your emotional state, the more effective you will be in beginning stress management early, before the stress has such a dramatic cascading effect. Many of the following healthy lifestyle choices will help you reduce stress and promote optimal health. The most significant is physical activity.

Movement as Medicine

The human body is meant to move. While it may benefit from intense bicycling, routine weight training, and running marathons, these are not required in order to use physical activity to reduce stress and gain better health. Even the simplest movements such as swinging your arms when you walk, doing stretches at your desk, or carrying the groceries up the stairs will benefit your body and your mind. Movement helps us maintain our freedom, our ability to seamlessly perform everyday tasks. But movement can be more than just making it through the day. It can be medicine—a healing balm for body, mind, and spirit. Here are just a few of the important and far-reaching benefits of physical activity:

● Enhanced immunity

● Improved mood and self-image

● Stronger muscles and bones

● Reduced pain

● Increased energy and vitality

● Improved circulation of blood and lymphatic fluid

● Improved ability to sleep

- Better digestion

- Decreased risk of developing cancer

- Increased survival after cancer diagnosis

When you think of exercising more, you may flash to images of spandex, step aerobics, and mirrors in front of weight machines. But not everyone is comfortable in that typical gym environment. Fortunately, exercise goes far beyond those stereotypes or a treadmill at the local YMCA. Exercise includes walking, gardening, movement classes, yoga, and much more.

According to the American Cancer Society, researchers at Stanford University School of Medicine found that "no matter when you start, exercise improves health. Even people who start exercising later in life appear to gain many of the same health benefits as people who've exercised their whole lives."

Research is confirming that people with cancer can benefit from exercise. Not that long ago, cancer patients were told to take it easy and not do anything too strenuous. Obviously, that's good advice in certain circumstances; for example, following a major surgery. However, recent research has begun to reveal that exercise can be an extremely effective part of any cancer treatment program—even for those who are undergoing chemotherapy or radiation therapy.

Research has repeatedly demonstrated an overall increase in immunity in people who exercise regularly, and exercise has been shown to be particularly beneficial to patients with breast, prostate, or colon cancer. In the case of colon cancer, the American Cancer Society says, "physical activity speeds up the digestive process, shortening the exposure of the bowel lining to harmful substances."

The Nurses' Health Study, which followed 85,000 women over a 16-year period, demonstrated that women who reported moderate to vigorous physical activity for at least seven hours a week had an 18 percent lower risk of developing breast cancer than those who were sedentary.

Researchers at Harvard Medical School found that exercise improved survival rates in women diagnosed with breast cancer. "We found the maximum benefit in women who walked the equivalent of three to five hours a week," says Harvard researcher Michelle Holmes, explaining that women who are physically active have lower levels of hormones that stimulate breast cancer growth. There was no additional benefit from walking faster or longer than the average pace of the study participants—two to three miles per hour. A 2008 study published in the *Journal of Clinical Oncology* found that women who did the equivalent of at least two to three hours of brisk walking each week in the year before they were diagnosed with breast cancer were 31 percent less likely to die of the disease than women who were sedentary before their diagnosis. The study also found that women who increased their physical activity after diagnosis had a 45 percent lower risk of death compared with women who were inactive both before and after diagnosis.

Exercise is also important for men with prostate cancer. In a 14-year study, men over 65 years of age who regularly exercised most vigorously experienced slower disease progression and had a lower risk of dying from prostate cancer. Previously, exercise was thought to weaken the patient and the patient's immune system. However, research has confirmed that not only is physical activity during cancer treatment safe, in most cases it will actually enhance immunity and increase energy levels. "The results of the clinical studies, in brief, show that exercise is not dangerous, but in fact improves your overall health and well-being," according to the authors of *The Healing Power of Movement: How to Benefit from Physical Activity during Your Cancer Treatment*. About the only downside of aerobic exercise is increased oxidative stress, or free radical–caused damage to cells. If you're exercising regularly, it's probably a good idea to increase your intake of antioxidant-rich foods or antioxidant supplements to counteract the oxidative stress.

Movement for Weight Management

Research has clearly demonstrated a direct link between excess weight and cancer development, so exercise can play a fundamental role in preventing and treating cancer by assisting with weight management. Another study involving participants of the Nurses' Health Study, featured in the *Journal of the American Medical Association*, identified obesity and inactivity as significant risk factors for pancreatic cancer. The researchers concluded that physical activity decreased the risk of pancreatic cancer, especially among those who were overweight.

Physical activity can help you maintain a normal, "anticancer" weight. The American Cancer Society reminds us that dieting isn't the only way to lose weight: "One pound of body fat equals 3,500 calories . . . To lose one pound per week, reduce total calories by 500 per day. You can do this by eating 250 fewer calories a day and burning an extra 250 calories through physical activity." Or you could avoid those calories in the first place. Here are some ways to burn off 250 calories:

● Walk for 50 minutes at a moderate pace.

● Run for 20 minutes.

● Cycle for 30 minutes.

● Dance for 60 minutes.

Exercise Can Complement Conventional Treatment

By Susan Ryan, DO

Exercise is a form of medicine. In recent years, interest in demonstrating the benefits of exercise has increased substantially. Certainly, some of the effects can be measured through biophysical standards such as blood pressure and the efficiency of the cardiovascular and pulmonary systems. There are some equally important benefits that may not lend themselves to such easily measured outcomes, such as improved sleep quality and self-esteem, and an overall sense of well-being. In the area of integrative oncology, adding exercise to the regimen can offer a broad range of benefits.

As a concomitant cancer therapy, exercise was previously suspect because it was presumed to adversely affect the immune system. While it is true that extreme bouts of intense and prolonged exercise do leave the immune system vulnerable, many more recent studies have refuted the belief that exercise should be avoided during conventional cancer treatment.

The physiological and psychological impacts of cancer treatments are numerous. Exercise can help manage many of them, including the maintenance of body composition, especially muscle and bone density. By engaging in repetitive physical activity, one's endurance can be preserved and the devastating fatigue that is associated with cancer and cancer treatments such as chemotherapy and radiation can be minimized.

One of the most important benefits of an exercise program is enhanced sense of self. While difficult to measure, the results are clear: those who exercise feel like they retain a sense of control and rebound faster from each round of chemotherapy. They feel like their quality of life isn't so compromised during treatment, and they return to improved health and wholeness faster following treatment.

Many of the early studies of the effects of exercise on cancer involved participants who had early-stage breast cancers. But since those studies, other researchers have looked at many different types and stages of cancer along with a myriad of treatment regimens. It is well documented but still not broadly accepted that exercise is quite safe for many people with cancer.

In general terms, moderate aerobic exercise that is sustained for periods up to 30 minutes is safe; however, it is important to check with your oncologist to make sure that exercise is safe for you. You can start off with merely

Here is some additional fitness advice from the American Cancer Society:

- If you haven't been active, start with moderate activities that you enjoy and gradually increase the duration, frequency, and intensity as you are able, with the goal of 30 minutes or more five or more days a week.

- If you are active, you can increase intensity, duration, or frequency to 45 minutes or more of moderate to vigorous activity five or more days a week, increasing even further as you become more fit.

- If you are active and want to maintain your current level of fitness, you may want to consider adding new activities to your routine or rotate activities throughout the week. This will not only make exercising more interesting and fun, but will also use different muscles.

If you want to exercise but feel too exhausted or weak from your illness or treatment, it is important to listen to your body and not overdo it. When you're feeling weak, you may obtain the most benefit from gentle

5 minutes of walking and build up by 5-minute increments each week. Bicycling or other activities can also be used to achieve the aerobic goal. Aerobic exercise strengthens the heart, which may help prevent the cardiovascular toxicity associated with some chemotherapy drugs.

In addition to aerobic training, it is essential to perform some weight or resistance training. This not only will target the prevention of chemotherapy-related osteoporosis but will maintain the muscle mass that gives a person their get-up-and-go. Doing weight or resistance training three times a week will allow time to recover and provide for flexibility in one's schedule.

Speaking of flexibility, nothing is more important as we age than preserving our flexibility—physically, intellectually, and spiritually. Balance is critically tied to flexibility, and yoga and tai chi regimens are incredibly beneficial in this regard. Given the neurotoxic effects of some chemotherapy agents, it is important to incorporate a flexibility program to help prevent these devastating side effects. Flexibility enhances blood and oxygen flow to the brain and muscles as well as other parts of the body, potentially helping to reduce neurotoxicity.

If you have been sedentary prior to your diagnosis or treatment, it is very important to discuss exercise with your doctor before embarking on a new exercise program. In addition, if you are significantly fatigued or debilitated by your cancer or your treatments, it is critical that you do not overexercise. During these times, it is important to reduce your intensity, duration, and frequency of exercise. Working with a sports medicine expert, an exercise trainer who has worked with cancer patients, or a physical therapist may provide additional benefit for those who are just getting started or have special physical needs associated with their illness.

Physical activity and consistent exercise can help manage or alleviate many of the side effects of cancer and cancer treatments. Exercise not only adds years to your life, it also adds life to your years.

Susan Ryan, DO, is board certified in both sports medicine and family medicine. She has been a team physician for Olympic, professional, and collegiate athletes in multiple sports. She is on this book's editorial advisory board.

stretches, from changing positions, or moving to a new resting location. Exercise may leave you feeling more tired temporarily, but it should never exhaust you—if it does, you are doing too much.

Movement for Mental Clarity

Adding movement to your cancer treatment program will provide many physical benefits; however, exercise has emotional and mental health benefits as well. Exercise releases endorphins. These powerful neurotransmitters (chemicals in the brain) are the body's own painkillers and can also enhance mood, resulting in that "exercise high" we so often hear about. In addition, exercise can improve self-image, increase confidence, combat depression and fatigue, and contribute to a sense of empowerment. Best of all, big gains are made with even modest efforts. A recent study featured in the journal *Cancer Nursing* demonstrated that a 12-week dance and movement program significantly improved quality of life for breast cancer survivors.

Another study followed 40 breast cancer survivors who exercised and 79 who were sedentary. Researchers Pinto and Trunzo found that those who exercised had higher body esteem and were in a better mood than the sedentary women. The regular exercisers "reported significantly more positive attitudes . . . significantly less confusion, fatigue, depression, and total mood disturbances."

Exercise will also help with insomnia. However, it's best to avoid strenuous exercise later in the evening because the release of those endorphins may actually get in the way of a good night's sleep. On the other hand, gentle movement such as yoga or tai chi before bedtime can aid you in falling asleep. A study from the University of Texas M. D. Anderson Cancer Center found that patients with lymphoma who practiced Tibetan yoga had better subjective sleep quality, could get to sleep faster, slept longer, and used less sleep medications than patients who were not practicing yoga.

Yoga is also a great physical activity to consider because it is less jarring on the body and incorporates other important healing practices such as deep breathing and relaxation. Using a series of body postures and breathing exercises, yoga helps loosen muscles, encourages flexibility, relaxes mind and body, and helps relieve stress and anxiety. If you are hesitant to do yoga because you have a mental image of seemingly impossible contorted positions, bear in mind this observation from the American Cancer Society: "Although some of the postures seem to be extremely difficult to achieve, a basic principle of yoga is not to push beyond one's limit."

Lorenzo Cohen, MD, director of integrative medicine at the M. D. Anderson Cancer Center, did a study of women who practiced yoga while undergoing radiation treatment for breast cancer. The women reported better physical functioning, less fatigue, and fewer problems with sleep. The average patient in the study was 52 years old.

Many scientific studies have demonstrated the effectiveness of yoga as part of an integrative cancer treatment plan. Many of the larger cancer treatment centers, even conservative ones, offer yoga instruction and encourage the practice of yoga. A recent study at the University of Calgary demonstrated improvement in a number of quality-of-life variables in breast cancer survivors who participated in a seven-week yoga program. Participants showed improvements in irritability, depression, and confusion, as well as in general fitness and physical symptoms, such as gastrointestinal disturbances.

A research review featured in *Cancer Control* revealed that the practice of yoga by cancer patients and survivors led to improvements in mood, stress, cancer-related distress, cancer-related symptoms, sleep, and overall quality of life.

Massage Therapy

When delivered by a trained professional, massage not only feels good, it is also good for you. This form of bodywork can provide many emotional and physical benefits. A recent study featured in the *International Journal of Neuroscience* demonstrated that there is a biochemical stress-reducing reaction that occurs in the body following massage. Researchers noted a significant decrease in cortisol (the hormone associated with stress) and a significant increase in serotonin and dopamine (feel-good hormones). The researchers concluded that massage therapy can be effective for a variety of stressful experiences and medical conditions, including cancer.

Another study demonstrated enhanced immune activity in women with breast cancer following massage therapy, as indicated by increased levels of natural killer cells and lymphocytes. These are important immune system cells that help the body kill cancer cells.

Some people wonder whether massage therapy is safe for people with cancer. A literature review by Lisa Corbin, MD, from the Center for Integrative Medicine at the University of Colorado Hospital concluded that "conventional care for patients with cancer can safely incorporate massage therapy . . . The strongest evidence for benefits of massage is for stress and anxiety reduction, although research for pain control and management of other symptoms common to patients with cancer . . . is promising. The oncologist should feel comfortable discussing massage therapy with patients and be able to refer patients to a qualified massage therapist as appropriate."

Studies are now evaluating massage as a complementary therapy during active cancer treatment. Recently, researchers from Copenhagen found that a six-week program featuring structured physical activity, relaxation, body awareness techniques, and massage reduced symptoms related to chemotherapy treatments. Italian researchers recently found that reflexology foot massage significantly reduced anxiety in hospitalized patients receiving chemotherapy compared to those who did not receive the foot massage.

There are a few important cautions regarding massage for people with cancer. All of the following should be avoided:

- The area directly over a known tumor

- Bone that may be affected by cancer (to reduce risk of fracture)

- Deep massage work in people who are prone to bleeding

- Lymph massage if lymphatic spread is possible

It appears as though the benefits of massage therapy often outweigh the potential harm. Discuss massage with your doctor and be sure to choose a licensed massage therapist, preferably one who has worked with cancer patients.

Meditation as Medicine

How many times have you driven along the same road and never noticed a unique tree or missed the rainbow after the rain because you were rushing to your next appointment? Why is it important to notice the rainbow? Because that awareness brings our awareness into the present moment and doing so strengthens the connection between mind and body. We are learning that heightened awareness allows us to tap into the healing potential of the mind. The way we think, feel, live, and act *in total* affects our physical health. There is a direct physiological and energetic link between awareness of our thoughts, feelings, and emotions and the body that encases us. Our senses—vision, hearing, taste, touch, and smell—work together to give us information. Beyond that there is the place of mindfulness, ultimate awareness, and consciousness, creating and defining mind-body-spirit medicine. Meditation is a way to practice and enhance everyday mindfulness, making it a cornerstone of mind-body medicine.

Research is demonstrating that by focusing on the here and now while gently redirecting anxiety-provoking inner thoughts and images, we can help stimulate the relaxation response and positively influence important body systems. One of the most studied forms of meditation is mindfulness meditation, which has been researched extensively by Jon Kabat-Zinn, PhD. The mindfulness-based stress reduction (MBSR) program that Dr. Kabat-Zinn promotes is available through the Center for Mindfulness in Medicine, Health Care, and Society, and in many hospitals and universities throughout the world. More than 20 years of published research on MBSR has shown it to increase relaxation, reduce pain levels, and fortify the ability to cope with pain, increase energy, and improve self-esteem. A study featured in *Psychosomatic Medicine* showed that a mindfulness meditation program positively impacts brain and immune function. MBSR involves being in a comfortable posture, with your eyes closed and your spine reasonably straight. Direct your attention to your breathing, and when thoughts, emotions, or external distractions appear, simply accept them—without judging or getting involved with them. When you notice that your attention has drifted off and you are focused on thoughts or feelings, simply bring your attention back to your breathing.

Because sleep disturbance is a big issue for many people with cancer, researchers at the University of Calgary designed a study to see whether an eight-week MBSR program could help with this. Participants reported a reduction in sleep disturbances and improved sleep quality, as well as significant reductions in stress, mood disturbances, and fatigue. Another study, involving prostate cancer patients, showed that MBSR improved overall quality of life, symptoms of stress, and sleep quality. And yet another study showed that a combination of massage and MBSR helped reduce and manage chronic pain.

A research review of mindfulness meditation for cancer patients found that most of the studies have been done with breast and prostate cancer patients. The researchers conclude, "Consistent benefits—improved psychological functioning, reduction of stress symptoms, enhanced coping and well-being in cancer outpatients—were found." A 2004 meta-analysis evaluated 64 studies. Although all of the studies were relatively small, they all showed a broad range of benefits. A research review by Drs. Smith, Richardson, Hoffman, and Pilkington with the Research Council for Complementary Medicine in London concludes that MBSR "has potential as a clinically valuable self-administered intervention for cancer patients."

Meditation is safe, and it's easy to learn. As it has gained popularity, there are many books, classes, retreats, and resorts devoted solely to teaching people different ways to meditate. Clearly, the scientific literature indicates it can have significant health benefits.

Creative License

It may be difficult to believe that participating in art therapy, writing in a journal, or listening to music could be healing. However, researchers have confirmed that creative activities such as these can have enormous physical benefits. A recent study at Northwestern Memorial Hospital, in Chicago, found that after a one-hour art therapy class, cancer patients experienced significant reduction in eight of nine symptoms, including pain, anxiety, and depression.

Alastair Cunningham, PhD, of the Ontario Cancer Institute in Toronto, studied 22 terminal cancer patients who participated in a complementary program that included art therapy. Dr. Cunningham, a cancer survivor himself, found the program prolonged life. While the prognosis for all the patients was one year, two patients experienced complete remission and several others lived more than three years. Dr. Cunningham told *CURE* magazine, "Changing behaviors changes thoughts and ultimately changes reality."

Art therapists specializing in cancer care believe the therapy can help people move from isolation to connection, powerlessness to empowerment, and eventually from hopelessness to feeling hopeful. Art therapist Shannon Scott, from the University of Michigan Comprehensive Cancer Center, explains in *CURE*, "So much of the cancer experience is out of the patient's

Spirituality and Health

By Reverend Pam Roberts

Spirituality is that which gives meaning to our lives. Our spirituality represents our highest values and beliefs. Thus, the practice of spirituality is as diverse as the people practicing it. For some, spirituality means religious practice and meeting regularly within a community, temple, sangha, or church. For others it means gaining perspective by taking a walk in nature. For still others it means putting priority and energy into family, friends, and causes that they believe are important to make the world a better place.

How can spirituality affect our health? Our spirituality gives purpose to our lives. It gives us a reason to live and engage more deeply with the pulse and source of life. It helps us live life more fully by connecting us with the sacred and the universal, so we feel less isolated and alone. Some of the early cancer studies revealed that isolation adds to our illness or dis-ease. Humans are basically "herd" animals; we are not meant to live without a sense of belonging and community.

So what does it mean to be spiritual? At its heart, it means deeply engaging in that which gives meaning to our lives. Some of us are spiritual through our daily prayers or meditations. Others express spirituality by giving produce we've grown to others or supporting community causes with time, energy, money, and talents. In a very concrete sense, to be spiritual means to delve into where our passion and yearning lead us.

Several years ago, I was incredibly sick. My husband encouraged me to stop working so hard and engage in a hobby. A friend encouraged me to take horseback riding lessons because it was something I had always wanted to do but had not allowed myself the luxury of doing. So I went to the stable for a lesson. When I saw the huge draft horse standing in the corral, it was love at first sight. The next thing I knew I bought the horse, then a ranch to go around him. Because of that horse, who gave me back my energy and passion for life, I now use horses in my work with clients. My life is dedicated to working with horses to help other people find that same joy and zest in their lives. My experience illustrates that nontraditional symbols can help us create meaning and connection in our lives.

How do we incorporate spirituality into our lives? We do this by following the yearning in our hearts. We not only trust the yearning, we trust our way of nurturing that yearning and passion. For some people that might mean beginning to do daily devotions or reflections

hands. Art therapy gives patients a sense of control to come to the studio and have the time and space to do what it is they want to do."

Similarly, writing, music, and even creative visualizations can help people heal while exploring their untapped creative potential. These activities provide people with a positive vehicle for expressing themselves. And when faced with a cancer diagnosis, incorporating positive activities and feelings into the daily routine is critical.

Cultivate Honest Emotional Expression

We don't think anyone would argue against the assertion that positive emotions such as love, joy, laughter, and contentment are good for you. Not many people wish for more anger, sadness, and resentment in their lives. While it may seem obvious, cultivating positive emotions, relationships, and circumstances in your life is worthwhile, even if it takes a little extra thought and

of some kind, or beginning a prayer or meditation practice. For others our yearning might lead us to become involved in a support group, study group, yoga class, hiking club, religious institution, or retreat center.

Spiritual direction is a long-held practice for many people. This involves monthly meetings with a person or group trained in listening for the movement of the Spirit in one's life. Spiritual direction can help us learn which kind of prayer or meditation practice may be meaningful for our personality type. It can also help us become more attuned to the ways in which the Spirit is at work in the events of our daily lives. Spiritual direction helps us create meaning out of experiences that might otherwise seem mundane.

Here are some practical reflections to prime your thinking about your own spiritual direction:

1. What matters most to me in my life? Do I live in a way that makes that obvious to those who know me?

2. Who matters most to me in my life? Have I taken the time to tell them how much their words, actions, thoughts, and presence mean to me?

3. When do I feel like I am part of the flow of life? How often do I give myself the luxury of participating in that activity or practice regularly?

4. Do I believe in God, a Higher Power, a Universal Force? How and when do I take time to develop my relationship with that?

5. Do I enjoy expressing my love in my actions? Do I enjoy expressing my love with quiet reflection or contemplation?

6. What does my life mean in the greater context of human society? Why am I alive?

7. At what times in my life do I have a sense of knowing that I was "created to do this"?

8. When do I know my compassion? How do I express it?

9. How and when do I find meaning in my life by helping to relieve the suffering of others?

Reverend Pam Roberts is executive director of Samaritan Counseling and Education Center in Colorado, a specialist in Equine Facilitated Learning programs, and a cancer survivor.

effort. Something as simple as laughter can cause health-promoting physiological changes in the body. According to research featured in *Alternative Therapies in Health and Medicine*, laughter not only helps reduce stress, it also improves natural killer cell activity, which is a key anticancer component of the immune system. This confirms older research by famed cancer patient Norman Cousins, who watched humorous videos to help heal his cancer.

We're not advocating that you be positive and cheery all of the time. We are suggesting that you strive to be authentic in your enthusiasm and that you look for ways to increase your experience of positive emotions. However, painful emotions are bound to occur, and they need expression, too. Find friends with whom you can safely express yourself when you're feeling down, and look for other ways to express and explore painful emotions. Part of emotional health is to be fully present and "real" with *all* of your emotions. While it is painful to experience depression or anger, it's even more hurtful not to let yourself feel these emotions. Sadness can bring you

Foundational Health Plan

Here is a quick review of the key aspects associated with our diet and lifestyle recommendations for people with cancer. This advice applies to all types of cancer and includes aftercare advice as well.

Diet

- Eat 7–10 servings of fruits and vegetables every day (serving = 1 cup raw or ½ cup cooked).
- Eat 6 servings of whole grains (serving = 1 slice bread or ½ cup cooked grains).
- Eat adequate protein (body weight in pounds times 0.45 – 0.9 = total grams/day).
- Drink at least eight 8-ounce glasses of purified water daily.
- Increase consumption of omega-3 (fish, flax, nuts, seeds).
- Take dietary supplements as indicated.
- Use spices and seasonings liberally.
- Eat organic, nonprocessed foods.
- Avoid saturated fat and completely eliminate trans fats.
- Avoid simple sugars and refined carbohydrates.
- Limit fat to 30 percent of your total calories.
- Reduce or eliminate alcohol.
- Avoid overeating.

Lifestyle

- Do not smoke and limit exposure to second- and thirdhand smoke.
- Avoid or reduce your exposure to environmental toxins.
- Get sufficient sleep (7 to 9 hours every night).
- Exercise regularly (if able, exercise for 3 hours per week).
- Engage in health-promoting stress reduction techniques (meditation, spiritual practice, journaling, hobbies, etc.).
- Love yourself and those you are close to.
- Practice deep breathing daily.
- Be your authentic self.

down into the depths of your own inner ocean, where treasures often lie. You need to occasionally dive down there to gather those riches. The key is to come back up before you run out of air and then to use what you have found to enrich your life experience at the surface.

In addition to being authentic and fully present, a cancer diagnosis may be the perfect time to do a little emotional closet cleaning. Cancer often encourages people to take stock and evaluate their life, particularly in regard to their goals and what's meaningful and important to them. Take an inventory and "throw out" any emotions and thought patterns that aren't serving you. Consider counseling or a support group to help you sort through your emotions and promote a peaceful and uncluttered internal space.

As well as going inward, it is equally important to explore outward. A thorough evaluation of your relationships and how you connect with others may be in order. Isolation and loneliness can become a part of the cancer experience and be a barrier to healing. Reaching out to loved ones, healing or letting go of toxic relationships, and engaging in healthy connection with others are all important in the process of healing from cancer. Numerous studies have linked healthy companionship, support groups, and fulfilling relationships to overall well-being, survival, and quality of life. Our relationships and how we connect with others can provide a rich dimension to our lives and to our healing process.

Making a Spiritual Connection

Spirituality has different meanings for different people. Some may view it as a means to connect with a higher power or one's inner wisdom. Others may feel attending a church and engaging in a prayerful practice represents spirituality. And still others may believe that being a good person, giving back to society, or communing with nature is spiritual. No matter how you define spirituality, research is demonstrating that it is an important component of the healing process. A recent study featured in the journal *Integrative Cancer Therapies* found that spirituality influenced all aspects of the cancer experience for a group of men with prostate cancer. Spiritual practices studied included unique ceremonies, indigenous healing rituals, prayer, meditation, and the use of spiritual imagery. Finding your spiritual core and ways to honor your individual spirituality will be a positive contributor on your healing journey. Spirituality can also help provide you with a greater context for your experience with cancer. Questions such as "Why me?" and "What is the lesson to be learned in this experience of cancer?" are often best answered within a spiritual paradigm. For more information on spirituality, refer to the sidebar "Spirituality and Health" on pages 82 and 83 by Rev. Pam Roberts.

A Special Note to Caregivers

We understand how difficult it can be to have a loved one diagnosed with cancer. As emotions stir, you try desperately to hold things together so you can care for your loved one. While you are not the one who is suffering physically from the illness, it is still very important that you pay attention to your own health. Follow the advice in this chapter along with your loved one. You will not only be supporting your loved one along their healing journey, you will also be ensuring that you stay well throughout the process. Pay close attention to your diet and lifestyle activities and to the best of your ability follow the advice outlined in the Foundational Health Plan featured on page 84.

Putting It All Together

A healthy lifestyle forges a seamless interconnection between body, mind, and spirit. The most important ways to enhance that critical connection are through movement, bodywork, meditation, creative activities, encouraging love and joy, creating community, and finding meaning in your life.

Along with diet, healthy lifestyle choices provide a foundation on which the healing process can securely rest. This foundation can help you tackle the integrative cancer treatment plan with strength and confidence.

five

Treatment Approach Overview

We know that cancer treatment is just part of the picture. However, if you have just been diagnosed with cancer, it's the only part you see. Your cancer treatment plan becomes the primary focus of your life. As life goes on for everyone else, your world comes to a grinding halt. You catch glimpses of everyday activities in your peripheral vision, but they seem like a sideshow—distractions to your process, your plan, your fight. Cancer has become your job, your obsession. A cancer diagnosis defines and disrupts your life in profound ways. Given that cancer treatment takes center stage, it is of utmost importance to understand as much as possible about the components of an integrative treatment plan. Let's start with conventional treatment.

Conventional medicine is based upon three basic treatment options. Although there have been improvements within each, these same options have been offered to cancer patients for decades. Surgery, radiation, and chemotherapy have all been shown to kill cancer cells. Unfortunately, they can also cause varying degrees of damage to normal tissues and they do not always cure cancer. The continued hunt for more effective treatments and treatment support options is the driving force behind current research and development in conventional cancer care. Targeted molecular therapies are one result of this search. While still falling short of eradicating cancer, conventional cancer therapies are powerful weapons in this fight.

A great deal of individualized thought and information gathering should go into determining a cancer treatment plan. To decide which conventional and/or complementary treatments are most appropriate, ask yourself these key questions:

- Where is the cancer?
- What stage is the cancer and has it spread?
- How old is the person and how is their overall health?
- What are the chances of survival and remission?
- Which treatment offers the best chance of destroying the cancer while causing the least harm to the person?
- What are the risks associated with the proposed treatment?
- What are the goals of the person with cancer?

Answering these questions will help you make educated decisions. This, in turn, will give you greater confidence in your treatment and will keep you focused on doing what you can to maximize its benefits.

Surgery

Typically, if the cancer is operable, surgery will be recommended. Removing the cancer, if at all possible, is considered paramount. For most people with cancer, surgery starts with a biopsy. If surgical removal of the cancerous tissue is possible, more extensive surgery will be recommended. Sometimes, surgery is all that is required. The cancer is removed and the person can develop a proactive plan to prevent a recurrence. In some cases, surgery is not the entire treatment but is the first part of an overall plan that may later include chemotherapy, radiation, or other treatments. The surgery can range from simple removal of a protruding lump, with a short recovery period, to extensive removal of cancerous tumors along with other tissue, requiring a long recovery time, possible rehabilitation, or even plastic surgery. Surgery to remove particular organs can affect health and well-being long after the person has recovered from the surgery.

While surgery is a common intervention among people with cancer, it remains frightening to most patients. The best way to ease fears associated with surgery is to develop a high level of comfort regarding the procedure, the surgeon, and the facility where the surgery is planned to take place. Ask a lot of questions prior to the surgery and understand the possible risks and what you can expect during the recovery period.

Radiation

Radiation is often recommended as a complement to surgery for cancers that are localized to one or several distinct areas in the body. The American Cancer

What Are My Chances?

By Heather Greenlee, ND, MPH, PhD

Oftentimes conventional oncologists speak in terms of statistical chances. One therapy may provide a better chance of survival than another. But how do we evaluate what it means to be statistically significant? How do we make sense of the math and apply those numbers to quality-of-life issues?

Both conventional oncologists and integrative practitioners aim to provide information to patients about the chances that different treatments will work for their cancer. People want to know many different kinds of information about their treatment: What are the chances it will shrink the tumor? What are the chances it will prevent the return of the cancer? What are the chances it will prolong my life? What will be the impact on my quality of life or how I feel? Oftentimes this information is presented in terms of statistics. In order to understand what these statistics mean and how to interpret them, it is helpful to understand the following concepts. (For more information on these terms, you can consult the National Cancer Institute's "Dictionary of Cancer Terms" at www.cancer.gov/dictionary/).

Clinical trial: Much of the information on the effects of specific cancer treatments comes from clinical trials. Clinical trials are research studies where patients with a specific type of cancer are assigned to different groups that can be compared. For example, the study could compare a new treatment to an old treatment, or a new treatment plus the old treatment could be compared to the old treatment alone.

Observational study: Observational studies are studies where patients are observed for outcomes but no specific treatment is given.

Statistical significance: Researchers use statistical tests to interpret the results of their research. For example, in a clinical trial they can compare participants who were selected at random to receive a specific treatment to those who were not selected to receive the treatment. Researchers want to know if there is a statistically significant difference between the groups. In other words, are the differences they see between the groups a result of the treatment, or might they have occurred by chance? This provides information about whether that treatment is better or worse than whatever it is being compared to (another treatment or no treatment at all).

P-value: This commonly used statistic tells us the probability that the difference between two groups is only coincidental. P-values are used to help conclude if any difference seen between groups is real or is due to chance. The standard limit for a significant p-value is anything that is equal to or less than 0.05. If a p-value is less than 0.05, this means that there is less than a 5 percent chance that the observed difference is due to chance.

Risk: This term is used to indicate how likely something is to happen. Risk statistics are often used for describing the effects of cancer prevention strategies and cancer treatments. Risk can also be used to evaluate other aspects of cancer treatment, including whether the treatment will shrink the tumor, cause side effects, or prolong life.

Risk of recurrence: This refers to the likelihood that a cancer will return after treatment, either to the same location (a local recurrence) or to a different location in the body (a metastasis). For example, when thinking about cancer treatment, risk can refer to the number of

---

Society reports that approximately 60 percent of cancer patients receive some sort of radiation therapy. Medically speaking, radiation is a form of ionizing energy most commonly delivered via a beam from a machine outside the body and targeted to a specific tumor or group of cancer cells. Ionizing radiation produces ions after interacting with cellular material. This process

people who have cancer recurrence after the treatment. Here risk is calculated as the number of people with cancer recurrence divided by the number of people in the total population treated for that cancer.

Risk ratio: Also known as relative risk or odds ratio, this statistic is often used to predict cancer risk, treatment benefit, and cancer recurrence. It provides a ratio of the risk of disease in the people who received a treatment compared to the risk of disease in the people who did not receive the treatment. It is calculated as the percentage of people receiving treatment who developed the disease divided by the percentage of people not receiving treatment who developed the disease. A risk ratio equal to 1 means that there is no benefit from the treatment. A risk ratio less than 1 means that the treatment helped to prevent disease. A risk ratio greater than 1 means that the treatment caused more people to get the disease.

Survival benefit: This refers to how many weeks, months, or years a treatment is expected to add to a patient's life after a specific cancer treatment.

Survival curves: Also known as Kaplan-Meier survival curves or Cox proportional hazards, survival curves are statistics used to predict survival time after cancer treatment. These are different from risk ratios and odds ratios in that they take time into account and examine how two groups who do or don't receive treatment differ in either having cancer recurrence or dying.

How Does This Apply to You?

These statistics are often generated when researchers study large groups of people. Therefore, these statistics can tell a population's risk, but not an individual's risk. This is important to understand when as a patient or a family member you are considering what

treatments to use or not to use. Few treatments work the same in 100 percent of the people who take them, and there are no guarantees that you will experience the positive (cure) or negative (side effects) of any given treatment.

When evaluating whether the results from a specific study apply to you, be sure you consider selection criteria and study intervention. Selection criteria describe what types of patients were eligible to enter the study. Consider whether the patients in the study were like you in terms of type of cancer, cancer stage, previous cancer treatments, other illnesses, age, gender, race, and ethnicity. Study intervention is the treatment that people in the study received for their cancer. Be aware of whether the same doses and schedule that are being offered to you were used in the study, and if there were other medications or treatments used.

Why Aren't There More Statistics about Integrative Oncology?

Many of the integrative oncology treatments have not undergone as much research as have conventional oncology treatments. This is partly due to lack of research funding and partly due to lack of researchers investigating these treatments. Clinical trials are expensive and time-consuming, and specially trained researchers are needed to conduct these studies. Due to the scarcity of research on integrative oncology treatments, conventional oncologists often have more statistics to share with patients than do integrative practitioners. However, this is slowly changing as more research is being conducted on integrative therapies. Stay tuned for more information!

Heather Greenlee, ND, MPH, PhD, is a postdoctoral research scientist with the Department of Epidemiology at Mailman School of Public Health of Columbia University. She is also on this book's editorial advisory board.

transforms cellular material into electrified particles that are unstable and reactive, making the cells susceptible to destruction. Radiation penetrates cells and kills them by activating the process of programmed cell death, known as apoptosis. Radiation damages cellular DNA in both cancer cells and healthy cells, although healthy cells are more resistant to radiation damage

What's New with Radiation?

Medical radiation can be defined as ionizing energy transmitted at the speed of light via oscillating electric and magnetic fields. The purpose of this radiated energy is to initiate cellular death. As the radiation travels through the patient, it deposits energy and breaks chemical bonds, damaging cells. "The deposition of radiation dose and the damage it induces is random and complex," according to the textbook *Clinical Oncology*, "and depends on many aspects of both the radiation and the biologic tissue."

Recent advances in the delivery of radiation can help reduce damage to surrounding healthy tissue while targeting the cancer cells. The goal of these advances is to concentrate the radiation in the cancerous tissue. Brachytherapy, for example, puts radioactive material into small pellets or seeds, or delivers radiation through a cathode within a tube. The radioactive material is then implanted inside a tumor or the space where a tumor has been removed. The radiation is delivered in such a way that it doesn't extend beyond the intended area of treatment.

Intensity-modulated radiotherapy, or IMRT, is a newer and more precise way to deliver radiation. IMRT varies the intensity of the radiation beam across the tissues in the field of radiation to spare normal tissues while concentrating radiation at the site of the tumor. IMRT is made possible by newer computer-based technology that creates three-dimensional images of the tumor and surrounding tissues and organs. Multiple radiation beams are then shaped to match the 3-D image, pinpointing the cancer while minimizing exposure of nearby healthy cells to radiation. Tomotherapy takes this one step further by using advanced spiral fan-beamed CT image-guided scanning technology to target cancer and then precisely modulate radiation intensity based on the location and type of cancer. Tomotherapy focuses IMRT treatments so precisely that even normal internal tissue movements can be taken into account, allowing for precise radiation of structures within body organs and tissues and allowing even tighter margins and more protection of normal tissue.

Although these new delivery systems make radiation therapy more tolerable for the patient, side effects still can occur. If radiation therapy is chosen, it is best to support the body during the process. For more information on how to offset the side effects of radiation, refer to chapter 6.

and they can repair themselves more effectively than cancer cells. Side effects of radiation therapy depend on the target, duration, and type of the radiation treatment. Some of the most common side effects are as follows:

- Anemia (low red blood cell count)
- Fatigue
- Nausea or vomiting
- Diarrhea
- Hair loss
- Skin irritation or burns
- Sterility

Radiation can also result in more serious side effects, including stiffening of lung tissue (fibrosis), secondary cancers, and the possibility of weakened bone strength or damage to the bone marrow, where red blood cells, platelets, and white blood cells are produced.

Radiation can be used alone as a primary therapy or in conjunction with other treatment options. Radiation is used to destroy cancerous tumors. Radiation is also used to prevent a cancer recurrence in the same tissue or organ as the original tumor by eliminating cancer cells that may have strayed some distance from the original tumor. Radiation therapy can also destroy metastatic tumors when those tumors are causing pain or significant organ dysfunction. The equipment and methods used to deliver radiation therapy have become more sophisticated over the years. While external beam radiation is the most common form, brachytherapy can provide an even more tightly focused radiotherapeutic effect. Brachytherapy delivers radiation into or near the tumor via a radioactive pellet (seed) or through a radioactive tube placed into the tissue. The goal with some of the newer methods of delivering radiation is to target the cancer cells even more narrowly and avoid exposing nearby healthy cells to the destructive doses of radiation.

(For more information on new developments in radiation therapy, refer to the sidebar opposite.)

Chemotherapy

Chemotherapy is used before, during, or after radiotherapy. Some cancers are not sensitive to radiation therapy or are too widely disseminated for radiation therapy to be effective. For these cancers, chemotherapy is often the primary treatment, especially in the case of lymphoma, leukemia, and metastasized solid tumor cancers. Chemotherapy can also be used to shrink tumors before surgery.

Chemotherapy involves giving the patient chemical agents that are toxic to cells. After being administered orally, intravenously, or by injection, these chemical agents circulate throughout the body. The goal with chemotherapy is to halt cell reproduction and growth, which leads to cell death. Most chemotherapy drugs are designed to attack rapidly dividing cells. Cancer cells are among some of the most rapidly dividing cells in the body.

There are five major classes of chemotherapy drugs:

- Alkylating agents bind to the DNA in cancerous cells, preventing the DNA from uncoiling in cell division.

- Antimetabolites replace nutrients needed for DNA synthesis with inactive substances, thus preventing cellular division.

- Antitumor antibiotics generate activated oxygen free radicals, which cause DNA breaks that in turn prevent DNA from uncoiling and cause eventual cell death.

● Mitotic inhibitors interfere with the architecture within a cancer cell, thus damaging a cell and triggering apoptosis while also preventing the cell from dividing.

● Topoisomerase inhibitors incapacitate topoisomerase enzyme, which is needed for DNA uncoiling and cell division. These drugs also trigger apoptosis.

(See the sidebar on page 94 for information about promising new chemotherapy drugs.)

There are more than 40 different chemotherapy drugs currently being used to treat cancer. Some of these drugs are so toxic that other drugs (known as co-medications) are used to help offset their side effects. Additionally, chemotherapeutic agents may be combined with one or more other drugs for a synergistic effect. Chemotherapy regimens may be well tolerated with minimal side effects, or they can be difficult to endure and produce considerable side effects.

Quality-of-life issues often arise during chemotherapy. Patients receiving chemotherapy can feel much worse during treatment than they did with the cancer alone. Side effects of chemotherapy vary depending on the chemotherapy agent used and the person's sensitivity to the drugs administered. These side effects can range anywhere from mild and manageable to severely debilitating and in some cases life threatening. Some of the most common side effects are as follows:

● Nausea and vomiting

● Hair loss

● Mouth sores or dry mouth

● Constipation or diarrhea

● Fatigue and weakness

● Difficulty swallowing or dental problems

● Taste impairment

● Loss of appetite

● Bleeding or blood count issues

● Anemia

- Infection

- Numbness and tingling (neuropathy)

- Cardiovascular damage

- Difficulty sleeping

Side effects occur when healthy, rapidly growing cells are affected by the chemotherapy. Because these drugs cannot distinguish between a rapidly dividing cancer cell and a rapidly dividing normal cell, many noncancerous cells are destroyed in addition to the cancer cells. Rapidly growing cells are found in the hair follicles, digestive tract, reproductive system, and bone marrow. Because ovarian and testicular tissues are sensitive to chemotherapy, infertility may result from certain chemotherapy drugs. Additionally, most chemotherapy drugs cannot be used during the first trimester of pregnancy, as the rapidly growing fetus will be damaged. Side effects can also occur as a result of certain cells concentrating the chemotherapy agent. For example, nerve tissue is uniquely susceptible to certain chemotherapy drugs. This toxicity manifests as cold sensitivity, numbness, and tingling, typically in the fingers and toes. Finally, chemotherapy treatments cause inflammation in the body, which, in turn, causes some of the side effects most commonly associated with chemotherapy, such as fatigue, lack of appetite, "chemo-brain" (difficulty concentrating or remembering), and weakness.

Side effects are usually unique to the type of drugs used. Certain chemotherapy drugs may cause nerve damage, while others might cause digestive toxicity or heart problems. The recovery of normal cells begins as soon as the treatment is discontinued. Nonetheless, treatment recovery time varies from one patient to the next depending on how the person is supported physically, mentally, and emotionally during chemotherapy.

In some cases, the primary goal of chemotherapy is to improve the patient's quality of life. Some patients feel better while on chemotherapy because their tumor burden is decreased, which then decreases some of the symptoms caused by the cancer, such as fatigue, loss of appetite, and weight loss. This improvement in symptoms can make chemotherapy a burden worth bearing.

Fortunately, in the last two decades there has been enormous progress in alleviating side effects of chemotherapy. Discuss side effects of chemotherapy with your doctor and ask about potential co-medications that may help make treatment much more tolerable. (For more information on how nutrients, herbs, and other natural therapies can help offset the side effects of conventional treatments, refer to the conventional cancer treatment tables on pages 140–172.)

New Drug Developments

According to the National Cancer Institute's online drug dictionary, more than 500 drugs are being used to treat cancer or cancer-related conditions. Chemotherapy drugs used to treat cancer are considered cytotoxic, which means they cause cell death. Cytotoxic agents are the most commonly used drugs in cancer treatment. But several new categories of anticancer drugs, described below, are either in development or already available.

Differentiation drugs: These compounds can stimulate the maturation and differentiation of immature cells into functional cells. (And as mentioned in chapter 1, cancer cells aren't as well differentiated as normal cells.) Drugs in this category may be more effective for prevention. The FDA has already approved one drug in this class to be used for colon cancer prevention in high-risk families. Another differentiation drug, all-trans-retinoic acid, is being tested for use in leukemia.

Gene therapy: This form of treatment injects specific genes into the tumor. No drugs have been approved in this class. "No proof of efficacy has been shown," according to the textbook *Clinical Oncology*, "and the technical hurdles are still daunting." Nonetheless, this is an exciting area of development that has the potential to correct the cancerous mutations within DNA in a relatively nontoxic manner.

Vaccines: The concept of using viruses to build up immunity to infectious organisms is not new. But only recently has this approach been considered for cancer. Researchers featured in the *Journal of Clinical Oncology* believe we are getting closer to using a tumor-specific antigen, fed to a partially disabled virus, which, when injected into the body, activates an immune response against the tumors that express that same antigen. Cancer vaccines can also be introduced to the body by creating a synthetic tumor antigen, removing some immune cells from the blood in order to expose them to the synthetic antigen, and then reinjecting them into the body to create a systemic immune response. These are known as cancer-specific vaccines. According to *Clinical Oncology*, "To date, no convincing clinical evidence exists for sufficient efficacy of cancer vaccines, and the ability to correlate immune response to a vaccine and clinical effectiveness have been elusive." Nonetheless, several cancer vaccines are in the last phase of clinical trial development and will be brought to market soon. The first cancer treatment vaccine to be introduced to the market may likely be for prostate cancer.

As with any pharmaceutical agent, all of these new treatments may have side effects and risks. A thorough risk-versus-reward analysis is always in order. Be sure all of your questions are answered and all options are weighed carefully before you make a final decision regarding any drug therapy.

Targeted and Hormonal Therapies

It is becoming much more common for cancer patients to receive targeted drugs with their chemotherapy regimen. Unlike older chemotherapeutic drugs, the actions of targeted drugs focus on molecular targets that are reliably expressed in cancer cells. The goal of targeted drugs is to interact with these specific targets and in doing so to prevent cell division or trigger cell apoptosis. There are three main types of targeted molecular therapies:

1. Tyrosine kinase inhibitors comprise a family of proteins that bind and deactivate certain receptors that exist on the cell membrane of the cancer cell and also block multiple proteins within the cell in the

tyrosine kinase pathways. Normally, activation of tyrosine kinase pathways results in cell proliferation and in the release of angiogenic factors. Tyrosine kinase pathways are overexpressed in cancer cells. Tyrosine kinase inhibitors bind to the membrane receptor or to one or more of the tyrosine kinase proteins within the cell and block the signaling of this pathway. The net result is to prevent cell division (tumor growth) and prevent angiogenesis (blood supply to the tumor). Examples of tyrosine kinase inhibitors are axitinib, bosutinib, cediranib (Recentin), dasatinib (Sprycel), erlotinib (Tarceva), gefitnib (Iressa), imatinib (Gleevec), lestaurtinib, nilotinib (Tasigna), semaxanib, sorafenib (Nexavar), sunitinib (Sutent), and vandetanib (Zactima).

2. Monoclonal antibodies bind to certain cell surface receptors and block the action of those receptors. This results in decreased signaling from the cell membrane to the cell nucleus. The cell surface receptors that are targeted by monoclonal antibodies are receptors that normally signal the DNA in the cell's nucleus to divide. Certain cancers express a large quantity of these cell surface receptors; for instance, certain breast cancer cells express HER-2/neu receptors. A monoclonal antibody known as trastuzumab (Herceptin) binds to HER-2/neu receptors, which prevents cell division and also triggers cell apoptosis. In addition to Herceptin, monoclonal antibodies include drugs such as alemtuzumab (Campath), bevacizumab (Avastin), cetuximab (Erbitux), edrecolomab (Panorex),gemtuzumab (Mylotarg), lapatinib (Tykerb), panitumumab (Vectibix), rituximab (Rituxan), trastuzumab (Herceptin), and tositumomab (Bexxar).

3. Hormonal therapies target specific enzymes that are required in the production of certain hormones or block the receptors on cell surfaces that bind these hormones. This is an effective therapy when certain cancers utilize hormones to stimulate their growth. For instance, certain breast cancers are categorized as estrogen receptor positive (ER+). This means the breast cancer cells have a significant number of estrogen receptors on their surfaces, and when estrogen binds to these receptors a message is sent to the cell DNA to divide. Hormonal therapies block the estrogen receptor (as in the case of Tamoxifen) or block the production of estrogen (as in the case of aromatase inihibitors). Hormone therapy will be discussed in more detail in chapter 10.

Targeted molecular therapies are not without side effects, and the side effects can be mild to major. Various side effects including rash, diarrhea, muscle cramps, nausea, and elevated blood pressure are common. While generally somewhat better tolerated than chemotherapy, these treatments are not benign. Fortunately, patients receiving targeted molecular therapies will also benefit from certain nutrients, herbs, and other natural therapies (see the "Targeted Therapies" chart on pages 158 to 159 for more information).

Clinical Trials

Depending on the type of cancer, enrolling in a clinical trial may be a treatment option for you. A cancer treatment clinical trial is the final stage of a lengthy research process. Cancer treatment clinical trials involve cancer patients who have voluntarily agreed to participate. These trials are designed to evaluate a new treatment such as a drug, surgery option, radiation, or other new method or combination of methods. There can be risks associated with clinical trials, so the decision to enter one should not be made hastily. Discuss your options with your doctor. For more information on clinical trials, visit www.cancer.gov/clinicaltrials/learning and for a list of current clinical trials presently taking place, visit www.cancer.gov/clinicaltrials/search.

Expanding Our Treatment Options

To win the cancer battle, we often must use more than the standard conventional treatment methods. Hope and power can come from having options and exercising the right to choose one or more of those options, as well as combining therapies for optimum success.

There are choices beyond surgery, radiation, and pharmaceuticals (chemotherapy and targeted drugs). There are new conventional therapies under development and there are also many therapies already in use to enhance conventional cancer treatments. Many of these healing methods can be used before, during, and after conventional treatments. Integrative healing brings the humanity back to cancer treatment. That's why more people than ever before are choosing a more integrative treatment approach.

Choosing Integrative Medicine

Nearly 70 percent of people diagnosed with cancer aren't satisfied with the three choices offered by conventional medicine—surgery, radiation, and chemotherapy—and an increasing number of people are exploring alternatives. Although we prefer the term *integrative medicine*, most of the data on patients' choices deems anything outside of conventional medicine as *complementary and alternative medicine* (CAM). While data regarding CAM use among cancer patients varies, a survey featured in the journal *Supportive Care in Cancer* (2005) involving newly diagnosed cancer patients receiving chemotherapy and radiation indicated that 91 percent used at least one CAM therapy. Sadly, only 57 percent of those surveyed discussed their CAM use with their oncologist. This disconnect is a clear indication that patients need to become more comfortable in disclosing all therapies to their physicians and physicians need to be more supportive of an integrative approach. In another study conducted by the University of Pennsylvania in 2006, 86 percent of recently diagnosed female cancer patients reported satisfaction with complementary and alternative medicine as a cost-effective approach. In 2004 the *Journal of Clinical Oncology* reported that 88 percent of 102 cancer patients at the Mayo Comprehensive Cancer Center (a conservative Midwest hospital and research facility) used at least one CAM therapy. An amazing 93 percent of those using CAM used dietary supplements, 53 percent used other CAM therapies such as prayer or chiropractic, and nearly 47 percent used both supplements and other therapies.

Given the high rate of complementary and alternative medicine use among cancer patients, it is important to clarify three key terms:

● **Alternative medicine** is used in place of conventional medicine.

● **Complementary medicine** is used along with conventional medicine.

● **Integrative medicine** combines conventional medicine with CAM practices that have been shown to be effective.

The National Center for Complementary and Alternative Medicine (NCCAM) has identified five CAM domains and four primary CAM systems of healing. The domains, or categories of therapies, are as follows:

1. Biologically based practices (which focus on the use of herbs, supplements, and foods)

2. Mind-body medicine (including support groups, prayer, and meditation)

3. Manipulative and body-based approaches (massage, chiropractic, and the like)

4. Energy medicine (such as qigong, Reiki, and use of magnets)

5. Alternative medical systems (complete systems of theory and practice)

NCCAM breaks down the fifth domain, alternative medical systems, into four primary systems of healing:

1. Ayurvedic medicine

2. Homeopathy

3. Naturopathy

4. Traditional Chinese medicine (TCM)

These five domains and four primary healing systems encompass a wide variety of therapies that can be used to complement cancer treatment, offset side effects of cancer treatment, and strengthen the body's natural healing ability.

A Brief Look at Selected Integrative Therapies

The best way to truly heal cancer is to use a comprehensive, multidimensional mind-body-spirit approach. Cancer is a complex illness, and treatment success is enhanced by supporting all aspects of the patient's health and well-being. If a patient finds a specific integrative therapy helpful and there are no dangers associated with its use, it's likely that it will enhance the person's quality of life and ability to heal.

When deciding on a treatment plan, whether conventional, alternative, or integrative, consultation with a licensed health-care practitioner who specializes in cancer care is absolutely critical. Do not discontinue medications or treatments without first discussing your options with your oncologist. If you aren't comfortable discussing your desire to use complementary therapies with your oncologist, you may want to choose another oncologist who will be more open to exploring an integrative approach with you.

Because the conventional treatments used to attack cancer can be toxic and extreme, complementary therapies can play an important role in helping to sustain or rebuild important body functions before, during, or after conventional therapy. (Chapter 6 is devoted to this important topic.) If you're working with an integrative health-care practitioner, your individualized treatment plan may include one or more complementary therapies in place of conventional treatment or to enhance conventional treatment.

Many of these therapies have been studied using conventional research methods, while others have stood the test of time and are supported by impressive historical and clinical evidence. It is important to note that very few of these therapies have been approved as stand-alone cancer treatments by the U.S. Food and Drug Administration. Following is a brief overview of some of the integrative therapies most commonly used by cancer patients.

- *Acupuncture*: This is a form of traditional medicine that originated in China more than 5,000 years ago. The premise of acupuncture is that health is determined by the balance of a vital life force energy called qi (pronounced "chi"), which flows along 12 major pathways in the body, called meridians. Small needles are inserted into one or more of the over 1,000 acupuncture points along the meridians in order to support optimal flow of qi throughout the body and thereby improve health in specific ways. Studies have demonstrated that acupuncture can relieve pain, nausea, fatigue, and other symptoms associated with cancer and cancer treatment.

- **Biofeedback**: Using electronic devices, biofeedback monitors certain bodily processes such as breathing, heart rate, and blood pressure and conveys this information to the person to help them learn to consciously influence those systems. Biofeedback can help ease headaches, improve breathing, help reduce stress and anxiety, and relieve pain associated with the cancer or conventional cancer treatment.

- **Constitutional medicine**: These healing systems begin by determining the person's constitution—their strengths, susceptibilities, metabolic status, or predisposition toward certain conditions. Examples of constitutional medicine include Ayurveda, traditional Chinese medicine, and Tibetan medicine. The focus of constitutional medicine is on helping the person achieve and maintain balance in accordance with their constitutional type. In these systems, internal harmony results in physical, emotional, and spiritual good health and may improve overall quality of life.

- **Creativity**: Many innovative researchers are confirming that creative endeavors enhance a positive connection between mind and body. In addition, creativity is believed to stimulate immune activity and help reduce the damaging effects of stress. Creative activities that can promote physical and emotional health include art, music, and writing (especially journaling).

- **Detoxification**: The body has systems in place to break down and eliminate harmful substances, a process known as detoxification. Detoxification therapies assist the body in eliminating or neutralizing toxins. For more information on detoxification, refer to chapters 7 and 12.

- **Diet and nutrition**: The healing power of foods has been borne out in numerous scientific studies, and there is no question that some foods can heal and some can harm. Tipping the scales in favor of healing foods and a health-promoting nutrition plan is the goal of diet and nutrition therapy. We discuss diet and nutrition throughout the book, especially in chapter 4.

- **Heat therapy**: Also known as hyperthermia, heat therapy artificially raises the body's temperature to help alleviate infection, inflammation, or other health conditions. Raising the body's temperature above 98.6°F stimulates the release of pyrogens (from bacteria), which, in turn, mobilize immune cells. In addition, localized hyperthermia treatment may be used to increase circulation of blood and lymph fluid in specific areas without inducing a change in core temperature. People with cancer should only use hyperthermia under medical supervision.

- **Herbal remedies**: Also referred to as botanical medicine or phytotherapy (phyto meaning "plant"), herbal medicine has been used throughout history to promote health and prevent or cure illness. Many pharmaceutical drugs originate from medicinal herbs, and these drugs are often used in ways that correspond with their traditional use in native cultures where they originated. Plants can have mild effects or pronounced activity depending on the herbs used, whether they're used alone or in combination, and the form in which they're used. There are many botanical therapies with great benefit to people with cancer discussed throughout this book.

- **Homeopathy**: This form of medicine uses highly diluted natural substances to bring the body back into balance. Homeopathy uses substances in infinitesimally small doses to help the natural processes of the body regain homeostasis. It is intended to create constitutionally based well-being as well as to relieve symptoms such as nausea, constipation, diarrhea, and peripheral neuropathy, among others.

- **Hydrotherapy**: Hydrotherapy is the use of water, ice, steam, and hot and cold temperatures to maintain and restore health. It is believed that hot water can stimulate the immune system and help detoxify the body by releasing heat and water-soluble toxins via sweat. Cold water is used therapeutically to relieve inflammation. Contrasting the two therapies is believed to reduce inflammation and pain and help with digestion.

- **Hyperbaric oxygen therapy**: This therapy involves pumping pressurized pure oxygen into a sealed chamber and having the patient breathe the concentrated oxygen for 30 to 120 minutes. In cancer care, hyperbaric oxygen therapy is used to stimulate healing of wounds that are not healing properly, typically following surgery. This application of hyperbaric oxygen therapy is scientifically documented.

- **Meditation**: This mind-body technique is designed to produce a calm, relaxed, nonreactive state of mind. Many mind-body experts believe meditation allows for greater awareness and clarity by anchoring the person in the present moment. It can also help alleviate symptoms of stress, anger, fear, anxiety, and depression. There are a variety of ways to meditate, but most methods fall into two categories: concentrative meditation and mindfulness meditation. Concentrative meditation focuses on breath, an image, or a mantra in order to still the mind. Mindfulness meditation involves turning off the mind's internal dialogue and simply receiving whatever exists in the environment without judgment; when distracting thoughts, memories, worries, or images arise, the person simply witnesses them without reacting to them or becoming involved with them.

- *Movement*: Aerobic and anaerobic exercise, yoga, tai chi, and dance are all considered movement therapies. Decades of research have confirmed that exercise is a powerful health intervention. The health-promoting and illness-preventing benefits of exercise are endorsed by the National Institutes of Health, the American Medical Association, and the Surgeon General, along with a variety of other organizations, institutions, and health pioneers. Exercise is particularly important for people with cancer in order to improve tolerance to treatment, reduce fatigue, and maintain lean body mass.

- *Naturopathic medicine*: Naturopathic physicians are doctors trained to provide family health care and to emphasize the use of natural therapies to stimulate the innate healing processes of each person, and in so doing to prevent and treat acute and chronic illnesses. Naturopathic medicine is used by people both as their primary health care and as complementary health care, particularly in the case of integrative cancer care. Naturopathic physicians utilize most of the integrative therapies covered in this book. For more information on naturopathic medicine, refer to the sidebar on page 105. To find a naturopathic physician in your area, visit www.naturopathic.org and for a board certified naturopathic oncologist, visit www.oncanp.org.

- *Psychotherapy*: Psychotherapy treats mental and emotional disorders using psychological methods such as counseling. It may take place in individual or group sessions and should always be conducted by a licensed practitioner. Psychotherapy can be used to help alleviate illness-related anxiety, which can be a particular problem with cancer because of all the unknowns the disease presents.

- *Reiki*: This form of energy therapy gently encourages balance on all levels by reducing stress, pain, and anxiety; restoring a sense of well-being; enhancing the body's innate ability to heal; and creating other benefits that are specific to the individual. The touch of a Reiki practitioner is light and noninvasive. Reiki is thought to work by means of a cascade of healing pulsations that flow spontaneously through the practitioner according to the need of the person receiving treatment.

- **Self-talk and visualization**: Can we talk ourselves into being healthy? Experts in self-talk and visualization believe these activities can influence health. Preliminary research indicates that you can positively impact your health and possibly change the course of disease by giving yourself positive messages or practicing techniques such as guided visualization. BlueCross BlueShield of California found that patients who used guided imagery tapes prior to surgery healed faster following the procedure. As we learn more about the connection between mind and body, self-talk and visualization techniques will likely become even more important to our healing process.

- **Supplements**: Intended to augment the diet and stimulate certain naturally occurring bodily processes, dietary supplements consist of vitamins, minerals, herbal extracts, or other nutrients. They may contain either a single nutrient or a combination of nutrients and are sold over the counter and regulated under federal dietary supplement guidelines. Supplement programs can be designed to promote the well-being of specific physiological systems, such as the immune system, or can alter specific cellular events in order to affect processes such as tumor growth, inflammation, and angiogenesis. In general, manufacturers are not allowed to make claims that their products can aid in treatment of specific diseases. (For more information on some of the supplements currently thought to play a role in treating cancer, refer to the "Integrative Cancer Care Supplement Guide" on page 161.)

You may find yourself wondering, as the researchers do, exactly how these natural substances work. The simple answer is that they work similarly to pharmaceutical agents—biochemically and physiologically in the body after we ingest or inject them. In fact, many over-the-counter and prescription drugs were inspired by or are derived from plants and other natural substances. Bark from the white willow (*Salix alba*) is the original source of aspirin, which is now produced synthetically. Digoxin, a heart medication, is derived from foxglove (*Digitalis purpurea*). Many chemotherapy drugs were originally isolated from plants or derived from natural compounds: vincristine and vinblastine were developed from compounds found in periwinkle (*Catharanthus roseus*); paclitaxel is derived from the Pacific yew tree (*Taxus brevifolia*); and irinotecan is derived from camptothecin, a compound from *Camptotheca acuminata*, a Chinese tree known in its native land as *xi shu*, which means "happy tree."

But if the natural substances work similarly to pharmaceutical agents and are so effective, why aren't they sold and prescribed like drugs? A big reason is that natural substances are often not as powerful as their drug counterparts. Drug developers seek to strengthen the naturally present compounds by isolating active chemicals from the natural source, then manipulating these compounds to create very specific effects that are stronger and that can be reliably reproduced from one person to the next. They can then patent the drug and have exclusive rights to its sale. These drugs, in contrast to the natural substances from which they were derived, are much more concentrated and contain one isolated chemical compound rather than a variety of chemical compounds. Because of this, natural substances are typically—although not always—safer and less toxic.

However, no matter how natural they are, certain supplements can interfere with medications. In those that have a variety of active ingredients, each constituent can interact with drugs in different ways. They can also vary quite a bit in potency and quality, and may even contain contaminants. For these reasons, it's important to read as much detailed information as possible on any supplement before you take it. It also underscores how critical it is to inform all of your doctors about any supplements you're taking.

Issues of Safety

A diagnosis of cancer brings with it an acute awareness that there are no guarantees in life. Though this can be most devastating in terms of facing your own mortality, it reverberates through many other aspects of the cancer experience, including uncertainty in regard to diagnosis, the effectiveness of conventional treatment options, and the safety of integrative therapies. While we cannot definitively guarantee the safety of all complementary therapies, we can make some generalized statements.

Mind-body techniques are generally safe. If meditation, stress reduction, counseling, relaxation, journaling, or any other mind-body approach appeals to you, it's worth a try, and it will assuredly enhance your sense of well-being. Exercise is also considered relatively safe, although you should ask your oncologist about any specific limitations. Acupuncture, biofeedback, constitutional medicine, and naturopathic medicine are all considered safe when offered by a licensed practitioner and when used as complementary therapies to conventional cancer treatments. Botanical and dietary supplements are safe and effective when used appropriately under the guidance of qualified licensed health-care practitioners. For more information about specific alternative treatment methods that we do not recommend for safety reasons, refer to the section on pages 173 to 176.

Ultimately, evaluating safety as it relates to cancer treatment is individualized based on the person, the cancer, and the information the person receives. A 35-year-old woman with stage IV lung cancer will view the safety of a particular herb or treatment differently than will a 65-year-old man with stage II prostate cancer, and they will also assess the pros and cons differently. In the end, you will make the best decision if you gather as much information as you can, consider it carefully, and clearly understand the risks versus the benefits. Remember, just because something is labeled "natural" doesn't mean it is safe. Then again, just because a drug is approved by the FDA doesn't guarantee its safety, either.

Even if supplements are safe on their own, their interactions with conventional medications may make them unsafe. This is one of the reasons why it is important to utilize the expertise of a licensed health-care provider such as a naturopathic physician or integrative physician when combining supplements with conventional treatments. This is particularly true in the case of cancer because the disease is complicated and the treatments are powerful. More information is being discovered at a rapid pace regarding interactions of herbs and supplements with drugs used in cancer treatment. Some of the interactions may decrease the effectiveness of conventional treatment, and some may increase the side effects. In addition, some herbs may be contraindicated for certain cancer types. (For more information, refer to the section "Nutrient and Herb Interactions with Conventional Cancer Treatments" beginning on page 140.) Given the substantial potential benefits as well as risks associated with supplements, we recommend that patients consult a naturopathic physician, and ideally a naturopathic oncologist. These doctors are trained in the scientific use of natural therapies and have extensive training in health and disease as well. (For more information on naturopathic medicine, refer to the sidebar opposite.) Unfortunately, due to the limited number of naturopathic physicians in the United States, access can be difficult. If a naturopathic physician is not available, it may be possible to find an integrative physician, integrative nurse practitioner, dietician, or doctor of pharmacy with some expertise in this area. Ultimately, people with cancer and their loved ones are often on their own when it comes to researching and evaluating CAM therapies. Accurate information is critical to optimizing chances for successful treatment. Providing that information and helping you learn how to find more information on your own is the purpose of this book.

Gathering Information

The key to determining the best integrative cancer treatment approach is understanding how to evaluate all of your options—conventional and

The Power and Principles of Naturopathic Medicine

Steeped in traditional healing methods, principles, and practices, naturopathic medicine focuses on holistic, proactive prevention and comprehensive diagnosis and treatment. Naturopathic physicians are experts in the scientific application of natural healing. Naturopathic medicine is one of the fastest-growing complementary health-care professions in the United States. Naturopathic physicians use scientifically based principles to guide their diagnosis and treatment, and provide individual and family health care, emphasizing the use of natural therapies.

According to the American Association of Naturopathic Physicians' Public Awareness Campaign, "In addition to the basic medical sciences and conventional diagnostics, naturopathic education includes therapeutic nutrition, botanical medicine, homeopathy, natural childbirth, classical Chinese medicine theory, hydrotherapy, naturopathic manipulative therapy, pharmacology and minor office procedures."

Naturopathic medicine excludes major surgery, therapeutic use of X-rays and radium, and use of most controlled substances. After completing undergraduate premedical training, naturopathic physicians attend a four-year graduate-level federally recognized naturopathic medical school. Naturopathic medical education consists of the same basic sciences as are taught in conventional medical programs, a scientifically based understanding of health and disease, and naturopathic philosophy and treatments. Naturopathic education includes four years of training in clinical nutrition, homeopathic medicine, botanical medicine, psychology and lifestyle counseling, drug-herb and drug-nutrient interactions and pharmacology, and requires supervised clinical training.

Naturopathic medicine embraces the medical oath "First do no harm." By using protocols that minimize the risk of harm, naturopathic physicians help facilitate the body's inherent ability to restore and maintain optimal health. It is the physician's role to identify and remove barriers to good health by helping to create a healing internal and external environment.

There are presently six naturopathic medical programs in North America accredited by the Council on Naturopathic Medical Education (CNME), which is the only professional accrediting agency for naturopathic medicine recognized by the U.S. Department of Education. These programs are at Bastyr University, Boucher Institute of Naturopathic Medicine, Canadian College of Naturopathic Medicine, National College of Natural Medicine, Southwest College of Naturopathic Medicine and Health Sciences, and University of Bridgeport. If you are considering seeing a naturopathic physician, be sure that their naturopathic doctorate is from one of these accredited colleges or universities rather than a correspondence or online course.

Currently, 16 states regulate (license or register) naturopathic physicians (Alaska, Arizona, California, Connecticut, Hawaii, Idaho, Kansas, Maine, Minnesota, Montana, New Hampshire, Oregon, Utah, Vermont, and Washington). In addition, Puerto Rico, the Virgin Islands, the District of Columbia, and the Canadian provinces of British Columbia, Manitoba, Ontario, and Saskatchewan also license naturopathic doctors. Licensing in other states is pending. "Legal provisions allow for the practice of naturopathic medicine in several of the unlicensed states," explains the American Association of Accredited Naturopathic Medical Colleges.

alternative. Having lots of choices can be positive, but it can also be overwhelming. For some people, black-and-white decisions are much easier; they prefer to avoid the gray areas. But when faced with a cancer diagnosis, avoiding the gray is nearly impossible. Complicating the cancer treatment evaluation process is the pressure to choose sides. Will it be conventional or complementary? It can be difficult to overcome this either-or dilemma and its attendant stress. If you, your loved ones, or your doctors have this sort of polarized view, remember that seldom is the situation with cancer black and white. It's perfectly fine to combine treatment approaches. As long as you're working with knowledgeable health-care practitioners and you are armed with trusted information about the pros and cons of each treatment, you can choose to utilize conventional and complementary treatments simultaneously, or you can alternate between them. You are a unique individual, and as such your cancer treatment should be individualized. Remember, these are ultimately your decisions to make.

Another difficulty that cancer patients and their families sometimes face is the desire to loyally or even blindly follow the advice of a single doctor. Most doctors will admit that at times even they are unsure what course is best. Cancer treatment is riddled with ambiguity, and oncology is one of the most emotionally and intellectually challenging specialties in medicine. Oncologists seldom have definitive answers; they're just doing their best to provide you with the information you need to make informed decisions. Don't be afraid to ask questions, and don't be afraid to leave the protective cocoon of your main oncologist. Most doctors are familiar with and even encourage second opinions. Relying on multiple sources to help you navigate will provide you with more perspective. And the more perspective you have, the better.

Some skepticism of both conventional and alternative treatment options is healthy. Suspicion can be particularly helpful when evaluating Internet information. Beware of the charlatan—the person, company, or organization aggressively trying to sell or promote the next "cancer cure." If you search the Internet for "cancer" and "cure," Google will quickly deliver more than ten million websites! Some of them are reputable, but most are not. That's why it is important to source other opinions when evaluating information—particularly when you find extraordinary claims that may indicate self-serving websites or commercial interests.

That said, there is an immense amount of useful information available online. PubMed, an open access online library of peer-reviewed and scientifically credible medical journals sponsored by the Library of Congress, contains a vast store of articles that provide helpful and trustworthy information. Though these are usually fairly technical, they can help you better understand various treatment options. Respected integrative cancer centers have websites, as do various nonprofit organizations. Many health-related government agencies have information about cancer on their websites, and it's encouraging to note how many of these have added information on CAM therapies in recent years. There's a great deal of information available on the Internet that isn't directly tied to product sales.

However, we are disappointed in the individuals, manufacturers, and organizations that irresponsibly push "natural alternatives" as cures for cancer for their own gain—and sometimes we find ourselves disgusted by the depths of their crassness. They do a great disservice to people with cancer, who face enough challenges without also having to wade through false claims and unsubstantiated hype. Their claims are also bad for integrative medicine, which can provide great benefit to people with cancer, and to people in general.

The following advice about red flags to watch out for when evaluating cancer information stems from our combined experience of nearly 40 years in the integrative health field and applies to information about both conventional and alternative treatments. (For more information on how to evaluate health-related information on the Web, refer to the sidebar on page 111.)

- *Information connected to product sales.* Sometimes a website's commercial intent is obvious, making it easy to be skeptical. But sometimes the product connection is more hidden. Here's a general rule for identifying commercial websites: if you can buy a product quickly and easily right after you read about how it or its ingredients will cure your cancer, you should leave the site, never to return. (In the case of printed literature, use it to start your next campfire.)

- *No author, author bio, or source of the information.* Every article, study, abstract, or other text should clearly indicate the source of the information. If there is no author or author biography, there should be an indication as to who was responsible for publishing the material. Assess this information carefully, because some publishers reap financial benefits from products mentioned in their literature.

- *No independent journal references.* If scientific information is presented, it should be backed up by references with full details on where the information was obtained (author, title of the book, journal or article, date and issue information, and other details of publication). References allow you to verify the information or learn more about the topic. You can then do an additional search to find the original abstract or journal article. No references means no good.

- *Not-for-profit—not automatically safe.* Just because a website or an organization claims to be nonprofit or has a Web address ending in .org does not mean that the information it provides is truthful and not financially motivated. Be aware that anyone can register a .org Web address; they need not be nonprofit. If the site is selling products and making unsubstantiated claims about them, nonprofit status is

continued on page 110

Questionable Alternative Cancer Treatment Theories

Effective medical treatments begin with a logical theory and sound science. Cancer treatment strategies must rest on a solid foundation—a framework of rules, ideas, and principles that make sense. The theoretical spectrum can be broad. Some cancer treatment alternatives sit on quicksand, some are a little less shaky, and others are as solid as a rock.

Integrated cancer treatment is designed to support key body systems, particularly the immune system, hormones (the endocrine system), and the digestive system, which encompasses elimination and detoxification. The integrative approach addresses deficiencies in those systems, as well as key conditions of ill health, namely, insulin resistance and chronic inflammation. Integrated cancer treatment includes a combination of healthful diet, nutritional supplements, lifestyle factors, and mind-body-spirit approaches, used in conjunction with conventional medicine, when appropriate. In contrast to integrated cancer treatment, some practitioners and people with cancer pursue only alternative treatments that do not embrace an integrative approach and are typically based upon theories and therapies that are scientifically unsubstantiated. The following are three theories that underlie most popular alternative cancer treatments:

1. Sugar feeds cancer.
2. Acidic pH promotes cancer.
3. Oxygen kills cancer.

While portions of these three theories may be valid, flawed logic and pseudoscientific reasoning invalidate them and their spin-off treatments. None of these theories have been scientifically validated and none are accepted by scientifically trained integrative medicine practitioners or by conventional medical establishments. A closer look at these three purported causes of cancer will expose their weaknesses as foundations for some alternative treatments.

Sugar Feeds Cancer

Cancer cells use glucose (sugar) for energy. A high-sugar diet combined with cancer has been compared to throwing gasoline on a fire. This theory springs from work done by Nobel Prize winner Dr. Otto Warburg. However, Dr. Warburg's findings are from 1931, and his statements are often taken out of context. Linking glucose metabolism within the cells to dietary sugar consumption is an oversimplification that leads to a misinformed conclusion.

We know that glucose is fuel for all cells, not just cancer cells. It is true that cancer cells do display a great number of insulin receptors on their cell surfaces, which helps draw proportionately large amounts of glucose into them because insulin receptors act like gates for glucose to enter a cell: insulin binds to glucose, then the insulin carries the glucose across the insulin receptor into the cell. Cancer cells require these extra insulin receptors because they are not very efficient at metabolizing sugar into energy and therefore require more of it than healthy cells. A cancer cell requires sugar in much the same way that a metabolically active cell (brain cell, heart cell, etc.) or a quickly dividing cell (intestinal epithelial cell) does. Despite the high sugar need of cancer cells, their demand for sugar cannot be selectively targeted away from the sugar needs of the rest of the body.

It is impossible to selectively starve a cancer cell by withholding glucose without starving healthy tissue as well. In fact, because cancer cells are loaded up with insulin receptors, they are particularly good at taking up scarce glucose. So, even if sugar intake is severely restricted and only a small amount of glucose is present in the system, a disproportionate share of the available glucose will be taken up by the insulin receptor–studded cancerous cells. Thus, avoiding all sugar will not starve cancer, but rather will deprive healthy cells of sugar needed for normal functioning. Additionally, all ingested foods—whether they start off as a fruit, vegetable, meat, or candy bar—are ultimately broken down into protein, sugar (glucose), and fat. The relative amounts of these three end products vary according to the food source, but even a diet of 100 percent vegetables will provide some glucose, albeit a smaller quantity. Ironically, someone who tries to reduce their sugar by relying on vegetables only may make their overall situation worse. The smaller quantity of sugar will be preferentially taken up by metabolically active cells and cells loaded with insulin receptors, such as cancer cells, leaving other tissues starving. This can result in a very fatigued, thin, and unwell person—with cancer.

There are, however, some significant benefits to avoiding or minimizing consumption of refined sugar. Consumption of refined sugar causes spikes in serum glucose, and over the long term, this can decrease insulin sensitivity, a condition called insulin resistance. Insulin resistance is a decrease in the sensitivity of insulin receptors on cells to the point where the receptors do not function properly to let glucose enter the cell. Insulin resistance in otherwise healthy cells creates other biochemical changes that promote cancer growth, and it can lead to excess levels of insulin and insulin-like growth factor—which might encourage some types of cancer to grow. Additionally, insulin resistance results in increased amounts of sugar in the bloodstream and creates a deficit of sugar inside healthy cells, where it is needed to make the energy that cells need to function. Excessive consumption of refined or simple sugars also impairs the function of some cells in the immune system, crippling their ability to survey and detect newly developed cancer cells and impairing their ability to extinguish cancerous cells once they are targeted.

At this point, there is no scientific evidence that sugar consumption directly causes cancer to spread. There is, however, much common sense behind the concept that a diet high in refined sugar impairs immunity and, over the long term, may create insulin resistance, a condition that favors the growth of cancer.

Acidic pH Promotes Cancer

The intracellular pH of some cancer cells is lower (more acidic) than the pH of a normal cell, which has led some to believe that you can kill cancer cells by raising cellular pH, and that improper internal pH balance can contribute to cancer. There is no scientific evidence, however, that suggests a direct link between alterations in pH balance and cancer prevention, or, specifically that a high pH (alkaline) environment will kill cancer cells. In fact, the converse may be true. Cancer cells and tumors tend to create an immediate milieu that is acidic. This is in part due to the fact that cancer cells require vast quantities of sugar because they are very inefficient at producing energy from glucose. In many cancer cells, glucose is metabolized anaerobically, which creates lactic acid as a by-product. Lactic acid is acidic. However, this very acidity and the elevated levels of lactic acid may actually be toxic to the cancer cell, ultimately contributing to its demise. Thus, trying to alkalinize the body (and the cancerous tumor) may be counterproductive at worst and irrelevant at best. The pH of cancer cells is the result of metabolic events within the cancer cell and is not reflected in the pH of other body fluids, such as urine, saliva, or blood.

Online information on high pH therapy cites a 1984 report claiming that high pH therapy for cancer has been studied with positive results on both animals and humans. The conclusions drawn from this report are highly suspect, as is the methodology of the study. The actual nature of the conclusions and the specifics of the intervention are left unexplained. It is also suspicious that any positive findings have not been duplicated in any subsequent study in more than 25 years. In fact, the only subsequent studies on humans are case reports of toxicity directly due to ingestion of cesium chloride as an alternative cancer treatment to raise the pH of cancer cells. One report described high levels of accumulated cesium in the liver, leading to liver toxicity.

On a more positive note, some early data from a mouse study indicates that oral administration of cesium chloride does, in fact, raise the pH of tumor tissue and sensitize the tumor tissue to the anticancer effects of vitamin D administered at the same time. This preliminary data may lead to future indications for cesium chloride along with vitamin D. However, at present, data in support of the pH theory is lacking.

Oxygen Kills Cancer

Promoters of oxygen therapy believe cancer cells and the microorganisms that purportedly

continued on next page

cause cancer cannot grow in an oxygenated environment. They believe that cancer thrives when oxygen levels are low. While it is true that cancer survives when deprived of oxygen, cancer also survives in an oxygenated environment, as evidenced by the very existence of lung cancer. Oxygen therapy entails bathing the body in oxygen, or exposing blood to ozone (three oxygen molecules combined to create O3), thereby theoretically creating an environment in which cancer cannot grow. However, there have been no studies confirming that oxygen therapy disrupts tumor growth, kills cancer cells, or enhances immunity.

Concentrated oxygen therapy, or hyperbaric oxygen therapy (HBO), has, however, proven to be effective in stimulating wound healing, and some researchers have explored how this might be helpful in cancer care. A 2006 research review by the Wilmer Eye Institute at Johns Hopkins Hospital featured in the *International Journal of Gynecological Cancer* evaluated the use of HBO for radiation-induced optic neuropathy, a devastating consequence of radiation exposure. The researchers found that although "there are case reports in the scientific literature of successful treatment with HBO, therapy with HBO has to be initiated soon after the onset of vision loss, and even then yields variable results at best." A 2006 animal study from the University of Texas featured in the journal *Brain Research* demonstrated that HBO "significantly decreased inflammation and pain" and should be considered "in situations where NSAIDs are contraindicated or in persistent cases of inflammation." Australian researchers demonstrated that HBO therapy reduced delayed radiation-induced injuries in patients with gynecological cancers. However, that study only featured 14 patients and more research is needed to confirm the results.

Ozone is another form of oxygen therapy. Ozone is created when ultraviolet light splits an oxygen molecule into two highly reactive oxygen atoms that recombine to form O3. Ozone therapy is used for treating superficial wounds and slow-healing ulcers. There is no scientific evidence that ozone therapy has any benefit as a cancer treatment.

irrelevant. Chances are they benefit from those product sales in some way, which automatically instills bias into the information they are presenting. If you can quickly click through a .org site to a for-profit website, the .org address may just be a front.

● *Unverifiable clinical trials and scientific information.* Some sites will claim that clinical trials and other research support certain products, but if you dig just a little deeper, you may find that their "clinical trial" or "research" has not been published anywhere else. If there is no reference or documentation for the clinical trial or research, chances are it hasn't been published and isn't valid. Until the information has been peer-reviewed and vetted by independent professionals, its soundness is questionable. There is probably a reason why the research hasn't been published, such as poor study design or inaccurate results, or, worst of all, it could be a fabricated study.

● *Borrowed science.* Some manufacturers use what is called "borrowed science" to make their product or information look valid. The problem with borrowed science is that it can be difficult to detect. For example, a product manufacturer for saw palmetto berry extract may claim the extract can reduce the size of an enlarged prostate as indicated by a recent study. However, upon further review, the study may have used a standardized extract of the oil of the saw palmetto berry, whereas the manufacturer's product is a different dosage of a crude extract, not standardized for a specific oil ingredient. Granted, this is not easy to detect. If the manufacturer is reputable, chances are their product is solid and will coincide with the research.

- **Site sponsorships.** In both the conventional and alternative realms, manufacturers of drugs and natural alternatives may pay for or run websites or produce the information other websites use. Such sponsorship and links should be clearly communicated and obvious to the reader. Full disclosure is important and a sign of credibility. You may have to dig deep into the website to find these hidden sponsorships. Be sure to review the entire site before making a decision regarding the site's accuracy and bear in mind that if the site is sponsored by a drug company, for example, the information may be biased.

- **Proprietary information.** Sites that claim proprietary formulas or do not list ingredients are essentially selling mystery products and refusing to tell you what is in their products. While it may be acceptable for a cook to keep a famous soup recipe secret, this is not acceptable with products that claim to cure or treat cancer, enhance the immune system, or have other health benefits. Chances are these products don't contain any special or medicinal ingredients, and they could even contain ingredients dangerous to your health.

Top 10 Tips for Evaluating Medical Information on the Web

1. The information should not be directly connected to product sales.

2. Articles and scientific information should feature a credible author and author biography or otherwise identify the source of the information. Ask yourself who or where the information is coming from.

3. Scientific information, including research, clinical trials, case studies, protocols, and medical opinions, should be supported by a list of references.

4. Be wary of outlandish claims and theories associated with cancer treatments.

5. Be sure the site and the information presented on the site are current.

6. Do not base your decision regarding credibility solely on patient testimonials.

7. Evaluate links just as critically as you evaluate the original site.

8. Find out who runs the site and who pays for it.

9. You should be able to easily contact the site manager, owner, or key representatives when you need clarification on issues associated with the site.

10. Do not give out personal information such as social security number, insurance information, credit card number, and so forth, unless you are convinced the site is safe and you are protected.

Studying the Studies

Conventional research has a variety of ways to evaluate whether a substance or treatment is effective.

- **In vitro studies** are done using isolated cells or tissue samples in a test tube or dish.

- **In vivo studies** use live organisms (typically animals).

- **Epidemiological studies** are large, population-based studies.

- **Clinical trials** involve observing or testing the effect of specifically identified treatments on a selected group of patients.

- **Observational trials** involve observing associations (correlations) between the treatments experienced by participants and the status of their health or disease.

- **Intervention trials** study the impact of a therapy on a group of subjects by applying that therapy in a controlled and regulated manner.

- **Double-blind clinical trials** are clinical trials in which neither the subjects nor the investigators know which subjects are receiving the test treatment.

- **Placebo-controlled tests** compare results in those subjects receiving the tested treatment to results in subjects receiving a placebo, or inert substance.

- **Phase I trials** evaluate the effect of a new drug or treatment on a small group of people (fewer than 100) to provide early indications of a drug or treatment's safety and safe dosage range, and to reveal any side effects. If a person with cancer has exhausted all other treatment options, they may be eligible for enrollment in a phase I trial for a new anticancer therapy.

- **Phase II trials** study the effect of a new or experimental substance at a safe dose, as determined in phase I. The therapy is tested on a larger group of people (with the same tumor type) to determine its effect on cancer growth, gauge patient tolerance, and to uncover side effects that may not have been evident in the phase I trial.

- **Phase III trials** compare the effects of a new or experimental substance to standard treatment in a controlled trial. This larger trial (usually 400 to 1,000 people) better determines the effectiveness of the drug compared to standard treatments,

It's important to learn to separate the wheat from the chaff. Although many "new" miracle products and novel theories are bogus, creative and innovative thinking has been the impetus for some of the most exciting and effective medical advances of our time. At some point, we have to trust the momentum and take a chance. Learn to rely on your intuition and the intuition of the people you love and trust, then try to validate that intuition with scientific information.

We understand the desperation that can come with a cancer diagnosis. And we understand the need to sometimes take a chance or a leap of faith. If you are considering taking such a leap, we hope you're tethered to solid science, sound advice, and a logical and effective evaluation of all the information you receive.

and reveals rarer side effects and other clinically relevant information important to understanding the indications and limitations for the new therapy. If there is no standard treatment with which to compare the new therapy, the subjects in the trial may be randomized to receive a placebo treatment. If clinical effect is shown in phase III trials, the drug is submitted to the FDA for approval.

- **Phase IV trials** are done after a new drug has been brought to market to assess for rare or long-term adverse effects that were not detected in the relatively short phase I through III trials.

- **Prospective study** determines the effect of a therapy using a clinical trial specifically developed to test the therapy.

- **Retrospective study** analyzes the impact of a treatment in a population by researching outcomes in a group of people who have used the treatment compared to those who did not use the treatment during the same time period.

- **Randomized trial** is a study in which patients are randomly assigned to receive the test treatment or to receive a placebo treatment. Randomized trials, also called comparison trials, help researchers determine if the test treatment exerts an effect that is more than the placebo effect.

- **Placebo effect** is when a patient experiences a beneficial effect following a particular treatment due to their expectations about the treatment, rather than from the treatment itself.

The pharmaceutical industry follows a standard that includes clinical, double-blind, and placebo-controlled trials. This research model is conducive to analyzing single substances or isolated treatments. But it is difficult to evaluate the effects of integrative treatments using this approach because of their multidimensional philosophy. Integrative medicine embraces multiple interventions that can impact disease progression and quality of life. We are only beginning to adapt our research methods to include evaluations of multiple substances, lifestyles, and treatments. In addition, quality-of-life issues have not typically been addressed within the conventional research model.

Using the gold standard of research—clinical, double-blind, placebo-controlled trials—as the sole measure of efficacy with CAM treatments is not always practical or effective. Many variables must be considered when evaluating these treatments.

Understanding Our Evaluation

The maze of information about complementary and alternative medicine can be so confusing it can become maddening. Sometimes it seems impossible to find the right path—the healing path. From this point forward, we will provide you with information about specific integrative cancer treatment options. We have based our conclusions on the following:

● Scientific, credible sources

● A combination of conventional gold standard clinical and preclinical research

● Practical risk-to-benefit ratios

The Journey through Cancer and the Seven Levels of Healing

By Jeremy R. Geffen, MD, FACP

As a medical oncologist, I have learned a great deal from many heroic people who have taught me about living courageously in the face of enormous challenges and the unknown. I have come to understand cancer as a journey—filled with ups and downs, periods of calm as well as tumult, and tremendous opportunities for healing and transformation. I have also seen how cancer can often challenge the mind, heart, and spirit of patients and family members as deeply—if not more deeply—than it challenges the physical body.

Over many years of clinical practice—and through the personal experience of cancer in my own family—I have observed that when patients and loved ones find themselves facing a cancer diagnosis, they generally focus their energy in a similar way. In their searching for meaningful and practical answers to crucial questions about healing, I saw an important pattern. I recognized that all questions and concerns encountered by patients and their loved ones fall elegantly into one of seven distinct but interrelated domains of inquiry and exploration. I call these the seven levels of healing and describe them in detail in my book *The Journey through Cancer*.

Level One: Education and Information

Level one provides basic knowledge about cancer and current treatment options, which is important to allow you to actively participate in and obtain the greatest possible benefit from your care. Feeling clear and confident about your treatment plan is important to put your mind at ease. It can also greatly enhance your ability to enter the deeper dimensions of healing. Find an experienced oncologist whom you trust, and who answers your questions fully. Take the time needed to make decisions based on knowledge and understanding, not fear.

Level Two: Connection with Others

Level two explores the importance of support on the cancer journey. The poet John Donne famously said, "No man is an island," and this is especially true when dealing with cancer. Connection with others is an enormously important component of the healing process. Studies have consistently demonstrated the numerous benefits derived from support groups and other psychosocial programs. Remember that family members can't satisfy all your needs. Seek support from friends, clergy, and self-help organizations. Join a support group. Talk with others who are navigating the journey through cancer and finding positive solutions.

Level Three: The Body as Garden

Level three invites patients and family members to regard the human body as a precious and wondrously complex garden—rather than a machine. This level explores the full spectrum of safe and effective complementary and alternative approaches to healing. Conventional treatments remain the foundation of leading-edge cancer care. However, taking an active role in caring for your body also includes good nutrition, exercise, massage, relaxation, and other non-

- Safety, side effects, and contraindications

- Types of studies available

- Input from our respected editorial board and other experts

We provide an evidence-based rating system to guide you in making safe and effective choices. (Refer to "Integrative Cancer Care: Our Rating System," pages 160–172.) We evaluate treatments based on their ability to halt disease progression, enhance quality of life, and ease side effects of the disease or conventional treatments (refer to "Nutrient and Herb Interac-

conventional therapies. Explore the myriad options available to soothe the body and mind and invigorate the heart and spirit.

Level Four: Emotional Healing

Level four enters the inner realm of the human heart. It explores the transformative power of releasing fear, pain, and anger on the journey through cancer. It also demonstrates the healing potential of self-love and forgiveness, and embracing all parts of one's self with compassion and tenderness. Keep a journal to explore and release hidden feelings. Work with a counselor or therapist. Don't neglect your emotional self.

Level Five: The Nature of Mind

Level five looks carefully at how our entire experience of life—including life with cancer—is profoundly influenced by our thoughts, beliefs, and the meaning we give to events. We can escape the tyranny of the mind and move forward consciously on our healing path. Anxiety is a common part of the cancer journey. To avoid feeling overwhelmed, examine the thoughts, worries, and beliefs that are troubling you the most. Once fear is replaced with knowledge and understanding, anxiety can be profoundly diminished. Focus on the positive. Ask yourself, "What are the blessings in my life? What am I learning? What am I grateful for?"

Level Six: Life Assessment

Level six explores the aspirations, goals, and purposes of our lives. It is deeply empowering to discover the real purpose of your life and move toward its fulfillment. Answering three essential questions can make your priorities clear and liberate enormous time, energy, and resources for healing:

1. What is the meaning and purpose of my life?

2. What are my most important goals for the coming year?

3. How do I want to be remembered by those whom I love and care about?

Level Seven: The Nature of Spirit

Level seven explores the spiritual aspects of life and healing. It embraces the nonphysical dimensions of our being that exist beyond time and space, and even beyond illness and health. There is no better time than now to fully honor and embrace your spiritual essence. It is the source of not only the love, joy, and fulfillment that we all seek, but physical healing as well. Explore this through meditation, prayer, reflection, time in nature, and sharing with loved ones. Remember that just as your body, mind, and heart need care and attention, so does your spirit.

Jeremy R. Geffen, MD, FACP, is a board-certified medical oncologist and the author of the highly acclaimed book The Journey through Cancer: Healing and Transforming the Whole Person *(Three Rivers Press, 2006) and the audio program* The Seven Levels of Healing *(Nightingale-Conant, 2001). He is also on this book's editorial advisory board.*

tions with Conventional Cancer Treatments," pages 140–172). Cancer can be a life-threatening illness, and we understand that it may not be prudent to wait for unequivocal scientific assurance of the effectiveness of a drug or therapy. Our goal is that our rating system will help you make some of your treatment decisions more easily, more safely, and with greater confidence.

Within conventional medicine, a treatment is typically not determined to be effective and safe until it has been demonstrated in at least three separate, successful, well-designed human clinical trials. This is the standard, for example, that Medicare uses to authorize coverage for a treatment. The randomized controlled trial is often considered the gold standard of medical evaluation because it reduces research errors and more clearly identifies whether the intervention being tested is effective by comparing it to a placebo (an inert substance). See the sidebar "Studying the Studies" on page 112 for more detailed definitions of study methodology.

Applying this gold standard to integrative treatments is not always possible. Randomized controlled trials are designed to study isolated pharmaceutical ingredients or single interventions rather than a multitreatment approach that may include combinations of herbs, nutrients, diet, and/or lifestyle changes. Although randomized trials have studied some complementary and alternative therapies, the majority of integrative therapies are not substantiated by definitive human clinical data.

Fortunately, there are many other types of research that can provide validation for an integrative approach. Thus, we can still apply high research standards to the evaluation of integrative medicine. Using findings from in vitro tests (those using cells and tissue samples), in vivo animal tests, and clinical data (vast population studies, small clinical trials, observational trials, randomized clinical trials, and so on), we can piece together a picture of the evidence for the effectiveness of a particular complementary therapy. When we combine that information with data on the safety of this therapy, we can make a reasonable determination about whether it should be used for specific indications.

Integrative Medicine Plan Overview

We've all heard the familiar adage "The whole is greater than the sum of its parts." This can be applied to many things, including the human body. To integrate is to bring different elements together to create a unified whole. This is the foundation of our integrative cancer treatment plan, and here, too, the whole is stronger than the sum of its parts. To view cancer as an isolated tumor or lone mass may be appropriate from an initial surgical perspective or crisis-management standpoint, but just as cancer can go beyond its original borders, so too must the treatment plan.

An integrative approach to cancer is built on a strong foundation of a healthy diet, positive lifestyle choices, and appropriate supplements. It devotes attention not just to cancer but to key bodily processes, particularly immune function, hormone status, insulin resistance, inflammation, digestion, and detoxification. Cancer can affect these critical biological processes, or it may spring from dysfunction in one or more of these bodily systems. Although some or all of these processes may, at first glance, seem to be unrelated to cancer, they are all interrelated, and each process must be realigned to a healthy status if the body is to heal. That is why all of our body systems are integral to a comprehensive plan, and we devote a chapter to each of these topics in part III of the book.

The integrative medicine cancer plan combines a healthy diet and lifestyle and the use of dietary supplements with the most appropriate and effective conventional treatments. The cancer patient deserves the most comprehensive treatment available, and that is the basis of the integrative medicine strategy.

Comprehensive Treatment

Conventional medicine has made incredible advances in the fight against cancer. However, true and deep healing is only possible with a multifaceted and integrative approach that revolves around the individual needs of the patient. We must find a way to address the whole as we consider the sum of our parts. According to Paul Reilly, ND, L.Ac., of the Seattle Cancer Treatment and Wellness Center, if we change the internal environment that allowed the cancer to grow, we can change the outcome. We need to tackle cancer using integrative and appropriate mind-body-spirit techniques to change our internal environment. An integrative treatment plan requires initiative, cooperation, and commitment from all parties involved and should always be focused on the patient's ultimate wellness.

six

Supporting Your Body during Conventional Treatment

Choosing the right direction can be frustrating, especially when you are drawn to different paths. Following a cancer diagnosis, many people feel compelled to go with conventional treatment over alternative therapies or vice versa. Or, they may choose conventional treatment, become frustrated, and then switch to a completely alternative approach, sometimes long after the cancer has progressed or side effects from treatment have become debilitating. The reverse is also true: someone recently diagnosed with cancer may choose a completely alternative path and only turn to conventional medicine after the disease has progressed.

None of these situations is optimal. We advocate using an integrative approach from the very start. Integrative medicine begins with prevention and continues into treatment and then restoration of health. If you choose conventional medicine, we highly recommend you augment that treatment with a variety of complementary strategies, including dietary changes, lifestyle modifications, and appropriate supplements. These strategies can help reduce or alleviate harmful and painful side effects from conventional treatments, enhance your quality of life during and after treatment, and in some cases, even enhance the effectiveness of the treatment.

To that end, part II of this book includes a comprehensive "Integrative Cancer Care Supplement Guide," as well as unique charts that profile conventional cancer treatments and helpful nutrients and herbs as well as ones to avoid. It is our hope that these resources, along with the detailed information in the cancer-specific chapters in part IV, will help you (and your health-care provider) create a custom integrative treatment plan to tackle your cancer.

In addition to recommending that you avoid an either-or approach, we also advocate letting go of the frantic and desperate need to find a cure. This is not to say we encourage you to throw in the towel and give up the fight. On the contrary, we strongly believe in and support the global march toward finding effective treatment strategies for cancer. We all want a sure-fire cancer cure to be discovered. But solely focusing on an as-yet-undiscovered cure will distract you from proactively and comprehensively managing your cancer now.

It may be time to look at cancer the same way we view diabetes or high blood pressure: as a chronic disease to be managed. Our focus could then shift to ways we can prevent, control, and manage the disease process and its physical symptoms. This kind of thinking shifts the focus away from death and toward quality of life.

"We sometimes work with patients not so much to focus on the need to eliminate all detectable cancer but more to accept the fact that the cancer is present," say the authors of *How to Prevent and Treat Cancer with Natural Medicine* (Michael Murray, ND, Tim Birdsall, ND, Joseph Pizzorno, ND, and Paul Reilly, ND). "Treatment is then designed to minimize symptoms and control the damage from the disease process." Integrative medicine works to support the body during treatment to not only ease side effects but also halt the disease process.

Whether you choose conventional cancer treatments or not, use the dietary and lifestyle recommendations in chapter 4 to help enhance your healing plan. If you have chosen conventional treatment, a healthier diet will help ease some of the more common side effects. Nutritional supplements will also be indicated in some cases. For example, researchers at Tufts University found that antioxidant nutrients (which are abundant in fruits and vegetables) improve tolerance to and recovery from chemotherapy and radiation. "Cancer treatment by radiation and anticancer drugs reduces inherent antioxidants and induces oxidative stress, which increases with disease progression," explains Dr. Carmia Borek of Tufts in *Integrative Cancer Therapies.* "Vitamins E and C have been shown to ameliorate adverse side effects associated with free radical damage to normal cells in cancer therapy," concludes Borek.

That's just one example of how dietary supplements can be important tools to help you manage cancer. Research has demonstrated that specific herbs and nutrients help ease cancer symptoms, manage side effects of treatment, enhance quality of life, and even assist in slowing down disease progression or help cause remission. The chart "Natural Management of Treatment Side Effects" on page 130 features a list of natural ways to ease side effects of conventional treatments.

Nutrients, Herbs, and Other Supplements

Before we explain how nutrients and herbs can help with cancer treatment, we must emphasize this precaution: It is critical to tell your doctors if you choose to use dietary supplements. It has been estimated that nearly 60 percent of those patients using complementary and alternative therapies for their cancer care do not disclose that use to their conventional doctors. Remember, your doctor does not have to agree with your choices; however, your doctor must know about your choices in order to provide you with safe and effective care. Certain supplements may have negative interactions with specific drugs and other medical treatments, but your doctors can't inform you of this possibility if they don't know what supplements you're taking. (See the sidebar "Are You Taking Warfarin?" on page 124 for an example of negative interactions to be aware of.)

While this admonition is important, we also realize that many conventional doctors aren't knowledgeable about integrative therapies, in particular dietary supplements. This can lead to two common assumptions, both of which are incorrect. (Uninformed patients may also hold these false beliefs.) One false assumption is that integrative therapies are essentially harmless, and therefore using them alongside conventional care is unlikely to be of benefit but also unlikely to create harm. The other common false assumption is that integrative therapies are harmful and likely to interfere with conventional therapies, and therefore must be avoided at all costs. Should your conventional doctor give you one of these responses, it is our hope that the information in this book will help guide you in making the best integrative choices for yourself—and hopefully you can educate your doctor in the process. If your doctor continues to be resistant, you may want to consider going to an integrative oncology hospital or clinic, or another oncologist who embraces a more holistic treatment plan.

To be fair, it must also be said that some alternative health-care providers are guilty of similar prejudices, dismissing conventional medicine with one fell swoop. They cannot fathom why anyone would want to subject themselves to what is often referred to as "cut, poison, and burn" (surgery, chemotherapy, and radiation). They're more likely to dismiss these forms of treatment if they don't understand the value of these therapies and the important role they can play in improving quality of life and extending survival. Extreme views on either side, conventional or alternative, are not in the best interest of the patient.

Nutrients and herbs can complement conventional cancer therapies, alleviate side effects of treatment, and even assist in directly treating cancer. Nonetheless, no matter how effective a nutrient has proven to be, there are no known natural substances that can replace conventional anticancer drugs. There are, however, many natural substances with significant anticancer actions or the ability to increase tolerance to conventional treatments. Melatonin is an excellent example. This hormone, produced at night by the pineal gland located in the brain and by our intestinal cells, helps to regulate our immune response. When used as a supplement, melatonin can influence sleep cycles, hormone balance, and cancer development. Animal studies have demonstrated that supplementation with melatonin can help stop cancer cells from growing and help the immune system kill cancer cells. Melatonin has also been shown in many trials of people with a variety of cancers to reduce a multitude of adverse effects from various chemotherapy drugs and radiation while improving overall survival.

Curcumin, found in the spice turmeric, is another good example. It has anti-inflammatory properties and has been shown in clinical studies to suppress inflammatory processes that can contribute to cancer development and progression. (The link between inflammation and cancer will be discussed at length in chapter 9.) Curcumin is a key ingredient in an herbal formula (Zyflamend) that, in a recent phase I clinical trial, demonstrated significant reduction in inflammatory markers in men with high-grade prostatic intraepithelial neoplasia (HGPIN) who are at increased risk for developing prostate cancer. Recent research involving colon cancer cells associated with abnormal cellular responses to inflammation demonstrated that curcumin helped to stimulate cancer cell death (apoptosis). Other studies have demonstrated anti-inflammatory, antiangiogenic, and antioxidant effects of curcumin with stomach, breast, prostate, and skin cancers. Interesting research from the Dana-Farber Cancer Institute at Harvard Medical School indicates that curcumin may help to prevent resistance to cisplatin (a chemotherapy drug) in cases of breast and ovarian cancer.

Curcumin is one of several natural substances thought to be chemopreventive, meaning it can prevent cancer or delay its growth. (Don't let the name confuse you. Chemoprevention means preventing or delaying cancer growth with natural substances. This is quite different from chemotherapy.) Curcumin and other natural chemopreventive agents can be used to prevent cancer, as well as to complement cancer treatment. In fact, most of the research on natural substances has been on prevention; however, this trend is now changing as promising nutrients and herbs are being studied to treat cancer, enhance other treatments, or offset side effects of conventional therapy.

Green tea is yet another excellent example of a natural dietary substance with a wide variety of anticancer properties. One of its active ingredients, epigallocatechin gallate (EGCG), has been proven effective in preventing and helping treat some cancers. "We have shown for the first time that EGCG, which is present in green tea at relatively high concentrations, inhibits the enzyme dihydrofolate reductase (DHFR), which is a recognized, established target for anticancer drugs," according to Roger Thorneley of the John Innes Center in Norwich, England. Professor Thorneley's research partner, Dr. Jose Neptuno Rodriguez-Lopez of the University of Murcia in Spain, explains, "We discovered that EGCG can kill cancer cells in the same way as methotrexate [a chemotherapy drug]." Studies have shown that EGCG works against cancer in a number of other ways: it can kill cancer cells by stimulating apoptosis, interfere with the liver's activation of cancer-causing substances, and reduce angiogenesis in tumor tissue. In addition, EGCG inhibits the enzymes that break down the connective tissue matrix. These enzymes can eat a pathway through connective tissue, allowing cancer to spread to other parts of the body. By inhibiting these enzymes, EGCG may help to prevent the spread of cancer. Finally, green tea has been shown in animal studies to support the tumoricidal activity of the chemotherapy drug adriamyacin, while reducing its toxicity to the heart and liver.

Certain natural substances can also support conventional cancer treatment by influencing hormone balance. Tamoxifen, raloxifene, and letrozole are examples of drugs used to influence hormone levels in women at risk of breast cancer. Tamoxifen and raloxifene reduce the activity of estrogen receptors, thus interfering with this receptor-driven proliferation signal on estrogen receptor positive cancer cells. Letrozole works by inhibiting the action of the enzyme aromatase, which is involved in estrogen production. This reduces production of estrogen in fat cells and conversion of adrenal hormones into estrogen.

Although natural substances cannot be substituted for these conventional medications, certain nutrients can support or augment the action of these hormonal therapies. Nutrients that can influence hormones include calcium D-glucarate found in some fruits and vegetables and as a supplement, and polysaccharides found in certain mushrooms and mushroom products. Calcium D-glucarate influences the breakdown of estrogen, creating less active (less estrogenic) metabolites. The polysaccharides from white button mushrooms are natural aromatase inhibitors.

B vitamins may also play a key role in complementary cancer treatment. Decades ago a connection between the amino acid homocysteine and heart disease was discovered. Although homocysteine is important in many metabolic pathways, when those pathways are functioning properly homocysteine is often converted into other compounds, keeping homocysteine levels low. However, too much methionine can lead to elevated homocysteine levels. Animal and human studies have demonstrated that both methionine and homocysteine will decrease when the diet has enough B6, B12, and folic acid. In the 1980s, researcher Kilmer McCully, MD, and others speculated that there may be a link between homocysteine and cancer. This spawned new research evaluating the use of B vitamins in conjunction with specific chemotherapy agents that elevate blood levels of methionine and homocysteine; it is believed that the B vitamins can enhance the effectiveness of these drugs.

Many of the natural substances that show promise as adjuvant cancer treatments are powerful antioxidants, meaning they can prevent and reverse oxidative damage caused by free radicals. Total antioxidant status declines during cancer treatment, so shoring up antioxidant status naturally may help reduce side effects of conventional therapies. In addition, antioxidant decline is correlated with decreased quality of life and decreased longevity. However, despite compelling reasons to use antioxidants along with chemotherapy and radiation, there are also times when this is ill advised. Radiation therapy and some chemotherapy drugs create free radicals and oxidation purposefully in order to damage the DNA of the cancer cells. Certain antioxidants, when present in high amounts, interfere with this tumor-killing effect, so it is inadvisable to use them while undergoing these conventional treatments. We have included some examples of antioxidants that may help alleviate the side effects of conventional treatment as well as antioxidants that are contraindicated with conventional treatments in the chemotherapy and radiation sections of this chapter. Also, refer to the section "Nutrient and Herb Interactions with Conventional Cancer Treatments," starting on page 140.

"In many instances the effect of an antioxidant compound with a certain therapeutic agent may be specific to a particular tumor type, or may vary with dosage of both antioxidant and chemotherapy," explain Davis W. Lamson, MS, ND, and Matthew S. Brignall, ND. Some studies demonstrate that specific antioxidants, for example, glutathione, can actually enhance the effects of certain chemotherapy agents. The body makes glutathione from the amino acids cysteine, glutamic acid, and glycine. Selenium increases the body's ability to produce glutathione, and supplemental N-acetylcysteine, alpha-lipoic acid, and selenium enhance glutathione production. Glutathione is ubiquitous in foods, but is concentrated in acorn squash, asparagus, avocados, broccoli, cantaloupe, grapefruit, okra, oranges, peaches, potatoes, spinach, strawberries, tomatoes, walnuts, watermelon, and zucchini. However, N-acetylcysteine can interfere with certain chemotherapy drugs, such as cisplatin, which probably gives you an idea of how complex this realm is and why good advice specific to your situation is needed. Again, the charts beginning on page 140 will also be very helpful.

In general, most antioxidants are safe to use after each dose of chemotherapy is metabolized and eliminated from the body. The time it takes for

Are You Taking Warfarin?

The anticoagulant drug warfarin (Coumadin) is often prescribed to cancer patients because of their increased risk of developing a life-threatening blood clot. Cancer, especially more advanced cancers, increase the risk of blood clots due to changes in the number and function of platelets—the cells responsible for forming blood clots. Warfarin is commonly prescribed to patients who have had a port implanted to receive repeated infusions of chemotherapy drugs. These implants can become a site for platelets to accumulate and form a clot; warfarin lowers this risk. It is also used in combination with other drugs to treat some forms of lung cancer.

While on therapeutic doses of warfarin, it is important to inform your doctor of any other prescription and nonprescription medications you may be taking, including any dietary supplements. There is a long list of medications, nutrients, and herbs that can interfere with the effectiveness of warfarin, including heart medications, antibiotics, aspirin and other NSAIDs, ibuprofen, naproxen, cimetidine, CoQ10, St. John's wort, curcumin, garlic, and ginkgo. Because iron, magnesium, and zinc can bind with warfarin, decreasing its absorption

and effectiveness, these minerals should be taken at least two hours apart from warfarin. Do not discontinue taking warfarin without first consulting with your physician.

Warfarin works by interfering with vitamin K's ability to promote blood clots. For this reason, once individuals start taking therapeutic doses of warfarin, they should not alter their consumption of foods containing vitamin K, which include green leafy vegetables, broccoli, cauliflower, and liver, and should aim for a consistent intake of those foods on a daily basis. Side effects of warfarin include headache, upset stomach, diarrhea, fever, and skin rash. If these side effects develop, there are several supplements that can help while not interfering with the warfarin. Among these are riboflavin or magnesium for headaches, chamomile tea or deglycyrrhizinated licorice (DGL) tablets for upset stomach, and lactobacillus probiotics or L-glutamine for diarrhea. Fever and skin rash side effects should be reported to your physician. Contact your doctor immediately if you experience unusual bleeding or bruising, black or bloody stools, blood in your urine, tiredness, or unexplained fever, chills, sore throat, or stomach pain.

the body to do this varies according to the chemotherapy drug. Consult a qualified complementary health-care provider with expertise in the area of cancer care if you plan to use antioxidants while receiving chemotherapy.

Support Before and After Surgery

A large percentage of cancer patients undergo surgery to either biopsy an area or remove cancerous tissue. Whether the surgery is minor or major, your body will still need support. The human body is amazing and when supported properly with healthy nutrients, it has the potential to rebuild and repair itself quickly.

Support before and after surgery involves shoring up wound-healing capabilities by controlling inflammation and fighting infection. You can do this by being well rested prior to surgery and eating health-promoting foods. You also need to avoid inflammatory foods and substances such as alcohol, tobacco, simple sugars, and processed foods. Meditating, using guided imagery and positive visualizations, or receiving acupuncture before and after surgery can also assist with recovery. (For more information on guided imagery, refer to the sidebar on page 126; for more on acupuncture, see the sidebar on page 127.)

Some nutrients and herbs can increase your risk of bleeding, something you do not want to encourage during surgery. Two weeks prior to surgery, stop taking vitamin E, and one week prior to surgery discontinue blood-thinning herbs such as garlic, ginkgo, red clover, and Panax ginseng. Herbs that may interfere with anesthesia should be discontinued at least three days prior to surgery; these include valerian, kava, echinacea, garlic, silymarin (from the herb milk thistle), and St. John's wort.

The authors of *How to Prevent and Treat Cancer with Natural Medicine* recommend modified citrus pectin (MCP) before having a biopsy or any other cancer surgery. Biopsy can cause seeding of malignant cells into the surrounding healthy tissue. This occurs in approximately 22 percent of breast cancer patients during core needle biopsies. This seeding is not associated with an increased risk of disease recurrence. This is likely due to the local immune destruction of those loose cancer cells. Nonetheless, extra protection can be achieved by taking MCP before and after surgery, as it has been shown to reduce cell adhesion and metastatic spread in several animal studies. "Having high levels of MCP in the bloodstream at these times can reduce the risk of the cancer being spread by the very procedure being done to treat it," explain the authors. The authors caution that MCP has been shown to interfere with the proper absorption of some oral chemotherapy drugs and should therefore not be taken simultaneously with those drugs.

Patients are often placed on an antibiotic prescription prior to or after surgery. Antibiotics can help prevent infection, but they also kill the body's own beneficial bacteria. For this reason, it's a good idea to take a probiotic supplement to restore those beneficial bacteria. Take a high-quality probiotic supplement with lactobacillus and/or bifidobacterium bacteria as soon after surgery as possible, but not before solid foods are allowed in the diet. Continue taking it daily for several weeks, even if you're also taking antibiotics during this time. Probiotics can be taken at any time, but may have the best effect when taken prior to, or in between, meals. You can also help restore beneficial bacteria with diet by eating foods that contain live cultures, such as yogurt, miso, and fresh sauerkraut.

Homeopathic Arnica Montana is an effective way to reduce the trauma associated with surgery. It can be taken both prior to surgery and for a couple of weeks afterward to reduce inflammation, bruising, and pain associated with surgery. It won't interfere with any other medications, and because it can be dissolved in the mouth, it is an ideal postsurgical supplement and may be used even before foods or liquids are allowed.

Going through Surgery? Just Imagine . . .

Guided imagery is emerging as a key mind-body form of healing. This technique involves using the imagination and mental images to promote relaxation and physical healing and achieve changes in attitudes or behavior. It can sometimes include listening to soothing music or verbal instructions that help the listener relax.

One of the most well-known proponents of guided imagery as a cancer therapy is O. Carl Simonton, MD, who first started using guided imagery with his patients in 1971. He has his patients imagine their cancer cells as something that can be easily destroyed and the body's white blood cells as warriors ready for battle.

But can our internal dialogue and the images we conjure positively influence our health? Even some of the most conservative organizations, including health insurance companies, are becoming interested in this idea. According to research by Blue Shield of California (as profiled in the PBS documentary "The New Medicine"), not only can guided imagery help patients cope with surgery, it can also save money. Blue Shield patients who practiced guided imagery by listening to a CD before surgery had significantly shorter hospital stays and lower expenses for pain medication. For the cost of a $17 guided imagery CD that Blue Shield provided, the company saved an average $2,000 per surgery. "The benefits were startling to us from a financial perspective," says Deborah Schwab, RN, NP, MSN, of Blue Shield in the PBS special.

New research is demonstrating that guided imagery can complement cancer treatment. According to researchers featured in the journals *Psychooncology* and the *Journal of Alternative and Complementary Medicine*, although there is no direct evidence that guided imagery will alleviate physical symptoms associated with cancer and cancer treatment such as pain and nausea, the research suggests it will increase patient comfort and enhance overall well-being.

The healing power of your mind is within your reach. You can tap into the health-promoting well of your imagination by using guided imagery and positive visualization techniques. Guided imagery recordings specifically for people with cancer are widely available. There's no downside to this inexpensive approach, and you may experience a world of benefit. Why not give it a try?

Supporting your connective tissue with nutrients that encourage healing can hasten surgical recovery. Vitamin C and zinc are required to help knit the collagen matrix of connective tissue together. Bromelain, a protein-digesting enzyme derived from pineapple, reduces inflammation that can otherwise delay wound healing. Flavonoids, such as proanthocyanidins derived from berries, also reduce inflammation and increase the strength of connective tissue.

Supporting Chemotherapy Treatments

At some point, most people with cancer will receive one or more of the 40-plus different types of anticancer drugs currently available. As discussed in chapter 5, chemotherapy can cause numerous side effects, including mouth sores, nerve damage, cardiovascular problems, decreased immune response, damaged salivary glands, hair loss, and digestive damage. Side effects can be short term, ceasing when chemotherapy is stopped, or can last longer, well after the therapy is completed. (Refer to the chemotherapy chart beginning on page 141 for more information on side effects.)

Can Acupuncture Help with Side Effects?

Acupuncture is a form of traditional Chinese medicine based on the premise that health is determined by a balanced flow of the vital energy known as chi. Chi flows along 12 major pathways, called meridians, linked to major organs. Small needles are inserted into one or more of the acupoints along the meridians.

Research into acupuncture in relation to cancer treatment has focused primarily on chemotherapy-induced nausea and vomiting. According to an evaluation of data from 11 clinical trials in the Cochrane Controlled Trials Registry (a government-funded database of controlled trials), acupuncture reduced acute chemotherapy-induced vomiting. Acupuncture has also been shown to alleviate cancer-related pain and dry mouth. Recent research indicates it can help relieve cancer-related menopausal symptoms as well. (Menopausal symptoms can occur following chemotherapy or can be surgically induced when the ovaries are removed.) Acupuncture is currently being studied in relation to immune enhancement, diarrhea relief, and shortness of breath in cases of advanced lung cancer.

Interest regarding use of acupuncture in anesthesia is also gaining momentum. Acupuncture can be used to reduce the amount of anesthesia medications needed before surgery, enhance the effects of anesthesia, or in some rare cases take the place of anesthesia for less complex surgeries. Acupuncture anesthesia research is in its infancy; however, this approach may become a viable option for people who can't tolerate anesthesia or who want to reduce the amount of anesthesia medication they're given.

It is important to work with a licensed acupuncturist with training equivalent to a master's degree. It is also a good idea to only work with acupuncturists who have experience working with people with cancer. Be sure the therapist uses disposable, single-use needles and a sterile technique to deliver the treatments.

For more information on acupuncture, visit one of these websites: www.acaom.org (Accreditation Commission for Acupuncture and Oriental Medicine); www.aaom.org (American Association of Oriental Medicine); or www.ccaom.org (Council of Colleges of Acupuncture and Oriental Medicine).

Thankfully, new developments in conventional medicine have helped to reduce chemotherapy's side effects. Some of the newer drugs are less toxic, and new delivery methods and dosing techniques can make some chemotherapy drugs more tolerable. No matter how severe or benign the side effects are, an integrative approach can help reduce them. This is important, as anyone who has undergone chemotherapy can attest. But certain supplements can do even more than reduce side effects; they can slow or halt cancer growth and enhance the tumor-killing actions of conventional drugs. Some of these substances can be classified as antioxidants, meaning they can neutralize free radicals (tissue-destroying reactive molecules), but interestingly, the benefits of antioxidants during chemotherapy are not always derived exclusively from their antioxidant actions. At high doses, most antioxidants stimulate apoptosis of cancer cells but not normal cells. This effect may be due to their ability to change expression of genes that control apoptosis. When taken at low doses, antioxidants tend to have no effect on cancer cells. Additionally, the manner in which antioxidants are administered alters their effect. For example, there is a difference between consuming antioxidant-rich foods versus supplementing individual antioxidants in higher doses. While eating antioxidant-rich foods is certainly healthful and can even help prevent cancer, the relatively low "doses" present in food don't seem to be effective antitumor agents. And single antioxidant supplements, as opposed to multiple antioxidants, tend to protect cancer cells instead of triggering their death. Thus, *high* doses of a *combination* of antioxidant supplements are likely to be of the most benefit in conjunction with chemotherapy as cancer-killing agents.

But again, more research is needed to figure out exactly which antioxidants in which combinations and at what doses are most useful for each type of cancer, especially for use alongside specific chemotherapy drugs. As mentioned previously, the use of antioxidants while on chemotherapy is controversial and must be considered very carefully. "The biggest issue is not whether to use an antioxidant, but rather which antioxidant offers the greatest benefits and what dosage should be used," conclude the authors of *How to Prevent and Treat Cancer with Natural Medicine*. That's the million-dollar question: which ones at what dose? The state of the evidence to date regarding this question for individual chemotherapy agents is presented in the "Nutrient and Herb Interactions with Conventional Cancer Treatments" charts starting on page 140. As with any medical program, a cautious and individualized risk-to-benefit analysis is important. But given the risks associated with many chemotherapy drugs, it makes sense to try to find ways to reduce those risks. Fortunately, there are many natural agents that are very effective in reducing some of the most debilitating and common side effects of chemotherapy. Refer to the "Natural Management of Treatment Side Effects" table on page 130.

One common side effect of chemotherapy that deserves special consideration is anemia. Chemotherapy-induced anemia is often not caused by low iron levels. While supplemental iron is very effective at correcting anemia due to iron deficiency, it won't be helpful if iron deficiency isn't the cause, and it may even be harmful. If you are undergoing chemotherapy, do not assume your anemia is due to iron deficiency; it is critical not to take supplemental iron unless recommended to do so by your oncologist. Too much iron can promote tumor growth and can worsen chemotherapy side effects. Supplemental iron is only recommended when iron deficiency has been confirmed by blood tests.

Clearly, use of supplements to support chemotherapy is both potentially very beneficial and extremely complex. To design a safe and effective supplement program, you need to work with a health-care practitioner whose knowledge in this area is up-to-date. The integrative treatment overview in chapter 5 also provides information about how to offset side effects of chemotherapy.

Supporting Radiation Treatments

According to the American Cancer Society, more than 50 percent of all cancer patients receive radiation therapy. It is believed that radiation is most effective against cells that are actively dividing. If radiation successfully hits dividing cells, those cells will either die or sustain injuries that prevent them from dividing, or from dividing more than one time. Because retinoic acid, a derivative of vitamin A, inhibits the repair of radiation damage in cancer cells, sufficient levels of retinoic acid can enhance the effectiveness of radiation therapy. Similarly, flavonoids such as genistein, apigenin, and quercetin may enhance radiation-induced cell death by decreasing the repair of DNA with radiation damage.

Like chemotherapy, radiation also kills healthy cells. But in contrast to chemotherapy, which is typically sent throughout the body, radiation is usually focused on the specific area of the body where the cancer is or was (when using radiation to prevent local recurrence). Side effects of radiation include local effects to the organs and tissues in the field of radiation, and systemic effects such as fatigue and loss of appetite. As with chemotherapy, radiation can cause secondary cancers.

Some nutrients, specifically vitamins A, L-glutamine, and honey, have been shown to help offset the side effects of radiation therapy without interfering with the intended effects of radiation. A clinical trial of individuals with glioblastoma demonstrated that melatonin improves survival and quality of life in individuals undergoing radiation therapy. Topically, a cream with the herb *Calendula officinalis* (marigold) can help soothe the skin side effects of radiation and assist with healing. Vitamin E cream may also help in the same way. The herb astragalus (*Astragalus membranaceus*) has been shown to increase white blood cells and their activity in patients undergoing radiation therapy. Because astragalus enhances white blood cell synthesis, it has recently been used to treat leukopenia (low white blood cell counts) due to chemotherapy or radiation therapy. Radiation to any area of the body that includes large bones (especially the pelvis and upper leg) will affect the bone marrow's ability to produce white (and red) blood cells. Thus, astragalus may help to prevent the immune deficiencies that can occur with radiation therapy.

As always, a healthy diet plays an important role and can help support the body before, during, and after radiation treatment. An interesting study featured in the *Journal of Clinical Oncology* demonstrated that dietary counseling significantly improved outcomes for colon cancer patients undergoing radiotherapy. The researchers concluded that this nutrition intervention not only improved the patients' nutritional status, it also improved their quality of life and lessened morbidity.

Helping Your Body Heal

The chapters in part III describe the important role that key body functions have on cancer prevention, development, and treatment. This will be helpful in understanding and appreciating the comprehensive and interdependent potential of the human body as we attempt to prevent and successfully treat cancer. As you work to alleviate cancer, it is important to look beyond the tumor and embrace a whole body approach advocated by integrative oncologists. This will give you the broad base needed to not only treat an existing cancer but also prevent a cancer recurrence.

Natural Management of Treatment Side Effects

The chart below lists a number of safe and effective natural strategies for managing common side effects of chemotherapy and other anticancer drugs. Conventional medications can manage these side effects in some individuals. Be sure to tell your oncologist about any side effects that you are experiencing and utilize the treatments that you find to be most helpful.

Side effect	Natural strategies (refer to Appendix: Dosage Ranges for dosing)
Nausea	Ginger—freshly diced ginger root tea, candied ginger, or ginger ale made from real ginger (all-natural brands)
	Acupuncture—ideally the day before and the day after each chemotherapy treatment
	Yarrow tea*/**
	Homeopathic remedies
Fatigue	Coenzyme Q10*
	Multivitamin
	Rest—as needed
	Exercise—to tolerance; goal is at least 30 minutes daily
	L-carnitine
Numbness and tingling in hands and feet (peripheral neuropathy)	L-glutamine
	Vitamin E*
	Vitamin B$_6$
	Acetyl-L-carnitine*
	Ginkgo biloba*

Side effect	Natural strategies (refer to Appendix: Dosage Ranges for dosing)
Taste changes	Zinc*
	Bland-tasting foods (oatmeal, potato, egg, yogurt, etc.)
Mouth sores	Honey
	L-glutamine—swish and swallow
	Vitamin E**—open soft gel onto mouth sores
	Zinc
	Chamomile tea**—swish and swallow
Lack of appetite	Zinc*
	Fish oil (omega-3 fatty acids)
Insomnia	Melatonin
	Chamomile tea after dinner
	5-hydroxy tryptophan
Constipation	Probiotics
	Slippery elm gruel**
	Flaxseed meal
	Water
	Coffee or black tea—in the morning
	Homeopathic remedies
Diarrhea	Probiotics
	Activated charcoal*
	Homeopathic remedies
Heartburn	Deglycyrrhizinated licorice (DGL) chewable tablet
	Calcium chewable tablet
	d-limonene
Headache	Vitamin B_2 (riboflavin)*
	Electrolyte replacement drink
	Magnesium
	Cold neck compresses and hot foot soak—for 20 minutes during headache

Side effect	Natural strategies (refer to Appendix: Dosage Ranges for dosing)
Hot flashes	dl-phenylalanine**
	Black cohosh*
	Vitamin E*
	Hesperidin**
Nail changes	Jojoba oil**—apply to nails daily
Excessive watery eyes and tearing	Vitamin A**—puncture soft gel and apply oil to eyelids and corners of eyes
Skin irritation	Apply one of the following immediately after each radiation treatment:
	Chamomile ointment
	Jojoba oil**
	Emu oil**
	Fresh aloe vera plant gel

*Refer to the "Chemotherapy Drugs and Their Nutrient and Herb Interactions" chart beginning on page 141 to make sure that this supplement is not to be avoided with the chemotherapy drug that you are receiving.

**Based on the clinical experience of naturopathic oncologists.

seven

Healing Support after Conventional Treatment

The chaos and emotions associated with a cancer diagnosis and treatment can be overwhelming. Just "getting through" the treatment becomes all consuming. Then, one day, conventional therapy is over. Now what? The transition from the completion of the intense and life-altering experience of cancer treatment to life after treatment is not always easy. While this is a welcome transition, many new issues surface. Cancer and its conventional treatments typically cause radical changes in a person's life and the lives of their loved ones. Schedules are turned upside down, work is often put on hold, and visits from caring family and friends can be emotionally and physically consuming. During this time, very little is the same as it was. Even our perspective on life changes. Perhaps the most common perspective shared by people undergoing conventional cancer treatment is the realization that each day is different and essentially unpredictable; thus, it really does help to focus on taking things one day at a time. This philosophy works well during treatment, and then, the much-anticipated last treatment arrives and brings with it an entirely new set of challenges and unknowns.

After the last chemotherapy infusion or pill or the last radiation treatment, people with cancer feel a variety of emotions. For some, it feels as if the dam that has held a torrent of emotions at bay finally breaks. There is a river of emotions such as fear, anger, depression, anxiety, frustration, gratitude, excitement, and confusion that rushes into our daily lives. Being physically exhausted from the treatment can add to the turbulence. And, yet, it is in the midst of all this that some of the most important decisions for long-term survival and quality of life must be made. Among these decisions are how to heal from the trauma of the disease and its treatments, how to lower the risk of recurrence and secondary cancers, and how to utilize the experience to live the most meaningful life possible.

Recovering from Cancer Treatment

Conventional cancer treatments can challenge the body, the mind, and the spirit. Restoring optimal health in all of these areas is important for a full recovery and a lifetime of being cancer free. Healing the body begins with a two-part process. The first process is to replenish the body with nutrients and to restore homeostasis (balance) in bodily processes. The significant cell destruction and damage caused by chemotherapy, radiation, and other conventional treatments tends to deplete the body of certain nutrients involved in cell repair and cleanup. Although the majority of conventional cancer treatments kill far more cancer cells than healthy cells, some healthy cells are destroyed as a part of the process. As a result, following treatment many people are overtly or functionally deficient in B vitamins, particularly folic acid, thiamine (vitamin B_1), and riboflavin (vitamin B_2). Bodily stores of certain minerals such as magnesium and zinc are also often diminished. Conventional treatments dramatically diminish antioxidant compounds such as vitamin C, vitamin E, and selenium, so replenishing these important immune-enhancing nutrients is crucial. Given the widespread and comprehensive depletion conventional cancer treatments can cause, one of the most important things to do after completion of therapy is to focus on a nutrient-dense diet and take a high-quality multivitamin/multimineral supplement. A diet high in organic fruits, vegetables, whole grains, nuts, seeds, vegetable oils, legumes, and lean meats will, over months, replenish these missing nutrients. Adding a high-quality multivitamin/multimineral supplement will also hasten the recovery process. Keep in mind that obtaining adequate sleep is a critical part of treatment recovery because it enhances the body's ability to utilize the nutrients you are replenishing.

The second part to the bodily recovery process is detoxification. After completing conventional therapy, in particular treatment with chemotherapy and/or radiation, many people say they feel "toxic" and feel the need to "detox" their bodies. In fact, there is a physiological rationale for this feeling. Both chemotherapy and radiation treatment create cellular damage, which, in turn, triggers the immune system to clean up the damaged and destroyed tissues. As you will learn in the next section, this cleanup process involves the release of large amounts of proinflammatory chemicals in the body. While the result of this inflammatory process is eventually to rid the body of the damaged and destroyed tissues, this process can also cause symptoms such as joint pain, muscle ache, headache, fatigue, constipation, and mood changes. Collectively, these symptoms can certainly be described as feeling "toxic." While this inflammation will typically subside over time, detoxification can facilitate the process. Proper detoxification support can speed up the process.

Detoxification after the completion of conventional therapy and after a period of nutrient repletion is an important part of overall recovery and healing. Ideally, detoxification should be supervised by a qualified health-care professional with expertise in safe and effective detoxification. For example, your doctor may want to request certain evaluations prior to beginning a detoxification program, such as an environmental toxicity assessment (identifies tissue levels of environmental toxins), a genetics test (to identify genetic alterations that affect detoxification pathways), a hormone metabolic profile (determines activities of hormone breakdown), and/or an assay of inflammatory markers in the blood (checks for abnormal levels of compounds associated with chronic inflammation). This information guides your doctor in determining an individually tailored detoxification program. While individually tailored detoxification is advantageous, a more generic detoxification is also most certainly beneficial.

Typically, detoxification should not be started until at least a month after the completion of treatment. If there is any residual ongoing treatment such as hormonal therapies, detoxification requires close monitoring by a qualified health-care professional to make sure that there is no adverse effect on the ongoing therapy. In general, effective detoxification can be achieved through the following:

- A plant-based whole foods diet that avoids processed foods, refined sugar, and alcohol

- Regular exercise that induces sweating

- Adequate sleep (7 to 8 hours every night)

- Regular bowel eliminations (1 to 3 times daily)

- 4 to 8 cups of green tea every day (or the equivalent in a dietary supplement)

Green tea is an important component of detoxification in that it supports the enzymes involved in the breakdown (metabolism) of toxins. Green tea also helps to collect fat-soluble toxins into the bowel for elimination. For more information about effective detoxification, refer to chapter 12.

The Gentle Detoxification Plan

The goal of gentle detoxification is to support gastrointestinal function and the formation and release of bile and other digestive secretions while minimizing inflammation. Gentle detoxification is most effective when it is done over several weeks to months. As you'll see from the pointers below, this is an approach that can be incorporated into your normal, day-to-day routine.

- Get enough sleep. Sleep is essential for restoration of digestive function. Plus, certain digestive functions are most active during sleep.

- Start each meal with a small glass of water with a squeeze of lemon. The sour taste of lemon stimulates the sour taste receptors on the tongue, which in turn stimulates the gustatory nerve and then the vagus nerve. The vagus nerve is the master nerve that turns digestive function on and keeps it on.

- Eat in a slow, relaxed manner. Chew thoroughly and enjoy the smell and taste of food; this stimulates nerves that trigger digestive function.

- Do not mix liquids with food. Allow your stomach and pancreas to digest food without diluting the digestive enzymes with too much liquid. Taking sips of liquid with your food will not be problematic, but avoid drinking large quantities of beverages once you have started eating.

- Avoid processed, chemically laden foods, which require additional detoxification.

- Avoid refined sugar and foods that contain simple sugar to reduce inflammatory potential and the burden on the liver and pancreas.

- Eat more organic vegetables, fruits, whole grains, seeds, nuts, and lean meat and fish, as they supply concentrated nutrients, thus reducing demands on the digestive system and detoxification pathways.

- Emphasize foods that naturally stimulate and support liver detoxification and bile flow, including beets, garlic, onions, parsnips, dark leafy greens, and even organic liver.

- If you have a tendency toward constipation, add a daily serving of oat bran or flax meal.

- Consider taking a good-quality multivitamin and an essential fatty acid supplement to provide nutrients essential for digestion and detoxification.

- Obtain gentle- to moderate-intensity exercise daily. Daily stretching will also improve the flow of blood and lymph fluid throughout the body and will support optimal liver function and minimize constipation.

- Find relaxing and joyful activities to do every day; a good mood improves digestion, just as a perpetual bad mood can cause many digestive woes.

In contrast to this approach, a prolonged fast is not appropriate detoxification for someone who has just completed cancer therapy. Prolonged fasting can cause rapid release of toxins stored in fat, which, in turn, can overwhelm detoxification pathways. In addition, fasting deprives the body of critical nutrients required to perform adequate detoxification. This will only aggravate inflammation and could cause more cellular and tissue damage.

Finally, a prolonged fast does not allow the body to obtain the important nutrients it requires after treatment, as explained previously.

Lowering the Risk of Cancer Recurrence and Secondary Cancers

Conventional therapy can be effective at destroying cancer. However, it is a healthy body and immune system that provide ongoing surveillance and destruction of cancer tumor regrowth. An important part of a posttreatment healing program is to support optimal health and to employ specific cancer prevention strategies. These strategies will support the innate healing capacities within each of us. Optimal health rests upon a foundation of healthy eating, adequate exercise, sufficient sleep, and meaningful and joyful living. The whole foods–based diet described in chapter 4 is the basis for healthy cells and healthy organs. In addition to food, movement is also healing. Our bodies are meant to move. The research on the importance of exercise in preventing cancer and its recurrence is substantial. At minimum, 30 minutes of moderately difficult exercise (brisk walking, jogging, bicycling, swimming, dancing, and so on) done every day is associated with a reduced risk of cancer and of dying from cancer. For instance, compared with women who were inactive both before and after a diagnosis of breast cancer, women who increased physical activity after diagnosis had a 45 percent lower risk of death, and women who decreased physical activity after diagnosis had a four-fold greater risk of death.

The idea is to change the environment to be the least hospitable to cancer. We do this with exercise but we also do this with sleep. Sleep is critical to optimal health. Sleep is critical for a well-functioning immune system. In fact, several key anticancer immune actions are most active during sleep. Stress reduction is also a big part of the anticancer plan. Finding ways to manage stress is of utmost importance. Elevated levels of stress-induced chemicals and hormones unravel immunity, cripple cell repair, and increase the susceptibility of our cells to cancer-causing DNA damage. While we cannot eliminate all the stress in our lives, we can certainly change the way we perceive stress. Meditation, yoga, tai chi, and hobbies are just a few ways to create more inner calm and less stress. It's important to make relaxation a part of your daily routine.

The last component of a cancer prevention plan is an appropriately tailored supplement program. This supplement program should include plant-based antioxidants such as green tea, turmeric, and proanthocyanidins (berries, grapeseed oil, or extracts). It may also include other cancer-preventive compounds such as melatonin, soy isoflavones, flaxseed lignans, essential

Attention: Caregivers

Having a loved one diagnosed with cancer can be devastating. As a caregiver, you are faced with your own set of challenges as you are physically and emotionally stretched to your limit. In fact, studies have demonstrated that individuals who are caring for a loved one with a serious illness can often succumb to physical and emotional issues as well, including

- Worsening of their physical health
- Impaired social and family quality of life
- Increased anxiety and depression

According to the U.S. Department of Health and Human Services, more than 50 million family caregivers are taking care of a loved one in the United States due to chronic illness, disability, and injury. Three of four families will find themselves caring for a cancer patient. The quality of life for these caregivers is often overlooked. Just as the patient's life changes dramatically during serious illness, so do the lives of their caregivers. Caregiver quality of life is influenced by the seriousness of the illness of their loved one, individual coping methods, social support, and many other factors.

From a diet and lifestyle perspective, caregivers can benefit from the same advice given to the patient. This includes eating a whole foods–based, healthful diet, performing consistent physical activity, taking dietary supplements when appropriate, and regularly engaging in proactive stress reduction techniques. In addition, caregivers will benefit from the following advice:

1. Develop an organizational system that helps you manage the details of your loved one's medical situation.

2. Ask for and accept help from family and friends.

3. Do not isolate yourself.

4. Remember that your feelings of fear, frustration, anger, or whatever they may be are valid and deserve to be recognized.

Psychological and social support including groups such as Gilda's Club, the Wellness Community, and others provide a wealth of benefit to families of people who have been diagnosed with cancer. Caring for a loved one with cancer is perhaps one of the most difficult things you will ever face. By taking care of yourself during the process, you will also be taking care of your loved one.

---

fatty acids, medicinal mushrooms, and vitamins C, E, and D. Finally, there are nutrients specific to lowering the risk for each cancer type (refer to the cancer-specific chapters in part IV). Implementing a reasonable and appropriate cancer recovery and prevention supplement program is an important part of healing from cancer.

Learning from Cancer

Cancer can be a door to greater health and life-affirming well-being. While not the easiest way to discover additional meaning and joy in life, the experience of cancer can certainly take us there if we allow it to. Life after cancer treatment is typically radically different than it was before cancer diagnosis. In addition to the direct challenges of the disease and its treatments, many other issues surface. People who have had cancer often experience a prolonged feeling of loss of control, which, in turn, can create anxiety and depression. The fear of recurrence can settle itself like a gremlin on the shoulder of the most confident survivor. Even after successful treatment, a cancer survivor's emotional states spin from hope to despair, gratitude to rage, confidence to fear. There may be financial challenges, relationship and intimacy issues, and career disruptions. All of these issues are real and without a magic fix. Without some attention paid to these issues, any physical healing will be incomplete and fragile. How people tackle the myriad of challenges faced after cancer is unique to each person. Successful strategies include psychotherapy, support groups, vacations, radical life changes, reprioritization of values, and daily healing activities. Whatever the solution, the cancer thriver must make time to heal. Healing on this level can, in turn, deliver a dimension of wellness never before experienced. Herein lies the gift of cancer.

From Survivor to Thriver

Surviving cancer and its treatments is no small feat. Cancer is a formidable illness and its treatments are among the most taxing in all of medicine. Emerging from this experience is something that every survivor should feel both proud about and grateful for. Turning this experience into one that enriches our lives with added clarity of purpose and wonderment allows us to accept cancer as a teacher. Cancer is not an easy teacher, but its lessons are valuable nonetheless. Whatever we each learn from our experience with this disease is uniquely ours. The willingness to let this disease transform our lives so that we honor and cherish life even more fully makes us more than survivors—it turns us into thrivers. We thrive on the feast of life, cherishing each and every morsel.

Nutrient and Herb Interactions with Conventional Cancer Treatments

The research on nutrient and herb interactions with conventional cancer treatments is extremely limited. These charts are invaluable for patients who want to use an integrative approach to treat their cancer.

The first group of charts features some of the most common chemotherapy drugs. Remember, herbs and nutrients should be taken under the supervision of a qualified physician during active treatment. Chemotherapy agents are often combined; any supplemental nutrients and herbs need to be evaluated and adjusted accordingly.

On page 155, we address helpful nutrients and herbs, as well as nutrients and herbs to avoid during radiation treatment. The hormone drug chart on page 156 will aid patients who are taking drugs in this category. Targeted therapies such as monoclonal antibodies and tyrosine kinase inhibitors are the newest category of drugs used to treat cancer. These drugs are so new that very little research on nutrient and herb interactions has been published. As a result, we had to rely on the clinical experience of naturopathic and conventional oncologists to help create the nutrient and herb considerations in that chart (see page 158). The "Integrative Cancer Care Supplement Guide" on page 160 offers a snapshot of the scientific validity associated with the use of a specific nutrient in the treatment of various types of cancer. Finally, we identify "Questionable Alternative Cancer Cures" on page 173. We evaluate these "cures" based on available scientific literature and then we give the "cure" a grade to help guide your use of these therapies.

Chemotherapy Drugs and Their Nutrient and Herb Interactions

Note: Generally, these herbs should not be taken within 48 hours of chemotherapy to avoid possible interference with the metabolism and effectiveness of the chemotherapy.

	Carboplatin
Trade name	Paraplatin
Cancers typically treated	Ovarian, head and neck, testicular, bladder, esophageal, sarcoma, lung
How administered	Intravenously (IV)
Side effects	• Decrease in blood cell counts • Hair loss (reversible) • Confusion • Nausea, vomiting, or diarrhea (usually a short-term side effect occurring in the first 24 to 72 hours following treatment) • Mouth sores • Numbness and tingling (peripheral neuropathy) • Hearing loss (rare) • Kidney toxicity (rare)
Helpful nutrients and herbs	• Vitamin C to support anticancer effects and improve overall tolerance • Vitamin E to support anticancer effects and to improve overall tolerance • Vitamin D to support anticancer effects • Silymarin to support anticancer effects, protect the liver, and help prevent kidney damage • Polysaccharides from the mushroom *Agaricus blazei* to support immune function, specifically natural killer cells (NK cells) • Alpha-lipoic acid to reduce nerve toxicity and protect hearing • Ginger to reduce nausea • Vitamin K (dietary sources only; not prudent to supplement with vitamin K) to support anticancer effects and to help protect bone marrow (caution when taking warfarin or other blood thinner medication) • Astragalus to reduce toxicity and support anticancer effects • Spleen polypeptides for immune support
Nutrients and herbs to avoid	• N-acetylcysteine could increase resistance to carboplatin. • L-glutathione could increase resistance to carboplatin. • Silymarin should be used with caution, as it may interact with other medications prescribed before, during, and after chemotherapy.

Cisplatin	
Trade name	Platinol, Platinol-AQ
Cancers typically treated	Bladder, ovarian, testicular, prostate, lung, esophageal, cervical, breast, stomach, sarcoma, lymphoma, myeloma
How administered	Intravenously (IV)
Side effects	• Decrease in blood cell counts • Hair loss (reversible) • Confusion • Nausea, vomiting, or diarrhea (usually a short-term side effect occurring in the first 24 to 72 hours following treatment) • Numbness and tingling (peripheral neuropathy) • Muscle cramping • Taste changes • Kidney toxicity • Loss of hearing • Visual changes • Allergic reaction
Helpful nutrients and herbs	• Vitamin E to reduce toxicity to nerves and support anticancer effects • Vitamin A to increase anticancer effect • Melatonin to enhance anticancer effect while improving overall tolerance • Magnesium to reduce kidney and muscle toxicity • L-carnitine to reduce damage to nerves and kidneys; may also help with fatigue • Ginkgo biloba to reduce damage to nerves and kidneys • Astragalus to help prevent decreased blood cell counts and support anticancer effects • Polysaccharide-K (PSK; from the fungus *Coriolus versicolor*) to reduce kidney damage • Silymarin to reduce kidney damage • Ginger for nausea • Quercetin to support anticancer actions • Spleen polypeptides for immune support
Nutrients and herbs to avoid	• Black cohosh may decrease the effectiveness of cisplatin. • N-acetylcysteine may interfere with the anticancer action of cisplatin. • High doses of B_6 (above 300 mg daily) may interfere with anticancer effects of cisplatin; vitamin B_6 up to 300 mg daily may help prevent peripheral neuropathy while not interfering with the efficacy of cisplatin. • Caution should be exercised in combining ginkgo with regular-strength aspirin due to potential risk of hemorrhagic stroke; ginkgo may also have interactions with medications used before and after chemotherapy. • Silymarin should be used with caution, as it may interact with other medications prescribed before, during, and after chemotherapy.

	Cyclophosphamide
Trade name	Cytoxan, Neosar
Cancers typically treated	Lymphoma, breast, ovarian carcinoma, leukemia, sarcoma
How administered	Intravenously (IV) or orally
Side effects	• Decrease in blood cell counts • Nausea and vomiting • Abdominal pain • Diarrhea • Decreased appetite • Headache • Hair loss (reversible) • Bladder damage • Infertility • Lung or heart damage (with high doses) • Secondary malignancies (rare)
Helpful nutrients and herbs	• Astragalus to help prevent decrease in blood cell counts • Ashwagandha to help prevent decrease in blood cell counts • Polysaccharide-K (PSK; from the fungus *Coriolus versicolor*) to help prevent decrease in blood cell counts • DHEA to support liver recovery from chemotherapy; however, DHEA not recommended as a supplement in women with breast, ovarian, or endometrial cancers because it is a precursor to estradiol (the main active form of estrogen) and could stimulate the growth of these hormone-sensitive cancers • Melatonin to support anticancer actions and reduce side effects • Ginger for nausea
Nutrients and herbs to avoid	• Curcumin may interfere with antitumor activity of cyclophosphamide. • Quercetin may interfere with cyclophosphamide.

	Doxorubicin
Trade name	Adriamycin, Doxil (liposomal Adriamycin)
Cancers typically treated	Breast, lymphoma, sarcoma, ovarian, bladder, thyroid, hepatoma, gastric, multiple myeloma
How administered	Intravenously (IV)
Side effects	• Decrease in blood cell counts • Mouth ulcers • Hair loss (reversible) • Nausea and vomiting • Heart damage • Facial flushing
Helpful nutrients and herbs	• L-carnitine to protect the heart • CoQ10 to protect the heart • Green tea (especially concentrated to theanine) to protect healthy tissue and enhance antitumor effects • Melatonin to support antitumor activity while reducing side effects • Vitamin D to support anticancer activity • Coriolus versicolor mushroom to support anticancer activity • Quercetin to reduce chemotherapy resistance • Sulforaphane to support antitumor actions and to reduce chemotherapy resistance • DHA from algal oil to sensitize cancer cells to adriamycin chemotherapy
Nutrients and herbs to avoid	• Avoid herbs during doxorubicin therapy because many herbs may interfere with conversion of doxorubicin into its active form in the liver. • N-acetylcysteine may increase resistance to doxorubicin.

	Etoposide
Trade name	VePesid or VP-16
Cancers typically treated	Lung, testicular, leukemia, lymphoma
How administered	Intravenously (IV) or orally
Side effects	• Decrease in blood cell counts • Hair loss (reversible) • Nausea and vomiting • Allergic reaction • Mouth ulcers • Low blood pressure (during administration) • Decreased appetite • Diarrhea and abdominal pain • Bronchospasm • Flulike symptoms
Helpful nutrients and herbs	• Vitamin E may increase anticancer activity. • Vitamin D may increase anticancer activity. • Vitamin C may increase anticancer activity. • Coriolus versicolor mushroom to support anticancer activity.
Nutrients and herbs to avoid	• Avoid herbs during etoposide therapy because many herbs may interfere with conversion of etoposide into its active form in the liver. • Vitamin K may reduce effectiveness. • Glucosamine may interfere with anticancer action.

	Fluorouracil, floxuridine, capcetibine
Trade name	Fluorouracil: 5-FU; floxuridine: FUDR; capcetibine: Xeloda
Cancers typically treated	Colon, breast, stomach, head and neck
How administered	Intravenously (IV)
Side effects	• Decrease in blood cell counts • Diarrhea • Mouth ulcers • Photosensitivity • Dry skin • Nausea • Headache • Malaise, confusion • Hand-foot syndrome
Helpful nutrients and herbs	• Melatonin to support blood counts and improve tolerance to treatment • Fish oil to support anticancer actions and reduce side effects • Vitamin A to increase anticancer actions • Vitamin B_6 to help protect against hand-foot syndrome • Vitamin C to increase anticancer actions • Vitamin E to increase anticancer actions • Panax ginseng to support anticancer actions and reduce side effects • Polysaccharide-K (PSK; from the fungus *Coriolus versicolor*) to increase response to treatment • Garlic to protect the digestive tract during treatment • Ginkgo biloba to increase tolerance of treatment • Curcumin to support anticancer actions • Green tea to support anticancer actions and reduce side effects • Lentinan from shiitake mushrooms to support anticancer actions and help preserve white blood cell count and function • Probiotics to help prevent digestive tract toxicity • Glutamine to help prevent diarrhea and changes in intestinal permeability • Fermented wheat germ extract (Avemar) to support anticancer actions • Ginger for nausea
Nutrients and herbs to avoid	• Beta-carotene may interfere with fluorouracil. • Probiotics should not be taken if white blood cell counts are low (less than 2.5) because of the risk of probiotic bacteria becoming a source of infection. • High doses of folic acid (greater than 15 mg/day) may increase toxicity.

Gemcitabine	
Trade name	Gemzar
Cancers typically treated	Pancreatic, bladder, sarcoma, breast, ovarian, lung
How administered	Intravenously (IV)
Side effects	• Decrease in blood cell counts • Nausea and vomiting • Fever and flulike symptoms • Rash
Helpful nutrients and herbs	• Melatonin to support anticancer actions, support blood cell counts, and reduce side effects. • Ukrain (thiophosphoric acid and chelidonine from *Chelidonium majus*) to support anticancer actions. (Note: Presently, Ukrain is only available in Europe, as an injectable product.) • Quercetin to support anticancer actions. • Curcumin to support anticancer actions. • Ginger for nausea.
Nutrients and herbs to avoid	None known

Ifosfamide	
Trade name	Ifex
Cancers typically treated	Sarcoma, testicular, lymphoma, lung, bladder, head and neck, cervical
How administered	Intravenously (IV)
Side effects	• Nausea and vomiting • Bladder irritation and inflammation and kidney failure • Decrease in blood cell counts • Hair loss (reversible) • Confusion, hallucinations • Diarrhea • Numbness and tingling
Helpful nutrients and herbs	• Ginger for nausea • Water-soluble fiber for diarrhea • L-carnitine to help reduce fatigue and toxicity to nerves (numbness and tingling)
Nutrients and herbs to avoid	• N-acetylcysteine and L-glutathione may decrease anticancer effects of ifosfamide.

Irinotecan	
Trade name	Camptosar, CPT-11
Cancers typically treated	Colorectal
How administered	Intravenously (IV)
Side effects	• Decrease in blood cell counts • Profuse diarrhea • Abdominal cramps • Hair loss (reversible) • Nausea and vomiting
Helpful nutrients and herbs	• Activated charcoal to help prevent diarrhea (effectiveness requires multiple doses for at least four days following chemotherapy) • Fish oil to reduce side effects • Melatonin to support anticancer actions • Polysaccharide-K (PSK; from the fungus *Coriolus versicolor*) to reduce side effects and increase anticancer actions • Theanine (from green tea) to increase anticancer actions • Sodium bicarbonate to help prevent diarrhea (effectiveness requires dosing throughout the day beginning the first day of chemotherapy for a total of four days)
Nutrients and herbs to avoid	• Avoid herbs during irinotecan therapy because many herbs may interfere with conversion of irinotecan into its active form in the liver. • St. John's wort interferes with irinotecan.

	Methotrexate
Trade name	Amethopterin, Folex, Mexate
Cancers typically treated	Breast, head and neck, bladder, colorectal, blood, bone, lymphoma
How administered	Intravenously (IV), intrathecally (into the spinal column), or orally
Side effects	• Decrease in blood cell counts • Nausea and vomiting • Mouth ulcers • Skin rashes and photosensitivity • Dizziness, headache, or drowsiness • Kidney damage (with a high-dose therapy) • Liver damage • Hair loss (reversible) • Seizures
Helpful nutrients and herbs	• Soy may protect against digestive tract toxicity. • Fish oil may increase anticancer effect. • Vitamin E may increase anticancer effect. • Folic acid (dietary sources only; not to be supplemented unless so advised by a physician) may protect against digestive tract toxicity. • Ginger for nausea.
Nutrients and herbs to avoid	• Kava may increase liver toxicity. • Willow bark may increase toxicity.

Oxaliplatin	
Trade name	Eloxatin
Cancers typically treated	Colon, metastatic rectal
How administered	Intravenously (IV)
Side effects	• Difficulty swallowing • Shortness of breath • Chest pressure • Numbness or tingling in hands and feet • Diarrhea • Mouth sores • Fatigue
Helpful nutrients and herbs	• Glutamine to help prevent nerve damage (numbness and tingling) • Astragalus to reduce toxicity and support anticancer actions • Vitamin E to support anticancer actions and to improve overall tolerance • Calcium and magnesium to decrease nerve toxicity • Alpha-lipoic acid to decrease nerve toxicity
Nutrients and herbs to avoid	• N-acetylcysteine may increase resistance to oxaliplatin. • L-glutathione may increase resistance to oxaliplatin.

Paclitaxel, docetaxel (taxanes)	
Trade name	Paclitaxel: Taxol; docetaxel: Taxotere, Abraxane
Cancers typically treated	Breast, ovarian, lung, head and neck, gastric, bladder
How administered	Intravenously (IV)
Side effects	• Decrease in blood cell counts • Allergic reaction • Nausea and vomiting • Diarrhea • Loss of appetite or change in taste • Thin or brittle hair • Joint pain (short term) • Numbness or tingling in the fingers or toes • Muscle aches and cramps • Fluid retention • Fatigue
Helpful nutrients and herbs	• Vitamin B_6 to help prevent nerve damage. • L-glutamine to help prevent nerve damage. • Melatonin to increase anticancer actions and reduce side effects. • Gamma-linolenic acid (GLA; from evening primrose or currant oil) to increase anticancer actions. • Fish oil to increase anticancer actions. • Panax ginseng may delay or decrease resistance to chemotherapy. • Green tea may increase anticancer actions. • Resveratrol to decrease chemotherapy resistance.
Nutrients and herbs to avoid	• Avoid herbs during paclitaxel therapy because many herbs may interfere with conversion of paclitaxel into its active form in the liver. • Quercetin may interfere with the anticancer activity of taxanes.

Topotecan	
Trade name	Hycamtin
Cancers typically treated	Ovarian, lung
How administered	Intravenously (IV)
Side effects	• Decrease in blood cell counts • Diarrhea • Hair loss (reversible) • Nausea and vomiting • Fatigue
Helpful nutrients and herbs	• Genistein (from soy) may increase anticancer effect; however, soy should be avoided as a supplement in women with ovarian or other estrogen receptor positive cancers. • Quercetin to support anticancer efforts. • Ginger for nausea.
Nutrients and herbs to avoid	None known

	Vinblastine
Trade name	Velban
Cancers typically treated	Lymphoma, testicular, head and neck, breast, kidney
How administered	Intravenously (IV)
Side effects	• Decrease in blood cell counts • Hair loss (reversible) • Loss of appetite • Nausea and vomiting • Constipation or abdominal cramping • Jaw pain • Headache • Numbness or tingling in the fingers or toes
Helpful nutrients and herbs	• Panax ginseng may delay or decrease resistance to chemotherapy. • Vitamin E may delay or decrease resistance to chemotherapy. • Carnosol (from rosemary) may delay or decrease resistance to chemotherapy. • Ginger for nausea.
Nutrients and herbs to avoid	None known

	Vincristine
Trade name	Oncovin, Vincasar PFS
Cancers typically treated	Leukemia, lymphoma, multiple myeloma, sarcoma, thyroid, brain
How administered	Intravenously (IV)
Side effects	• Numbness or tingling in the fingers or toes • Weakness • Loss of reflexes • Jaw pain • Hair loss (reversible) • Constipation or abdominal cramping • Diarrhea • Loss of appetite • Dizziness, weakness
Helpful nutrients and herbs	• Panax ginseng may delay or decrease resistance to chemotherapy. • Vitamin C may decrease resistance to chemotherapy. • Fish oil may increase anticancer effect. • Quercetin to suppress chemotherapy resistance.
Nutrients and herbs to avoid	None known

Radiation and Nutrient and Herb Interactions

Helpful nutrients and herbs	Nutrients and herbs to avoid
Honey to reduce mouth sores	*High-dose supplemented antioxidants* should be avoided during radiation to avoid potential interference with radiation
L-glutamine to reduce mouth sores and diarrhea	*Vitamin E* greater than 200 IU may interfere with radiation
Probiotics to reduce diarrhea	*CoQ10* may interfere with radiation
L-carnitine to reduce fatigue	*N-acetylcysteine* may interfere with radiation
Curcumin (from turmeric) to sensitize tissues to radiation	*Alpha-lipoic acid* may interfere with radiation
Cranberry extract to reduce urinary infections	
Melatonin to support immunity and to improve radiation anticancer effects	
Mushrooms to support immunity and to reduce fatigue during radiation	

Hormone Drugs and Their Nutrient and Herb Interactions

Drug category	Potential side effects	Helpful nutrients and herbs	Nutrients and herbs to avoid
Antiestrogens: • tamoxifen • raloxifene • toremifene	• Hot flashes • Vaginal dryness • Menstrual changes • Weight gain • Uterine cancer • Stroke • Pulmonary embolism • Muscle cramps • Painful intercourse • Increased risk of clots • Liver toxicity	• Avemar (fermented wheat germ extract) may enhance the action of antiestrogens. • Black cohosh may help relieve hot flashes, although the response is variable. Black cohosh does not interfere with antiestrogens. • Vitamin E may relieve antiestrogen-induced hot flashes and help prevent the high lipid levels antiestrogen therapy can cause. • Green tea may reduce liver toxicity caused by antiestrogens, while supporting the cancer prevention and apoptotic actions of tamoxifen. • CoQ10 supports the action of antiestrogens. • Gamma-linolenic acid (GLA) from evening primrose oil enhances the action of antiestrogens. • Riboflavin supports the action of antiestrogens. • Niacin supports the action of antiestrogens. • Omega-3 fatty acids may reduce side effects caused by tamoxifen and may support tissue sensitivity to tamoxifen. • Vitamin D may increase the apoptotic activity of antiestrogens. • Flaxseeds and high-lignan flax oil support the actions of antiestrogens. • Melatonin may increase the benefits of tamoxifen. • Individualized homeopathic remedies may reduce side effects. • Selenium may increase the antiestrogenic effect of tamoxifen. • Intake of CoQ10, riboflavin, and niacin together with tamoxifen normalizes liver function, cholesterol, and lipids, which are otherwise altered with tamoxifen alone.	• Indole-3-carbinol (I3C) may increase the breakdown of tamoxifen, making the tamoxifen less active. • Licorice root has potent estrogenic activities and may stimulate estrogen receptors on breast cancer cells. This makes licorice extract contraindicated during antiestrogen therapy, despite the fact that licorice extracts can be effective treatments for hot flashes and other antiestrogen-induced side effects. • Long-term use of phytoestrogenic herbs such as alfalfa, red clover, black cohosh, and ginkgo should be avoided during antiestrogen therapy.

Drug category	Potential side effects	Helpful nutrients and herbs	Nutrients and herbs to avoid
Aromatase inhibitors: • letrozole • anastrozole • exemestane	• Hot flashes • Menstrual changes • Weight gain • Ovarian tumors • Infertility • Reduced bone density • Fatigue • Dizziness	• Black and green tea polyphenols have aromatase inhibitory activity. • Citrus fruits contain naringenin chalcone, a flavonoid with aromatase inhibitory activity. • Polyphenols from red wine exhibit some aromatase inhibition activities. • Mushrooms and mushroom extracts have aromatase inhibitory activity.	• Soy isoflavones in low doses have aromatase inhibitory activity but in high doses stimulate estrogen receptor positive breast cancer cells. • DHEA is estrogenic and DHEA levels are correlated with disease progression in women taking aromatase inhibitors, suggesting that DHEA supplements are contraindicated for these women.
Luteinizing hormone–releasing hormone (LHRH) agents: • leuprolide • goserelin • triptorelin	• Osteoporosis • Incontinence • Reduced libido • Hot flashes • Mood swings • Nausea	• Black cohosh may be helpful in reducing hot flashes. • Zinc may increase libido.	
Antiandrogens: • bicalutamide • flutamide	• Hot flashes • Weight gain • Constipation • Pain • Irritability • Heart disease • Liver toxicity • Osteoporosis	• Black cohosh may help relieve hot flashes, although the response is variable. Black cohosh does not interfere with antiandrogens. • Omega-3 fatty acids may reduce side effects caused by anti-androgens and may support tissue sensitivity to antiandrogens. • Individualized homeopathic remedies may reduce side effects. • Soy is beneficial for men with prostate cancer taking bicalutamide to reduce drug-induced hot flashes and as an additional cancer preventative.	

Targeted Therapies

The three classes of drugs featured in this chart represent newer drugs that have not been on the market for that long. As a result, natural substances such as nutrients and herbs have not been studied in combination with these drugs. The information featured in the "Nutrient and herb considerations" column is not based on published clinical studies; rather it comes from clinical experience. More research regarding the interactions and benefits of natural substances is required.

Targeted therapy	Cancers treated	Side effects	Nutrient and herb considerations
Monoclonal antibodies:			
Cetuximab (Erbitux)	Head and neck, colorectal	Rash, fatigue, malaise	• Tea tree applied topically may decrease rash
Panitumumab (Vectibix)	Colorectal	Rash, diarrhea, low levels of magnesium and calcium	• Tea tree applied topically may decrease rash • Consider magnesium and calcium supplementation if blood levels are low • Probiotics may reduce diarrhea
Trastuzumab (Herceptin)	Breast, ovarian	Body pain, weakness, nausea	• Gamma-linolenic acid (GLA) may increase anticancer actions • Green tea, especially EGCG, increases anticancer actions and decreases drug resistance
Lapatinib (Tykerb)	Breast	Diarrhea, hand-foot syndrome, anemia, nausea/vomiting, elevated liver enzymes	• Digestive enzymes may reduce diarrhea • Probiotics may reduce diarrhea
Bevacizumab (Avastin)	Colorectal, non-small-cell lung cancer, breast, kidney, ovarian	GI perforation, decreased wound healing, hemorrhage, hypertension, congestive heart failure	• Proanthocyanidin flavonoids may reduce tendency for hemorrhage • Folic acid and B$_{12}$ may increase tolerance
Tyrosine kinase inhibitors:			
Erlotinib (Tarceva)	Non-small-cell lung cancer, pancreatic	Diarrhea, acne, nausea, vomiting, headache, mouth sores	• Caution with herbs due to possible interference with metabolism • Probiotics may reduce diarrhea

Targeted therapy	Cancers treated	Side effects	Nutrient and herb considerations
Tyrosine kinase inhibitors, *continued*			
Imatinib (Gleevec)	Leukemia, Gastrointestinal Stromal Tumor (GIST)	Nausea, vomiting, diarrhea, fluid retention, skin reactions, muscle cramps, headache	• Ginger may reduce nausea • Electrolyte drinks may reduce muscle cramps and headache • Vitamin D (if low) • Vitamin C may interfere with anticancer actions • Probiotics may reduce diarrhea
Sorafenib (Nexavar)	Kidney	Diarrhea, rash, fatigue, hand-foot syndrome, skin reactions, nausea	• Vitamin K may enhance anticancer actions (requires medical supervision) • Probiotics may reduce diarrhea
Sunitinib (Sutent)	Kidney, Gastrointestinal Stromal Tumor (GIST)	Fatigue, nausea/vomiting, abdominal pain, hand-foot syndrome, diminished appetite, skin discoloration, anemia, decreased white blood cells, low thyroid function	• Ginger may relieve nausea • Vitamin B_6 may reduce hand-foot syndrome • Electrolyte drinks may reduce fatigue and nausea
Other:			
Bortezamib (Velcade)	Myeloma, lymphoma	Fatigue, neuropathy, nausea/vomiting, diarrhea, fever, anemia, constipation	• Green tea, especially EGCG, inhibits anticancer action • Flavonoids may inhibit anticancer action • Probiotics may reduce diarrhea

Integrative Cancer Care: Our Rating System

We have developed a detailed alphabetical rating system to help you evaluate specific cancer treatments. Our unique rating system encompasses the quantity and type of evidence as well as safety contraindications and toxicity risks. The best rating is an A, which means that the supplement has excellent scientific evidence backing up its use and it is safe to use. The worst rating is an F, which means that there is a lack of any sound evidence and/or there are serious safety concerns associated with its use. The level of evidence for each supplement increases as you move from in vitro studies to randomized control trials (RCTs), so a supplement that has only been studied in vitro will be rated lower than a supplement with positive RCT evidence, for example. Here is how we ranked the research for each treatment:

Exceptional = a minimum of three RCTs or at least four well-designed smaller trials of ten or more people

Strong = two or fewer RCTs, other human data, pilot studies, epidemiological studies (studies of populations), or phase I human studies (the first phase of studying a treatment in humans)

Moderate = in vivo (animal) trials

Weak = in vitro (test tube) trials

Poor = theoretical or anecdotal (testimonial) evidence only

The four categories for the safety part of the equation are as follows:

Safe = no evidence of toxicity and demonstrated to be safe for human consumption

Limited = unsafe in some cases

Unknown = not enough evidence to conclusively demonstrate safety or toxicity

Unsafe = dangerous and harmful to humans

By combining values for quality of research and safety, we developed the following final rating system:

A = therapies backed up by exceptional scientific studies with a safe or limited safety rating and proven cancer applications

B = therapies supported by strong scientific evidence with a safe or limited safety rating and known cancer applications; or those with exceptional scientific studies but unknown safety

C = therapies with only moderate or weak scientific evidence, a safe or limited safety rating, and known cancer applications; or those with strong scientific evidence and an unknown safety rating

D = therapies with moderate or weak scientific support and a limited or unknown safety rating; or those with poor scientific support, a safe or limited safety rating, and limited cancer applications

F = therapies with poor scientific evidence and unknown safety; or therapies that have been demonstrated to be dangerous or have no cancer applications

Our rating system is a guide, a distillation of the information we have gathered and evaluated. It is one more tool you can use to help you determine what is best in your individual situation. You will notice that the descriptions of our "grades" do not rely on testimonials. Testimonials are stories, not studies, and as such their completeness, accuracy, and relevance can vary dramatically. Just like stories, testimonials can create a sense of hope and inspiration. It is important, however, to balance this emotional appeal with a critical analysis. Is the story complete? Are alternative explanations given? Has the question of potential harm been discussed? How old is the story—what has happened to the author now?

While it's true that individuals can benefit from products or therapies that don't have the strictest scientific validation, it's equally true that you will benefit from incorporating a healthy dose of skepticism in regard to testimonials.

Given the inherent challenges using testimonials as evidence for a therapy, we have excluded these as a way to judge the efficacy and safety of complementary therapies.

Rating system for cancer treatments				
	Exceptional science	Strong science	Moderate science	Weak science	Poor science
Safe	A	B	C	C	D
Limited safety	A	B	C	C	D
Unknown safety	B	C	D	D	F
Unsafe	F	F	F	F	F

Integrative Cancer Care Supplement Guide

This Integrative Cancer Care Supplement Guide should help you make safe and effective choices in your integrated cancer care by giving you an overview of the supplements that have been, or will be, discussed as part of our integrated cancer treatment plan. Some of these supplements are mentioned once in relation to a particular type of cancer; others are mentioned multiple times as part of general prevention as well as for use with specific cancers. This overview will help you learn more about these supplements by providing concise information about the rating the supplement earned (see "Our Rating System" on the facing page to learn more about the criteria we used in the rating process) and what kind of research has been done on its effectiveness: in vitro research represents studies done on cells in the laboratory; in vivo research refers to studies done in organisms, usually animals; epidemiological,

or retrospective, studies are large population studies that have investigated the use of the supplement with regard to the cancer; human trials encompass all trials done on humans, including small phase I studies; and randomized control trials (RCTs) are clinical intervention trials where the supplement is compared to a placebo in a randomized subject group. (For a more detailed review of these terms, refer to the sidebar "Studying the Studies" on pages 112 and 113.)

If you are currently being treated, it is important to know the generic names for your drugs, as this overview uses generic names, not brand names. The "Concerns and comments" column includes additional information important to the safe use of each of these supplements. Finally, this overview is not exhaustive. You should refer to the appendix for dosages or if a supplement you're interested in is not included here.

Natural substance	Specific cancer	Overall rating	In vitro studies	In vivo studies	Epidemiological/retrospective	Human trials	RCTs	Concerns and comments
Active hexose correlated compound (AHCC)	Liver	B	●	●			●	
Aloe vera	Bladder	C	●					
	Brain	B	●			1		One preliminary human study demonstrated that aloe enhanced disease stabilization and survival in glioma patients. Aloe vera may interfere with cisplatin.
Alpha-lipoic acid	Kidney	C	●	●				Reduces oxidative damage and may interfere with radiation to the kidney
	Pancreatic	B	●	●		●		May interefere with radiation. Caution with chemotherapy. caution with drugs that lower blood sugar. Supplement thiamin if taking high doses.
Anthocyanidins (also known as proanthocyanidins)	Breast	C	●					Theoretical possibility of stimulating ER-induced cell proliferation.
	Colon	B	●	●	●			
	Gastric	C	●					
Arabinogalactans	Colon	B	●	●		●		
	Liver	C		●				
	Sarcoma	C		●				
Artemisinin (*Artemisia annua*)	Head & neck	C	●					Artemisinin is not safe the first trimester of pregnancy due to possible toxicity to the fetus.
Ashwagandha (*Withania somnifera*)	Lung	C	●	●				Caution with chemotherapy. May have additive effects with other sedative drugs.
	Breast	C	●					

1 = limited   2 = preventive   3 = with IL-2 therapy   4 = mixed results   5 = theoretical

Natural substance	Specific cancer	Overall rating	In vitro studies	In vivo studies	Epidemiological/retrospective	Human trials	RCTs	Concerns and comments
Astragalus (Astragalus membranaceous)	Bladder	B	•	•	•			Human data exists for prevention only.
	Gastric	B	•	•	•	•		
	Leukemia	B				•		Astralagus improves immune defenses (dendritic cells) when given concurrently with chemotherapy in acute lymphoblastic leukemia.
	Lung	A	•	•	•	•	•	
Beta-glucans	General	A	•	•	•	•	•	
Black cohosh (Actea racemosa)	Breast	B		•				
Bromelain (enzyme therapy)	General	C	•	•	•			Caution with anticoagulant medications. Caution with gastrointestinal ulceration.
Carnosol	Melanoma	C	•					
Coenzyme Q10	Breast	B	•	•	•	•		May interfere with some chemotherapy drugs.
	Cervical	B	•		•			
	Melanoma	B	•	•	•			
	Thyroid	C	•		1			
	Ovarian	C			•			Only one human study, which included CoQ10 along with other antioxidants. May interfere with some chemotherapy drugs.
	Prostate	B	•		•			May interfere with some chemotherapy drugs.

1 = limited   2 = preventive   3 = with IL-2 therapy   4 = mixed results   5 = theoretical

Natural substance	Specific cancer	Overall rating	In vitro studies	In vivo studies	Epidemiological/retrospective	Human trials	RCTs	Concerns and comments
Curcumin	Bladder	B	●	●		●		
	Brain	C	●					
	Breast	C	●	●				
	Cervical	B	●	●	●	●		
	Colon	B	●	●		●		
	Leukemia	C	●	●				Not to be taken with cyclophosphamide, anastrozole, exemestane, letrozole, or erlotinib, or therapeutic doses (usually greater than 1 mg daily) of warfarin.
	Lung	C	●					
	Melanoma	C	●	●				
	Ovarian	C	●	●				
	Pancreatic	B	●	●		●		
	Prostate	C	●	●				
	Skin (not melanoma)	C	●	●				
	Stomach	B	●	●		●		
DIM (diindolylmethane)	Breast	B	●	●		1		
Ellagic acid	General	B	●	●			●	
Fermented soy products	Multiple	C	●	●	●			Caution in ER+ cancers
Fermented wheat germ (Avemar)	Breast	C	●	●				
	Lung	B		●		●		
	Melanoma	B					●	
	Multiple; colorectal	B	●	●	●	●		
Flavonoids	Cervical	C	●					
	Colorectal	B					●	
	Prostate	C	●	●				

1 = limited   2 = preventive   3 = with IL-2 therapy   4 = mixed results   5 = theoretical

Natural substance	Specific cancer	Overall rating	In vitro studies	In vivo studies	Epidemiological/retrospective	Human trials	RCTs	Concerns and comments
Flaxseed lignans (enterolactone)	Breast	B	•	•	•	•	•	
	Colon	B	•	•	•			
	Prostate	B	•	•	•	•		
Folic acid	Cervical	A[2]	•	•	•	•	•	Studies link folic acid with treatment of dysplasia (a precancerous condition). Trials show mixed results and suggest that a subgroup of women with dysplasia respond to folate therapy.
	Colon	A	•	•	•	•	•	Supplementation may mask vitamin B_{12} deficiency. High doses may be contraindicated with certain chemotherapy drugs.
Gamma oryzanol	General	C	•	•				
Garlic	Colon	B	•	•	•	•		Obtain medical supervision and monitoring when also taking anticoagulant medications. May interfere with some chemotherapy drugs. May interfere with hormonal drugs.
	Gastric	B	•	•	•	•		
Genistein	Bone	C	•	•				
	Lymphoma	B	•	•		•		Caution with ER+ cancers.
	Pancreatic	C	•	•				
	Prostate	A	•	•	•	•	•	
	Uterine	D	•	•				Conflicting reports; one animal study showing benefit.
Ginger	Bladder	C		•				
	Liver	C	•	•				
Ginkgo biloba	Gastric	B	•	•		•		Not to be taken with chemotherapy. Avoid prior to surgery because it can act as a blood thinner. Caution with ER+ cancers.
	Ovarian	C			•			

1 = limited   2 = preventive   3 = with IL-2 therapy   4 = mixed results   5 = theoretical

Natural substance	Specific cancer	Overall rating	In vitro studies	In vivo studies	Epidemiological/retrospective	Human trials	RCTs	Concerns and comments
Ginsenosides (in *Panax ginseng*)	Brain	C	•	•				May interfere with some chemotherapy drugs. Caution with ER+ cancers.
	Gastric	B	•	•	•	•	•	
	Kidney	C	•	•				
	Liver	B	•	•		•		
	Melanoma	C	•	•				
Goji (*Lycium barbarum*)	General	B	•	•		•		
Green tea (*Camellia sinensis*)	Bladder	B	•	•	•	•		
	Brain	C	•					
	Breast	B	•	•	•	•		
	Colon	B	•	•	•			
	Gastric	B	•		•	•		
	Head & neck	C	•	•		•		
	Kidney	C	•	•				
	Liver	C	•	•		•		
	Lung	B	•	•	•	•		
	Lymphoma	C	•					
	Melanoma	C	•	•				
	Ovarian	B	•	•	•			
	Pancreatic	B	•	•	•			
	Prostate	A	•	•	•	•	•	
	Sarcoma	C		•				Rhabdomyosarcoma

1 = limited   2 = preventive   3 = with IL-2 therapy   4 = mixed results   5 = theoretical

Natural substance	Specific cancer	Overall rating	In vitro studies	In vivo studies	Epidemiological/retrospective	Human trials	RCTs	Concerns and comments
Honey	Head & neck	A					●	Randomized trials have demonstrated a reduction in mouth sores during radiation therapy.
Indole-3-carbinol	Breast	B	●	●	●	1		Not to be taken with tamoxifen; best used as a preventative; may have harmful estrogenic effects; consider DIM (diindolylmethane) as an alternative.
	Colon	C	●					
Inositol hexaphosphate (IP6)	General	C	●	●				
Iodine	Breast	C	●					
L-carnitine	Leukemia	C	●					
L-glutamine	Breast	A	●	●		●	●	
	Esophageal	B					●	
	Colon	A				●	●	
	Sarcoma	C		●				Rhabdomyosarcoma
Limonene	Liver	C	●	●				
	Pancreatic	C	●	●				
Lutein	Leukemia	C		●				
Lycopene	Gastric	B	●	●	●	●		
	Head & neck	C	●					
	Prostate	A	●	●	●	●	●	

1 = limited   2 = preventive   3 = with IL-2 therapy   4 = mixed results   5 = theoretical

Natural substance	Specific cancer	Overall rating	In vitro studies	In vivo studies	Epidemiological/retrospective	Human trials	RCTs	Concerns and comments
Melatonin	Brain	B	•	•			•	May cause sedation and drowsiness. Avoid in bipolar disorder. Not to be taken with high-dose IL-2.
	Breast	A	•	•	•	•	•	
	Colon	A	•	•	•	•	•	
	Kidney	B	•	•	•	•		
	Lung	A	•	•	•	•	•	
	Lymphomas	B	•	•	•	•		
	Melanoma	A	•	•	•	•	•	
	Ovarian	B	•	•	•	•		
	Pancreatic	C		•				
	Prostate	B	•	•	•			
	Sarcoma	C		•				Leiomyosarcoma
	Thyroid	B	•		•	3		
	Uterine	B	•	•	•	•		
Mistletoe *(Viscum alba)*	Bladder	B	•	•		•		Use must be supervised by a licensed health-care practitioner.
	Breast	B	•	•		•		
	Colon	B				•		
	Leukemia	C	•	•				
	Lymphoma	B	•	•		4		
	Melanoma	B	•	•		•	•	
	Myeloma	C	•					
	Pancreatic	B	•	•		•		
Modified citrus pectin	Melanoma	C	•	•				
	Prostate	B	•	•		•		

1 = limited   2 = preventive   3 = with IL-2 therapy   4 = mixed results   5 = theoretical

Natural substance	Specific cancer	Overall rating	In vitro studies	In vivo studies	Epidemiological/retrospective	Human trials	RCTs	Concerns and comments
Mushroom polysaccharides	Breast	A				•	•	PSK, an extract from the *Coriolus versicolor* mushroom, is the subject of study in the trials of women with breast cancer.
	Colon	A	•	•	•	•	•	
	Gastric	A	•	•	•	•	•	
	Liver	B	•	•		•		
	Uterine	B	•	•		•		
N-acetylcysteine	Sarcoma	C	•	•				Kaposi's sarcoma.
Omega-3 fatty acids	Breast	B	•	•	•	•		
	Colon	A	•	•	•	•	•	Studies demonstrate prevention effects.
	Esopha-geal	B				•		A human trial demonstrated preservation of lean body mass after esophageal cancer surgery.
	Lung	B	•	•	•			
	Pancreatic	B			•	•		
	Prostate	A	•	•	•	•		
Pau d'arco	General	C	•	•				
Pomegranate	Prostate	B	•	•		•		
Probiotics	Bladder	A				•	•	Probiotics should not be taken when white blood cell counts are below normal, to avoid potential infection.
	Breast	D				5		
	Colon	B					•	
	Gastric	C	•					
Pycnogenol (pine bark extract)	Liver	C		•				

1 = limited   2 = preventive   3 = with IL-2 therapy   4 = mixed results   5 = theoretical

Natural substance	Specific cancer	Overall rating	In vitro studies	In vivo studies	Epidemiological/retrospective	Human trials	RCTs	Concerns and comments
Quercetin	Colon	C	•	•				Not to be taken with taxanes, dacarbazine, tamoxifen, anastrozole, exemestane, letrozole, or erlotinib
	Leukemia	C	•	•				
	Melanoma	C	•	•				
	Ovarian	B	•	•		•		
	Prostate	C	•					
	Sarcoma	C	•					Liposarcoma
	Thyroid	C	•					
Resveratrol	Colon	C	•	•				
	Leukemia	C	•	•				
	Skin (not melanoma)	C	•	•				
	Thyroid	C	•					
	Uterine	C	•	•				
Selenium	Bone	C	•	•	•			Caution in individuals with significant liver and kidney insufficiency
	Gastric	A	•	•	•	•	•	
	Liver	A	•	•	•	•	•	
	Lung	A	•	•	•	•	•	
	Pancreatic	B	•	•	•			
Shark cartilage (Neovastat liquid extract)	Kidney	A				•		
	Lung	B				•		
Silymarin (from milk thistle, *Silymarin officinalis*)	Liver	C	•	•				May interfere with some chemotherapy drugs.
	Lung	C	•	•				
	Prostate	C	•	•				
	Skin	C	•	•				
St. John's wort	Bladder	C	•					May interfere with other medications and chemotherapy drugs. Photosensitizing effects.

Natural substance	Specific cancer	Overall rating	In vitro studies	In vivo studies	Epidemiological/retrospective	Human trials	RCTs	Concerns and comments
Vitamin A	Bladder	A	●	●	●	●		Caution with liver disease. Caution with radiation therapy.
	Cervical	B	●	●		●		
	Kidney	B	●	●		●		
	Ovarian	A	●	●	●	●		
	Sarcoma	C	●					Rhabdomyosarcoma.
	Skin (not melanoma)	A	●	●	●	●		
	Thyroid	A	●	●	●	●		
Vitamin B$_6$	Bladder	B	●	●	●	●		Conflicting human trial data
Vitamin C	Bladder	B	●	●	●			Studied with vitamin E and zinc. Caution in individuals with a history of kidney stones.
	Bone	C	●	●	●			
	Breast	B	●	●	●	●		
	Cervical	B	●	●	●		3	
	Colon	B	●	●	●	●		Trial evidence is for prevention.
	Liver	C	●	●				
	Lung	B	●	●	●	●	●	Trial evidence for prevention and complementary therapy; one RCT did not show benefit.
	Ovarian	B	●	●		●		
	Skin (not melanoma)	B	●	●		●		Trial evidence is for prevention.
Vitamin D (continues on next page)	Breast	B	●	●	●			Use under medical supervision if parathyroid disease is present. Use of high doses for more than 2 months should be under the guidance of a licensed health-care professional.

1 = limited   2 = preventive   3 = with IL-2 therapy   4 = mixed results   5 = theoretical

Natural substance	Specific cancer	Overall rating	In vitro studies	In vivo studies	Epidemiological/retrospective	Human trials	RCTs	Concerns and comments
Vitamin D (continued)	Colon	A	•	•	•	•	•	Trials done with calcium. Use under medical supervision if parathyroid disease is present. Use of high doses for more than two months should be under the guidance of a licensed health-care professional.
	Kidney	C	•	•				Use under medical supervision if parathyroid disease is present. Use of high doses for more than two months should be under the guidance of a licensed health-care professional.
	Lung	B				•		
	Melanoma	C	•	•	•			
	Ovarian	B	•	•	•			
	Prostate	A	•	•	•	•	•	Calcitriol used in majority of clinical studies. Use under medical supervision if parathyroid disease is present. Use of high doses for more than two months should be under the guidance of a licensed health-care professional.
Vitamin E	Breast	C	•	•	•			Caution with anticoagulant medications. May interfere with radiation therapy.
	Cervical	C	•	•	•			
	Colon	B	•	•	•	•		A human trial demonstrated an increase in NK cell activity in patients with advanced colorectal cancer.
	Esopha-geal	B			•			A human trial showed a protective effect of vitamin E in the development of esophageal cancer.
	Kidney	C	•					
	Liver	B	•	•		•	•	
	Ovarian	B	•	•		•		
	Thyroid	C	•		•			
Zinc	Kidney	C	•	•	•			
	Prostate	B	•	•		•		

1 = limited   2 = preventive   3 = with IL-2 therapy   4 = mixed results   5 = theoretical

Questionable Alternative Cancer Cures

The fear that comes with a diagnosis of cancer can motivate people to try anything. This, coupled with the daunting prospect of undergoing relatively toxic conventional treatments that don't always work, may leave a person susceptible to the promises and claims of treatments with "a good story." And there is no shortage of such stories of miracle cures and lifesaving treatment regimens based on pseudoscientific explanations and claims of discovering the missing link in cancer treatment. Some of these stories are designed to prey upon the legitimate feelings of fear and hope that people fighting cancer naturally experience.

Because there are so many cancer treatments available—both conventional and alternative—it would be impossible to feature all of them in this book. Plus, cancer prevention and treatment is an ever-changing field. Progress is ongoing, and you should remain alert to new and legitimate advancements. Unfortunately, bogus cures also surface and resurface regularly. If you're considering therapies we don't address, see the sidebar "Top 10 Tips for Evaluating Medical Information on the Web" on page 111 to help you analyze information—especially information on the Internet. Asking the right questions will help you distinguish fact from fiction.

Following are descriptions of some currently popular products or treatments that we feel are questionable. They are not listed in the "Integrative Cancer Care Supplement Guide" due to safety issues, and all of them rate a "D" or "F" using our system.

714-X: Rating = F

The formula for 714-X includes camphor, nitrogen, ammonium salts, sodium chloride, and ethanol. It is typically given via injection into a lymph node. Proponents believe tiny living particles called somatids circulate in the bloodstream. Disease is diagnosed and monitored by noting the number and form of somatids in the blood. By interfering with the flow of these somatids, 714-X is believed to stimulate a positive immune response and cause cancer to regress. It is also believed that the nitrogen can help strip tumor cells, making them more vulnerable to the immune system response. No evidence exists to support these claims, and 714-X is not an approved cancer treatment in the United States. Canada allows its use by prescription only under the Emergency Drug Release Program of Health Canada. No scientific evidence exists supporting the concept of somatids in the blood, and there have been no clinical studies demonstrating the effectiveness of 714-X.

Cancell/Entelev/Cantron: Rating = F

Created in the 1950s, Entelev was believed to balance the vibrational frequency of cancer cells to return them to their normal state and thus be recognized by the immune system. Now sold under a variety of brand names, this product contains a variety of ingredients, typically including nitric acid, sodium sulfite, potassium hydroxide, sulfuric acid, inositol, minerals, vitamins, and possibly others. There are no published animal or human studies to substantiate the claims associated with this product. While the manufacturers claim many studies have been conducted, none of them have been published in peer-reviewed professional journals. On two different occasions the National Cancer Institute evaluated Cancell/Entelev. Both studies demonstrated no positive effect and were not published. It is highly unlikely that this product has any significant anticancer effect. The manufacturers discourage the use of this product along with conventional treatments, which could be dangerous because it could lead people to avoid or delay receiving potentially helpful conventional treatments.

Cancer Salves: Rating = F

Cancer salves are commonly referred to as black salve. Purveyors of these products claim the salve can cure any type of cancer by killing the cells topically or drawing the cancer out of the body. This theory is entirely lacking in scientific merit. In fact, these products may harm you. There have been reports of scarring and burns associated with cancer salves, which have varied ingredients but usually consist of herbs such as sanguinaria (bloodroot) and the chemical dimethyl sulfoxide (DMSO). There are also many cases of ulceration associated with the use of black salve. These ulcerations are the result of tumor growth that is so substantial that the tumor grows through the skin. To date, there have been no scientific studies done to confirm the effectiveness of any of the cancer salves currently on the market. Recently, some websites have advocated oral ingestion of black salve, which could be quite dangerous.

Carnivora: Rating = D

Carnivora is the trade name for a product made from the liquid extract of the Venus flytrap plant (*Dionaea muscipula*). Proponents assert that Carnivora can cure skin cancer and other cancers, as well as a host of other illnesses, through oral administration, injections, vaporized inhalation, or direct application to lesions. There is currently no scientific evidence, however, to support these claims. Carnivora is not approved by the FDA and doctors cannot prescribe it. Possible side effects include vomiting, nausea, skin irritations, and allergies.

Cesium Chloride: Rating = F

Radioactive cesium chloride (cesium-137) is used in conventional cancer treatment. Nonradioactive cesium chloride is available as a dietary supplement for use in high pH therapy. Cesium chloride is the salt form of cesium, a naturally occurring metal with a similar structure to lithium, potassium, and sodium. Cesium chloride became popular when it was observed that populations in certain regions with high concentrations of alkali metals in the soil had low rates of cancer. However, there is no scientific documentation of a direct link between dietary cesium and the prevention or treatment of cancer. According to the American Cancer Society's *Complementary and Alternative Cancer Methods Handbook*, "The acute and chronic toxicity of this substance is not fully known. Relying on this type of treatment alone, and avoiding conventional medical care, may have serious health consequences." Nausea and diarrhea are common side effects of cesium chloride consumption. One study performed by the Mayo Clinic found rapid heart rates in patients who had independently chosen to take cesium chloride in combination with other treatments for brain cancer. Cesium can also cause decreases in potassium levels, which can be dangerous for people with dehydration or heart conditions.

Chaparral: Rating = F

According to the American Cancer Society and the Food and Drug Administration (FDA), use of chaparral is dangerous and may cause irreversible, life-threatening liver damage. Claims that chaparral can treat cancer have not been substantiated in any human clinical trials, and other research on its effectiveness is limited. Chaparral should be avoided as an alternative cancer treatment.

Coffee Enemas: Rating = D

Coffee enemas are considered a part of colon hydrotherapy (described below). They are typically a component of an overall regimen that includes a special diet, dietary supplements, and other therapies. Coffee enemas stimulate liver function, emptying of the gallbladder, and overall detoxification. As tumors break down, toxic debris is produced, which is processed in the liver. It is believed that coffee enemas help support the detoxification of this debris. However, there is very little scientific documentation to support this claim. If used in excess, coffee enemas can cause electrolyte imbalance, dehydration, colitis, constipation, and even death. Coffee enemas are not approved as a cancer treatment.

Colon Hydrotherapy: Rating = D

Colon hydrotherapy is an ancient healing method of using water or other liquid substances to irrigate the colon and, in the process, stimulate peristaltic contractions and elimination. This practice may be of benefit to a patient with cancer for the relief of constipation, as a method of hydrating the body, or as a way to stimulate the release of water-soluble toxic waste compounds via the bowels. However, there are no direct anticancer actions from colon hydrotherapy. Colon hydrotherapy can be problematic for a person who is significantly depleted or who has diarrhea.

Coral Calcium: Rating = F

Makers of coral calcium products claim that it will alkalinize cells, and that alkalinization increases their capacity to absorb oxygen. Based upon a faulty interpretation of Otto Warburg's 1932 statement that cancerous tissue cannot survive in aerobic conditions, the theory behind coral calcium states that if oxygen content is increased, an aerobic intracellular environment will develop, which in turn will kill cancer cells. There is no scientific validity to this theory, and there are no studies demonstrating the effectiveness of coral calcium as an anticancer agent. In 2004, the Federal Trade Commission (FTC) took legal action against the makers of coral calcium products because they were making unsubstantiated claims, including that their products could cure cancer, multiple sclerosis, lupus, heart disease, and chronic high blood pressure. The FTC won that battle, and the manufacturer was directed to remove products from the market that featured those unsubstantiated claims. The National Center for Complementary and Alternative Medicine warns that the "claims [for coral calcium supplements] go far beyond the existing scientific evidence regarding the recognized health benefits of calcium." In fact, the calcium content of these products is composed primarily of calcium carbonate—the same form of calcium that is present in most inexpensive calcium supplements and over-the-counter calcium medications. In addition, an independent assay of coral calcium products revealed the presence of dangerous heavy metals, which are known carcinogens. Coral calcium is not recommended as a cancer treatment.

Exotic Fruit Juices and Extracts: Rating = D

Noni juice and mangosteen juice are examples of exotic tropical fruit juices that are being marketed by some sellers as natural cancer treatments. The theory is that the concentrated flavonoids in these exotic fruits can stimulate immunity and help kill cancer cells. While the manufacturers of most exotic fruit drinks make no claims as to any specific healing powers, advocates say that drinking it has led to miraculous recoveries from a variety of cancers. Mangosteen juice is claimed to have high concentrations of antioxidants, and in vitro studies do suggest that it may have anticancer properties. However, no human or animal studies have supported the effectiveness of mangosteen or noni juice as cancer treatments. Our low rating of exotic fruits and their extracts doesn't reflect a low opinion of the category of flavonoids. While more research is needed, a growing body of evidence indicates that specific

isolated flavonoids, such as quercetin, delphinidin, and anthocyanidins, do have anticancer and immune-stimulating properties. The problem with these branded fruit juices and extracts is that the exact amount and type of flavonoids they contain are unknown and unstandardized. Noni does contain potassium in amounts similar to orange juice and tomato juice, and while potassium is an essential mineral that's beneficial in most cases, there is a case report of hyperkalemia (excessive amounts of potassium in the blood) in a person with chronic renal insufficiency who was consuming noni juice daily. Because cancer patients are susceptible to electrolyte imbalances, the daily use of these extracts with concentrated electrolytes should be done with caution so as not to aggravate these imbalances.

Graviola: Rating = F

The leaves and stems of the graviola tree (also known as the pawpaw or soursop) are known to be toxic to cancer cells. Proponents claim that graviola, when taken as a supplement, is useful in reducing the body's resistance to chemotherapy. In moderate doses graviola is not known to induce side effects. As with many popular alternative treatments for cancer, however, claims of its effectiveness are extravagant and probably exaggerated. There are no human or animal clinical trials demonstrating its effectiveness in treating cancer in human or animal subjects. Additionally, there is concern that healthy cells may be more susceptible to the killing effects of graviola than cancerous cells, so this supplement could cause widespread tissue dysfunction, including immune suppression.

Hydrazine Sulfate: Rating = F

Commonly used in industrial processes, hydrazine sulfate also occurs naturally in tobacco plants and mushrooms. It is primarily used in advanced cancers to help relieve cachexia (a wasting syndrome marked by muscle atrophy). Hydrazine sulfate is believed to shut off the energy supply to tumors by disrupting their ability to obtain sugar. Although research results have been mixed, a report on the American Cancer Society website says that "most carefully designed studies have shown it does not help people with cancer live longer or feel better. It can also cause potentially serious side effects." There has also been a reported case of fatal liver and kidney failure associated with hydrazine sulfate. This chemical is not an approved cancer treatment in the United States; however, it is available by prescription in Canada and is widely used in Europe.

Hydrogen Peroxide: Rating = F

Most of us are familiar with the use of hydrogen peroxide to clean and disinfect wounds. In this application, a fairly dilute form is used. Hydrogen peroxide in higher concentrations is being used to treat cancer. It can be taken orally, injected, or used to soak specific body parts. However, medical researchers have been studying hydrogen peroxide for more than a century and have found no scientific evidence that it can effectively treat cancer. In fact, highly concentrated hydrogen peroxide can be harmful if swallowed. It is considered to be toxic at concentrations higher than 10 percent. When taken orally, hydrogen peroxide at concentrations higher than 35 percent can cause vomiting and burn the throat and stomach. Injection is even more dangerous: "High blood levels of hydrogen peroxide create oxygen bubbles that can block blood flow and cause gangrene and death," according to the American Cancer Society website.

Laetrile: Rating = F

Also known as amygdalin or vitamin B_{17}, laetrile is made from naturally occurring chemicals found in almonds and the kernel inside the pits of apricots and peaches. It also contains small amounts of cyanide, which is poisonous in amounts above the quantity found naturally in the occasional apple seed or other fruit kernel. Some proponents believe the cyanide component is what kills cancer cells. Laetrile is typically delivered intravenously along with high doses of other vitamins. It can also be used orally as apricot kernels, extracted for use in an enema, or in solutions applied topically. Due to the popularity of laetrile, the National Cancer Institute performed its own studies to evaluate its effectiveness. They found no scientific evidence indicating effectiveness as an anticancer treatment. A recent review of the Cochrane Central Register of Controlled Trials led researchers to conclude, "The claim that laetrile has beneficial effects for cancer patients is not supported by data from controlled clinical trials." Laetrile ingested in the form of apricot kernels or administered intravenously can be linked to cyanide toxicity in susceptible individuals. Cyanide toxicity can cause severe heart rate disturbances, breathing problems, and coma. While there are antidotes to these side effects, treatment usually requires intensive care hospitalization. Taking laetrile along with conventional treatment can increase the potential for cyanide poisoning. Laetrile treatment is illegal in the United States.

Poly-MVA: Rating = D

Developed by Merrill Garnett, DDS, PhD, Poly-MVA is a proprietary complex of palladium, alpha-lipoic acid, vitamins B_1, B_2, and B_{12}, and specific trace minerals and amino acids. Sold as a dietary supplement, its manufacturers claim that it demonstrates antitumor properties and that it raises energy levels by changing the electrical potential of human cells and increasing the charge density of DNA within the cell. Many claims also suggest that Poly-MVA is an effective treatment—and even a cure—for advanced cancer. However, there is no research confirming the underlying basis of Poly-MVA treatment. Additionally, no objective clinical studies exist that support Poly-MVA's effectiveness in either preventing or treating cancer. Potential side effects are unknown. Unpublished clinical observations have indicated that the palladium component may increase side effects of radiation therapy.

Part III

Key Body Functions

eight

Immune System

The immune system is often compared to an army—soldier cells fighting battles against invading microorganisms. The immune system is the body's first and last line of defense. The organs and cells of the immune system are on the front line, protecting us and fighting off microscopic enemy invaders, such as bacteria, viruses, toxins, fungi, and parasites, and defending us against traitors from within, including cancer.

"Coated with protein and sugar, the human body is a feast to microscopic life—and the only thing standing between 'us' and 'them' is the immune system," explain Robert Rountree, MD, and Carol Colman in their book *Immunotics*. "It allows us personal space on a planet teeming with hungry microorganisms."

Foreign antigens are microorganisms tagged by the immune system as "nonself." The initial scouts of the immune army, macrophages and dendritic cells, identify the antigens and send a message back to the rest of the immune system in order to create an organized defense. The identification of a foreign antigen launches the immune system into a flurry of activity. As the immune army springs into action, it sends out specialized troops to identify, kill, and clean up foreign invaders. Two major lymphocytes—B cells and T cells—carry out the bulk of the activity during this second phase. T cells, which mature in the thymus gland, have clusters of proteins on their surfaces that differentiate them into various groups.

One large group is CD4 T cells, which secrete cytokines (immune-regulating molecules) that stimulate the rest of the immune system into action. CD8 T cells, also known as cytotoxic T cells, are another important group of T cells. These cells directly kill viruses and cancer cells and secrete gamma interferon, which stimulates activity of macrophages and other immune cells. The immune system has the capacity to continually create and train new T cells, so more T cell troops can always be sent to the war zone depending on the size of the battle. There are even T cells that store information about antigens just in case the body encounters them again. This cellular memory allows for a faster response the next time the immune system encounters that antigen, and this function is especially impressive in regard to allergic responses.

B cells, which grow and mature in bone marrow, also respond to T cell signals. The job of B cells is to produce antibodies matched to specific antigens for the purpose of identifying invaders and marking them so they'll be easy targets for the rest of the immune cell army. Once foreign cells and organisms are marked for destruction, cells known as phagocytes—specifically, neutrophils and macrophages—are sent out to engulf and digest the antigens.

Natural killer cells (NK cells) are another important type of immune cell. They destroy cancerous cells and cells that are infected with viruses by releasing toxic substances directly into these cells. The NK cells are an elite squad of cells that can effectively recognize cancerous and infected cells and destroy them immediately.

B cells and T cells circulate within the lymphatic system. Lymph fluid bathes the body, transferring nutrients to cells, removing waste products, and transporting vital white blood cells to specific battlegrounds. Immune system cells congregate in various lymph nodes strategically positioned throughout the body. The spleen, located in the upper left part of the abdomen, is one of the central command centers for the immune response. The spleen manufactures lymphocytes and traps foreign antigens in order to initiate the B cell response. The spleen also filters the blood and lymphatic system of cell debris, microorganisms, and old or damaged cells. The immune system army fights on your behalf day in and day out, winning battles both small and large on a regular basis.

While this all sounds straightforward enough, there is still a great deal we do not know about the immune system. In fact, much of what is known today about immunity and how to enhance it has only surfaced within the past few decades, and the pace of new research and advances is accelerating. While it may not be possible to unlock all of the mysteries of the immune system and understand how to maximize its potential, we are certainly making progress. We are also learning more about tumor biology and the immune system's role in the prevention and treatment of cancer.

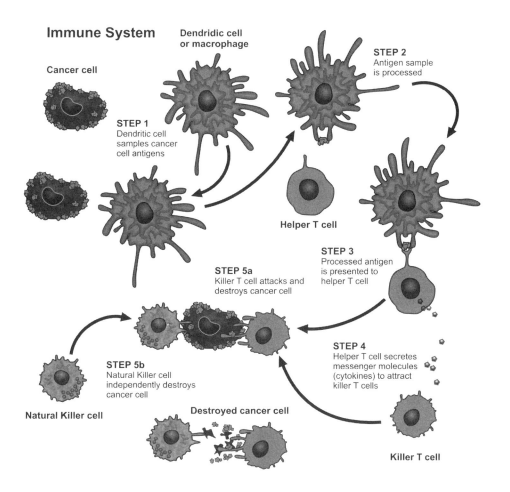

Immune System

Cancer cell

Dendridic cell
or macrophage

STEP 2
Antigen sample
is processed

STEP 1
Dendritic cell
samples cancer
cell antigens

Helper T cell

STEP 3
Processed antigen
is presented to
helper T cell

STEP 5a
Killer T cell attacks and
destroys cancer cell

STEP 5b
Natural Killer cell
independently destroys
cancer cell

STEP 4
Helper T cell secretes
messenger molecules
(cytokines) to attract
killer T cells

Natural Killer cell

Destroyed cancer cell

Killer T cell

Cancer and the Immune System

A healthy immune system can quickly and easily identify foreign cells. In the case of cancer, a cell that is dividing abnormally and showing other unnatural signs can be identified and tagged just like a genuinely foreign cell. Theoretically, a healthy immune system can destroy cancerous cells before they get a chance to multiply and become dangerous. We all have cancer cells circulating in our bodies all the time, and yet not everyone develops cancer. When cancer does not develop, it is because the cancer cells are disorganized, uncoordinated, and spread out, making them easily defeated by a strong, organized, well-fed, and well-rested immune army. Sometimes, however, the cancer is stronger and more organized than the immune system and can evade the immune response.

Not that long ago, cancer was thought to be simply an immune deficiency. If a person got cancer, it was believed to be caused by a weakened immune system that allowed the cancer to develop and spread. While decreased immunity is certainly a contributing factor, we now know that cancer is not merely the result of immune deficiency. In fact, a fast-growing cancer can coexist with a strong immune system. As cancerous tumors grow, they can develop features that camouflage them from the immune system's surveillance. Cancer can also scramble the messages between immune cells and even send out its own messages in the form of cytokines that confuse the immune system and prevent it from responding effectively. However, despite these cunning tactics, the influence and the power that a healthy immune system has on cancer cannot be underestimated.

As cancer grows, its evasion tactics become even stronger and more challenging for the diligent immune system. In this scenario, big weapons are called for. Chemotherapy can be likened to a large bomb that is lobbed into enemy territory. The bomb destroys the majority of the enemy, but it is unlikely to destroy every cancer cell. The foot soldiers of the immune system must be healthy and strong enough to swarm in and kill any last cancer cell that remains. Just as with all bombs, sometimes our own soldiers can become wounded. When this happens, more immune system foot soldiers must be mobilized from the lymph nodes, and more must be created in the bone marrow. This is why it is so important to focus on immune system health before, during, and after conventional treatment.

As mentioned previously, the immune system features many powerful players: T cells, B cells, neutrophils, macrophages, natural killer cells, and others work together to keep us healthy. T cells and natural killer cells are significant when it comes to both prevention and treatment of cancer. Natural killer (NK) cells are especially important in preventing damaged cells from continuing to divide and grow into cancer cells. "The average cell suffers 10,000 free radical assaults per day," explains Mitchell Gaynor, MD, in his book *Dr. Gaynor's Cancer Prevention Program*. "Good antioxidant protection saves most of the cells from serious damage." However, cells that sustain serious damage can become malignant and replicate into cancerous tumors. These seriously damaged cells are typically hunted down and destroyed by NK cells, thus averting the development of cancer (see the illustration on page 181).

Unfortunately, cellular damage caused by free radicals is constant and can overwhelm NK cells. Free radicals are in the air we breathe, the water we drink, and the foods we eat. They are also generated through exercise, converting food to energy, or battling an infection. These reactive molecules can damage cells through oxidation, a destructive process similar to the way oxygen can cause an apple to turn brown once it's cut. When the antioxidative system is depleted and the immune system is deficient, the body can't counter the cellular damage, tissue destruction, and tumor growth initiated by free radicals. This is why antioxidant foods and dietary supplements are so critical: additional antioxidants quench free radicals, averting cellular damage. As we discussed in chapter 4, antioxidants are present in many healthy foods such as fruits and vegetables. Popular antioxidant supplements include vitamins C and E, as well as selenium and zinc. Garlic, green tea, and curcumin are examples of herbs with antioxidant properties.

If antioxidants fail to adequately quench free radicals, these free radicals will cause cellular damage. And if these damaged cells are not targeted and destroyed by NK cells, they will replicate and can develop into cancerous tumors. Once a cancerous tumor has formed, other cells in the immune system become critical components of our defense. T cells carry out a variety of vital tasks. Different groups of T cells are trained to attack specific antigens. Damaged, or malignant, cells have antigenic proteins that T cells recognize on their cell surfaces. Upon recognition, the T cells initiate cellular destruction. In addition, T cells ensure that the entire immune system is operating at peak capacity. They are important in orchestrating the immune response and executing immune system strategies.

When T cell function is suboptimum, the body's ability to fight cancer is jeopardized. Several studies have demonstrated that cancer patients who have low numbers or low activity of T cells will not fare as well as those who have high T cell counts. Researchers at the University of Pennsylvania in Philadelphia found a direct link between poor survival and low T cell counts in women with advanced ovarian cancer. Women whose T cells were able to penetrate the tumors were 38 percent more likely to live for five years or longer, while those patients whose tumors did not contain T cells only had a 4.5 percent chance of living five years. Scientists believe that T cell infiltration of tumors enhances conventional treatment (chemotherapy and radiation) and improves the person's prognosis. (Research into T cell function may eventually play a role in the development of immune-boosting vaccines to enhance a patient's T cell response.)

Regulatory T cells (also known as suppressor T cells) are a specialized subpopulation of T cells that act to suppress activation of the immune system and thereby maintain immune system balance and tolerance of self. Body tissues secrete chemicals that stimulate regulatory T cells so that the immune system does not attack the body's own tissues. Cancerous tumors secrete enormous amounts of chemicals that stimulate regulatory T cells. This essentially shuts down the immune response at the site of the tumor. Cancerous tumors are therefore very effective at immobilizing the immune system's reaction to the tumor.

"Therapeutically targeting regulatory T cells is a direct and powerful means to manipulate the immune system to achieve beneficial effects on various disease pathologies, including allergy, autoimmunity, and cancer," according to a research paper featured in *Evidence-Based Complementary and Alternative Medicine*. "This powerful target for immunoregulation is of much concern to practitioners and researchers of complementary and alternative medicine because it allows a great deal of control and certainty in dealing with the prevalence of debilitating immune system–related disorders." Developing ways to inactivate regulatory T cells with immunologically based conventional and integrative techniques will play an important role in the continued fight against cancer.

Phagocytes are a category of cells that engulf and consume foreign invaders and cellular debris. They include monocytes, which circulate in the blood; macrophages, which are found in tissues throughout the body; dendritic cells, which are more stationary, monitoring their environment from one spot, such as the skin; and neutrophils, cells that circulate in the blood but move into tissues when they are needed. Phagocytes are called to action in response to toxic compounds, inflammatory chemicals, aberrant cells, cells that have undergone apoptosis, and various biochemical signals released by foreign invaders. Once activated, phagocytes (along with natural killer cells) produce potent chemicals such as gamma interferon and tumor necrosis factor (TNF). These chemicals directly kill these aberrant cells. Phagocytes are a critical component of our overall immune response to malignant cells.

Enhancing Natural Immunity

The immune system is a complex system that involves powerful players communicating and working in concert to keep the body healthy. Sometimes, however, this sophisticated internal defense mechanism can become overwhelmed, disorganized, handicapped, and in dire need of support. Because cancer is so directly related to immune function (or dysfunction), supporting the immune system on a variety of fronts is critical for both prevention and treatment.

There are five key ways to enhance healthy immune function:

1. Making healthful dietary choices

2. Getting enough (and not too much) physical activity and exercise

3. Reducing stress

4. Taking certain dietary supplements

5. Avoiding or reducing exposure to pathogens and other environmental toxins (discussed at length in chapter 2)

Be sure to review the "Foundational Health Plan" sidebar on page 84 of chapter 4 for an overview of essential diet and lifestyle strategies to support immune function.

Exercise

As with eating a healthy diet, regular exercise has a wide range of health benefits, including enhancing immune function. Many clinical studies have shown that a consistent, balanced program of diverse exercise enhances immune activity. Additionally, regular exercise causes the large muscles of the body to contract and act like a pump for the lymphatic system. This helps circulate lymph fluid through the body's filtering process, which destroys toxic compounds. Some studies have demonstrated, however, that too much of this good thing can have the reverse effect. But can you really exercise too much? For most of us, it's a moot point. We have to start exercising in the first place, or be exercising enough, before that could ever be a problem. However, research does show that excessive exercise can actually impair immune function. Although the benefits of exercise are far-reaching, the physiological processes of exercise produce free radicals and can stress the system. As is usually the case, balance is the key.

"Heavy, long-term exercise (such as marathon running and intense gym training) could actually decrease the amount of white blood cells circulating through the body and *increase* the presence of stress-related hormones," according to the National Institutes of Health (NIH). But most people have the opposite problem—not exercising enough. Research involving exercise and enhanced immunity is gaining momentum.

Shifting to a moderately active lifestyle will help improve immune function. A moderate exercise program consists of 20 to 30 minutes of physical activity daily, which can include activities such as walking, biking, hiking, playing a sport (such as golf or tennis), lifting weights, yoga, or other exercises. Be sure to increase the duration as your body becomes accustomed to the activity. In a personal interview, sports medicine specialist Dr. Susan Ryan concluded, "Exercise-enhanced immunity does not increase with intensity, it increases with consistency."

Stress and the Immune System

When we are exposed to stress, physiological alarms are triggered and cortisol levels rise. Prolonged elevation of cortisol also leads to impaired immunity. A review in the journal *Lancet Oncology* found that external stressors, as well as depression, decrease activity of cytotoxic T cells and natural killer cells. The researchers conclude that "the persistent activation of the hypothalamic-pituitary-adrenal (HPA) axis (and thus cortisol) in the chronic

Stress, the Mind, and Immunity

By Alex Concorde, MBBS, PhD, FRSM

Dr. Hans Selye was the first to describe the connection between stress and health. A remarkable and independent thinker, Dr. Selye encapsulated his theories and ideas on stress in what he called the general adaptation syndrome (GAS). He described stress as "the non-specific response of the body to any demand that is made on it."

Dr. Selye concluded that our daily lives are influenced by two kinds of stress: pleasant stress that contributes to wellness and unpleasant stress that contributes to illness. He believed the difference between positive and negative stress really depends on the individual's own perception of what constitutes a demand.

According to his theories, both positive and negative stress create a similar physical response. Our heart begins to race, our palms may sweat, and our attention heightens. This is how we can pull an all-nighter to study for an exam, have energy to celebrate after winning a long race, or manage sleepless nights as we stay up with a sick child. Our stress response keeps us on alert so we are ready to take on the challenge that faces us. And even positive, happy challenges produce a similar response.

Ever since Dr. Selye's work, health professionals have struggled to guide patients on whether a stressor could be positive or negative for them as individuals. The customary paradigm is that the nature of the stressor is significant. Intensity, duration, type, and repetition will determine whether a stressor will become a problem. For example, although planning your wedding may be fun and exciting, imagine if you had to plan your wedding every weekend. In this case, even a positive stressor if repeated too often could contribute to health problems. But is that the whole story?

Since Dr. Selye put forward his theories of stress in the 1950s, stress and stress-related conditions seem to have multiplied, while fresh theories to help advance the field have been few. What we are starting to appreciate is that stress is an imbalance between demands and resources. Anything that continually taps into your resources is depleting. This is why repetitive demands—especially without reinvigoration or a sense of "winning"—cause big health issues. And more than anything else, chronic stress-induced depletion is the predecessor of severe immune system dysfunction—the greater and more longstanding the relative depletion, the greater the risk of developing cancer. Even though all depletion and stress is negative, there are different types of stress. The two main types are current stress and legacy stress.

Current stress seems like an obvious thing: too much to do! But that is only a small part of it, because that is usually only about not having enough time. In fact, issues of self and spirituality stress response and in depression probably impairs the immune response and contributes to the development and progression of some types of cancer."

Physical symptoms of raised cortisol, or a prolonged phase II of the stress response, can include the following symptoms:

- Insomnia and/or daytime fatigue

- Loss of bone mineral density

- Hypothyroidism

- Mood disturbances, especially depression and anxiety

- Memory impairment

are the most potent current stresses as they cut away at the very core of being (which is about you, rather than your activities). So losing sight of who you are, feeling fractured as an individual, losing faith or trust in "bigger things" or in others—these issues create infinitely greater demands and consume infinitely greater resources than having too much to do.

Consequently, in preventing and treating cancer, addressing issues of individuality and spirituality are very important. Although the value of ongoing exercise and system support through diet and supplements are appreciable, individuality and spirituality are the "longest levers," meaning they're the most powerful tools, exerting the greatest force for gaining and maintaining health. Having fun should delight you and light you up as an individual, not just distract you from your worries.

However, even more than that there is legacy stress, which refers to all those demands and resources tethered to your emotional baggage and undesirable or adverse life experiences. I believe at least 80 percent of current stress has legacy attached to it. The problem with this is that the hormones and the immune system continue to be tilted toward disequilibrium by a mind anticipating, perceiving, creating, defending against, and reacting to threats that are real, huge, and current to the individual, but that in truth no longer exist.

You should view stress differently if you are trying to prevent or treat cancer. In prevention you can afford to set up your life, your personal focus, and your mind to maximally offset stress and constantly fill the bank with resources. This means minimal stress, rare adverse physical impact, and maximum biological bounce.

However, in people who have cancer and are receiving treatment, the equation is tilted—often drastically. Cancer itself can consume huge resources (including nutritional), the emotional stress of cancer can prove to be an enormous demand, and all forms of conventional treatment, while necessary, increase system stress. That being the case, it is important to clear as much legacy stress as possible as quickly as possible, with as little effort as possible, thereby rapidly tilting the imbalance back toward equilibrium by dramatically reducing demands and maximally increasing resources. This can be done through a combination of introspection, psychological therapy, counseling, and other activities. Professional assistance may be required.

Dr. Alex Concorde is head of research and development for the Concorde Initiative, and president of the International Association of Transformational Change. She is also on this book's editorial advisory board.

- Gastrointestinal problems such as ulcers and irritable bowel syndrome (IBS)

- High blood pressure

Several studies have confirmed the link between stress and immune dysfunction in both healthy people and those with cancer. One way stress is thought to favor cancer growth is by impairing DNA repair and/or apoptosis of damaged cells. And, as mentioned earlier, prolonged elevation of cortisol decreases NK cell and cytotoxic T cell activity. Researchers from the Ohio State University Comprehensive Cancer Center suggest that psychological or behavioral approaches to reducing psychological stress may reduce the development or progression of cancer. They conclude in the journal

European Society for Medical Oncology that "therapeutic interventions could be beneficial in the reduction of both the stress associated with cancer and the concomitant stress-related immune down-regulation."

The immune system is most affected when the stress is repetitive, intense, and sustained. In addition, the body's reaction to stress and its impact on immunity is dependent upon many variables, including the following:

- Genetic predisposition

- Psychological, spiritual, and emotional state (both historical and current)

- Physical health

- Lifestyle habits

- Hormonal status

Fortunately, there's much you can do to enhance your ability to cope with stress or, even better, reduce the amount of stress in your life. Tune in to what causes you stress in your day-to-day life, and try to figure out where you can make changes to avoid that stress. Of course, some stress is unavoidable, so spend some time exploring different stress reduction methods to find which work best for you. De-stressing is an individualized and ongoing process. It may take some time just to figure out exactly what will most help you to create that sense of calm and rhythm that occurs when you move out of a prolonged resistance phase of stress response and back into homeostasis. Make a habit of using these techniques regularly, both to cope with stress and to develop more equanimity. The mind-body approaches discussed in chapter 4 will be helpful. It's important that you choose methods that work for you. Additionally, numerous herbs and nutrients can support a healthy stress response (see the sidebar "Natural Substances to Alleviate Stress" on page 191 for information about specific substances).

Immune-Enhancing Supplements

Healthy immune function requires a multidimensional approach. Eating a healthy diet, getting consistent physical activity, and reducing stress can be immensely helpful, but a beleaguered immune system may need some additional sparks to get the engine started.

Numerous vitamins, minerals, herbs, and other nutrients can elicit a positive immune response. Although some of the natural substances we discuss below have not been studied directly to prevent or treat cancer, all of them have demonstrated impressive immune-enhancing properties, and they are our top choices for this purpose. (For dosage information, see the appendix.)

- **Astragalus**: This herb enhances the cytotoxicity and activity of natural killer cells and macrophages and protects against reductions in blood cell counts induced by chemotherapy.

- **Coenzyme Q10**: This potent antioxidant nutrient enhances natural killer cell and T cell activity. It also increases cellular production of energy and prevents cellular damage by neutralizing free radicals.

- **Curcumin**: Derived from the spice turmeric, this antioxidant phytochemical enhances the phagocytic activities of macrophages in the immune system. It also inhibits the production of inflammatory cytokines that stimulate tumor growth.

- **Echinacea**: This widely used herb stimulates the activity of macrophages, natural killer cells, and lymphocytes; increases production of interferon and tumor necrosis factor alpha; and neutralizes free radicals.

- **Flavonoids**: There are dozens of flavonoids present in fruits and vegetables, each of which has unique effects on immune function and tumors. These antioxidant nutrients protect the body by stimulating natural killer cells and by inhibiting critical enzymes that direct the inflammatory response, actions that work together to reduce inflammation and inhibit tumor growth.

- **Garlic**: Garlic enhances natural killer cell function and may increase tumor cells' antigenicity (the capacity to induce an immune response). Supplementing with garlic, particularly aged garlic extract, is inversely correlated with the incidence of all cancers, and garlic has been demonstrated to inhibit carcinogenesis by helping repair damaged DNA.

- **Green tea**: This powerful antioxidant promotes repair to DNA and encourages apoptosis of damaged cells. It also has antiangiogenesis properties, meaning it can prevent tumors from creating their own blood supply. Green tea polyphenols, namely, epigallocatechin gallate (EGCG), also inhibit overuse of the chemicals the body uses to regulate inflammation.

- **Lycopene**: This phytochemical is abundant in tomatoes, watermelon, pink grapefruit, papaya, and rosehips. Lycopene has been shown to increase the cell-killing actions of NK cells. Low serum levels of lycopene are correlated with an increased risk of prostate cancer.

- **Melatonin**: This potent antioxidant increases the cytotoxic activity of lymphocytes and also helps prevent chemotherapy- and radiation-induced bone marrow suppression. Melatonin reduces inflammation by inhibiting the action of a variety of proinflammatory cytokines, for example, interleukins and tumor necrosis factor alpha. Melatonin also increases cytotoxic T cell immune actions.

- **Mushroom polysaccharides**: Components in this common food stimulate lymphocytes and NK cells to secrete cytokines and interferon, which activate immune-mediated cytotoxicity, an important pathway for cancer cell death.

- **Omega-3 fatty acids**: Animal studies have shown that supplementation with omega-3 fatty acids increases macrophage function and is associated with tumor inhibition.

- **Plant sterols and sterolins**: Sterols and their glucosides, sterolins, are found in the fibrous parts of all plant-based foods. Sterols and sterolins are poorly absorbed when used in their natural form. Supplemental sterolins, which are extracted from plants, are absorbed better and exert immune-regulating actions. These compounds stimulate NK cell activity and increase counts of CD4 T cells, which are important in immune regulation. Sterols and sterolins have also been shown to decrease levels of cortisol and IL-6, a proinflammatory cytokine secreted by immune cells in response to stress.

- **Probiotics**: These supplements restore beneficial intestinal bacterial flora, which enhances the activity of immune cells located in the intestines. Probiotics improve the intestines' immunologic barrier, particularly by stimulating the antibodies produced in the intestines. These antibodies sample the food that we ingest for microorganisms and other disease-causing substances. If the intestinal antibodies find pathogens, they bind to them until they are excreted in the stool. This process is critical to keeping us disease free and also alleviates intestinal inflammation. Healthy intestinal bacteria metabolize nutrients needed for immune function (B vitamins, vitamin K). Healthy intestinal flora will also help prevent infections originating in the gut by creating an environment that is not hospitable to disease-causing, or pathogenic, bacteria. Friendly probiotics metabolize some of the fiber components of the food that we eat and alter the pH of our intestines in the process. Pathogenic bacteria cannot thrive in the pH generated by our friendly bacteria. Probiotics are also associated with anticarcinogenic effects, particularly via the detoxification of compounds in the gut that can cause genetic damage.

- **Spleen polypeptides**: These glandular extracts of spleen tissue (usually derived from cows or pigs) enhance cytotoxic T cell and macrophage

Natural Substances to Alleviate Stress

Many herbs and nutrients have been shown in scientific studies to possess antistress properties. These herbs and nutrients can help the body rebound from stressful situations or help support body organs and tissues associated with the stress response.

Herbs that may help counter some of the adverse effects of stress include the following:

- Siberian ginseng is considered an adaptogenic, meaning it has a normalizing effect and helps bring the body back to homeostasis. Siberian ginseng improves the body's nonspecific stress response, which is a general biological response rather than a response that relates to a specific stressful event. It also improves immune function and overall well-being.

- Panax ginseng can enhance immune function, physical stamina, and mental acuity and increases resistance to toxic environmental substances. However, Panax ginseng can also create overstimulation if used improperly. Panax ginseng should only be used under the supervision of a qualified health-care provider.

- Ashwagandha (*Withania somnifera*), also known as Indian ginseng, protects against stress-induced ulceration, lowers chronically elevated cortisol, enhances energy, reduces anxiety, and can counteract stress-induced hyperglycemia.

- Other adaptogenic and sedative herbs include schisandra (*Schisandra chinensis*), Indian tobacco (*Lobelia inflata*), vervain (*Verbena officianalis*), and lemon balm (*Melissa officinalis*).

Specific nutrients that can help the body manage the internal stress response include the following:

- Vitamin C helps normalize levels of cortisol and ACTH (adrenocorticotropic hormone; another stress hormone) in situations of severe stress.

- Vitamin B$_1$ protects the adrenal glands from functional exhaustion.

- Vitamin B$_5$ enhances adrenal function and helps regulate cortisol levels.

- Alpha-lipoic acid helps prevent toxin accumulation in tissues. (However, caution is advised with certain chemotherapy drugs and radiation therapy).

- L-theanine is an amino acid found in green tea leaves that has been shown to promote relaxation, improve sleep quality, and heighten mental clarity and focus.

- L-tyrosine helps restore the ability to perform tasks under stress.

- Phosphatidylserine prevents oversecretion of cortisol and ACTH in response to stress.

function, while also stimulating increased filtration of cellular debris in the blood.

● *Vitamin A*: Vitamin A deficiency impairs immunity by preventing normal regeneration of mucous membranes damaged by infection, and by decreasing the function of neutrophils, macrophages, and natural killer cells. Vitamin A is required in the development of both helper T cells and B cells.

● *Vitamin C*: This powerful antioxidant nutrient supports the phagocytic and cytotoxic activity of lymphocytes and natural killer cells.

- *Vitamin E*: Vitamin E increases T cell cytotoxic immune reactions, likely by reducing immune suppression caused by free radicals. Higher serum levels of vitamin E are correlated with lower risks of cancer development.

- *Zinc*: Zinc is associated with decreased rates of cancer, and this is attributed to its antioxidant and immunostimulatory actions. Destruction of cells by natural killer cells and production of interleukin-1, an immune-regulating protein, are two immune functions known to be zinc dependent.

Some systems of traditional medicine, such as Ayurveda, Tibetan medicine, and traditional Chinese medicine, employ combinations of natural substances designed to stimulate the immune system. In most of these systems, a particular formula is chosen to match the constitutional and individual characteristics of the person. Traditional formulas address underlying imbalances in the person's body that are identified according to the diagnostic principles of each system of healing. Homeopathy is another system of healing based on constitution and individual characteristics. Homeopathic remedies are chosen for a person based upon their totality of symptoms, even if the primary objective is to stimulate their immune system responses. To get the full benefit from any of these traditional healing systems, you need to work with a health-care professional trained in that system.

Immunity and Beyond

No matter where you are along the cancer spectrum—prevention, undergoing treatment, or recovery—supporting and enhancing your immune system is critical. But the immune system is not the only body system fighting the battle against cancer. It may be on the front lines, but it requires support in the form of proper inflammatory responses, balanced hormone function, optimal insulin metabolism, and healthy digestion, detoxification, and elimination. Effective cancer treatment requires a comprehensive systems approach that goes beyond immunity, and any successful treatment plan requires that all systems be involved in the process.

The systems biology approach that we advocate can and should be applied to cancer. There are many important biological systems in the body that are available to help us treat cancer. Now that we have looked at the immune system's influence on cancer development, the next step is inflammation. Its influence on cancer prevention and development is often misunderstood and underestimated. In the next chapter, we will explore how chronic inflammation can contribute to cancer.

nine

Inflammation

When we think of inflammation, we usually think of an injury or an illness such as arthritis. To many people, inflammation means a swollen joint, a painful contusion, or a red, irritated infection. We rarely associate inflammation with cancer. However, as researchers connect the dots of this complex disease, they have now drawn a clear line between the two.

Inflammation is the outcome of a complex internal response that involves the immune and endocrine systems. This coordinated response normally defends the body against a dangerous infection or injury. However, an overly exuberant and chronic inflammatory response can do just the opposite—it can cause illness, including cancer.

Inflammation is the immune system's first response to injury. It is the body's internal emergency medical team, first to the scene to flood the area with specialized cells trained to act quickly to resolve the crisis—the injury, infection, or illness. As the immune system sounds the alarm, important inflammatory cells move into action. Blood vessels dilate as white blood cells and antibodies are sent to the inflammatory emergency—*stat!* White blood cells, or leukocytes, filter out bacteria and debris. Neutrophils, the most common white blood cells, are responsible for much of the body's protection against infection and inflammation. Neutrophils arrive on the scene first and remove foreign particles by ingesting them, but their efforts only last a couple of days. Reinforcements arrive in the form of macrophages and lymphocytes. Macrophages clean up the debris of inflammation and help direct the body's overall response by secreting chemical messenger molecules. The lymphocytes (T cells and B cells) could be considered middle managers in the immune response, since they produce cytokine molecules that deliver messages to the immune system, turning it on or off depending on the demands of the situation.

Resolution of an inflammatory situation involves a massive and cohesive cellular team effort. No matter how large or small the crisis, the inflammatory emergency crews will work day and night until the issue is resolved. How can such an impressive response system lead to cancer? That depends largely on whether the inflammatory response is acute or becomes chronic.

Constant Chaos

Have you ever been in a meeting that was intended to resolve a problem, but just the opposite occurred? We have all experienced those unproductive, frustrating meetings that seem to do more harm than good. Imagine if you had meetings like that every week, or every day! And what would happen if even more people and more problems were added to the mix? Instead of crisis management, there would be chaos. Chronic inflammation is like those repeated chaotic meetings. In this situation, the internal emergency response team is no longer functioning as a cooperative unit. Instead, rogue cytokines and other inflammatory proteins take over.

When the immune system is operating smoothly, the inflammatory response is a controlled commotion similar to any emergency situation. There is a surge of activity managed with the shared goal of killing infectious agents, neutralizing foreign substances, or containing the injury. The hectic pace of the emergency responders can cause discomfort. The hallmarks of inflammation are redness, heat, swelling, and pain. Swelling occurs as blood vessels packed with white blood cells flow to the area. This increased blood flow causes tissues to puff up and compress nerve endings, resulting in pain.

What happens when the inflammatory response is not functioning smoothly? That's when the crisis management meeting is officially deemed out of control. Powerful chemical messenger molecules (cytokines, enzymes, interleukins, and prostaglandins) released by inflamed tissue or responding immune cells disrupt the coordinated response. What began as an efficient response to an emergency situation turns into a free-for-all.

The link between inflammation and cancer begins with a trigger—a bacteria, virus, injury, or oxidative damage—any of which can activate the production of a protein known as nuclear factor kappa B (NF-kB). NF-kB engages the inflammatory response, in part, by stimulating cell division, which allows injured tissue to repair itself. Another proinflammatory effect of increased NF-kB is to decrease apoptosis, which gives individual cells time to repair themselves. However, if the inflammatory response is prolonged, the influence of NF-kB extends beyond this acute response. Interestingly, as we age, we are more prone to prolonged NF-kB activation.

In the prolonged presence of NF-kB, apoptosis of cells, including cancerous cells, is decreased (so they survive longer) and their cell division is increased (which leads to tumor growth). Obviously, to prevent and treat cancer, we want the opposite to occur: *increased* apoptosis and *decreased* division of cancerous cells. In addition to doing exactly the opposite of what we want, NF-kB also activates COX-2 enzymes and powerful cytokines, including interleukin-1 (IL-1), interleukin-6 (IL-6) and interleukin-8 (IL-8). COX-2 enzymes make prostaglandins, which are lipid-like hormonal agents that influence dilation of blood vessels, clotting, stimulation of pain receptors, and cellular proliferation. IL-1 is a cytokine that activates the growth and function of neutrophils, lymphocytes, and macrophages. It is also involved in inflammation-induced fevers.

IL-6 is a lymphokine secreted by many cells, including adipose cells (found in fat tissue), endothelial cells (cells lining blood vessels), phagocytes, and T cells. IL-6 mediates the acute inflammatory response and enhances B cell production and function. While IL-6, IL-1, and COX-2 enzymes are critical for mounting an adequate acute inflammatory reaction, when they are secreted continuously they disrupt the checks and balances that control cellular activity and growth. Continuously secreted IL-6, for instance, stimulates the invasion and migration of breast cancer cells. High blood levels of IL-6 are correlated with shorter survival among women with metastatic breast cancer. High IL-6 blood levels are also associated with shorter survival in patients with leukemia, kidney cancer, and prostate cancer. In addition to stimulating invasion, IL-6 also stimulates the release of another molecule, vascular endothelial growth factor, or VEGF. VEGF is responsible for angiogenesis (development of increased blood supply) to tumors. VEGF is necessary for tumor growth, and people with high levels of VEGF have more aggressive cancers. IL-8 is another inflammatory lymphokine that is correlated with increased angiogenesis, increased metastasis, and worse survival in breast cancer, colon cancer, gastric cancer, non-Hodgkin's lymphoma, leukemias, lung cancer, melanoma, ovarian cancer, prostate cancer, and squamous cell head and neck cancers. Unfortunately, one of the characteristics of metastatic cancer is the ability of the cancer cells to produce these inflammatory molecules themselves. Thus, the cancer perpetuates the inflammatory milieu, which, in turn, stimulates their continued growth. This is the vicious cycle of inflammation and cancer and is why naturopathic oncologist Dr. Dan Rubin refers to cancer as an "unhealed wound."

Controlling Inflammation with Conventional Drugs

Conventional drugs used to manage acute inflammation are effective at controlling some of the symptoms. However, the side effects of these drugs can outweigh their benefits when treating chronic inflammation. Prescription and over-the-counter drugs used for symptoms associated with inflammation include nonsteroidal anti-inflammatory drugs (NSAIDs), such as ibuprofen, naproxen, and aspirin, and a subset of NSAIDs called COX-2 inhibitors, such as celecoxib and rofecoxib. Chronic NSAID use is associated with severe ulcers and many other side effects.

NSAIDs block COX-1 and COX-2 activity, and taking a COX-2 inhibitor blocks the activity of the COX-2 enzyme. Blocking COX enzymes impedes production of prostaglandins, the promoters of the inflammatory response. While blocking COX-2 activity and prostaglandin production is an effective way to interfere with the body's inflammatory response, when used long term this approach has some downsides. In addition to their role in inflammation, prostaglandins influence blood flow, digestion, and wakefulness. Thus, prolonged use of NSAIDs and COX-2 inhibitors may create problems in these areas, including ulceration in the digestive tract.

Conventional medicine also falls short in effectively managing or even detecting a chronic inflammatory internal environment that has not yet manifested in acute symptoms of inflammation. Systemically, inflammation may be percolating under the surface, not yet bubbling over with overt symptoms such as muscle swelling or joint pain. But this biochemical environment of inflammation can be a precursor to many illnesses, including cancer.

Antioxidants as Anti-inflammatories

One ever-present component of inflammation is the generation of free radicals. These highly reactive compounds and the cellular havoc they create play an integral role in maintaining and perpetuating the inflammatory response. Free radicals both result *from* inflammation and lead *to* inflammation by causing direct oxidative damage to cells and tissues. Each molecule in our cells is made up of atoms. One component of an atom is circulating negatively charged particles called electrons. Free radicals are molecules that are missing electrons and they are desperate to replace them. They are so hungry for electrons that they literally rip them off other molecules with which they have contact. After this "robbery" takes place, the molecular victim is left both damaged and hungry for electron replacement. They, in turn, may rob their neighboring molecule of their electrons and the cycle of free radical–induced cellular damage has begun. This damage amplifies inflammation by increasing the activity of several key enzymes and proteins, such as NF-kB, that are involved in the inflammatory response.

"Think of free radicals as small sparks in a forest," explain Robert Rountree, MD, and Carol Colman in their book *Immunotics*. "Extinguished early on, they pose no threat. Left to spread, they can cause a catastrophe." One consequence of free radicals is damage to cellular DNA. When DNA mutation occurs and these cells replicate, the process of carcinogenesis begins. As discussed previously, too many free radicals can also initiate and sustain chronic inflammation with consequent reductions in apoptosis. Thus, these mutated cells are unlikely to undergo apoptosis. The combined result of all of these events caused by free radicals is unregulated division of damaged cells, which can lead to cancer formation. So, you can see the importance of finding ways to neutralize free radicals or reduce their activity. This is the role of antioxidants.

"Oxidative stress is a condition that occurs when the body has too many free radicals and too few antioxidants," according to *Immunotics*. As expected, the way to prevent and reverse oxidative stress is to increase antioxidant stores and neutralize excess free radicals. As their name implies, antioxidants are compounds that can prevent or reduce oxidative damage caused by free radicals. Antioxidants do this because they are electron donors. By donating electrons to the electron-hungry free radicals, they prevent electron robbery from cellular molecules. Antioxidants can come from the diet or from dietary supplements. Antioxidants are very helpful at breaking the cycle of chronic inflammation. They can also help prevent the damage to DNA that contributes to the development of cancer and other illnesses, as evidenced by many studies demonstrating that key antioxidant supplements can help prevent cancer. Some important antioxidants to reduce chronic inflammation and potential cancer risk are listed below.

- Alpha-lipoic acid has been shown to enhance the effects of other antioxidants, specifically vitamins C and E.

- Coenzyme Q10 is especially beneficial in reducing oxidative stress; it also works synergistically with vitamin E.

- Curcumin, a compound found in turmeric, reduces lipid peroxidation from free radicals.

- EGCG (epigallocatechin gallate), a flavonoid found in green tea, is a potent antioxidant and also promotes apoptosis of cancer cells.

- Folic acid, an antioxidant B vitamin involved in DNA repair, has been demonstrated to be especially beneficial for those who consume alcohol.

- Garlic has antioxidant and anticarcinogenic effects substantiated by animal and human trials.

- Selenium supports antioxidant activity and promotes the body's production of its own antioxidants.

Pain? Try Acupuncture

For many people, managing acute pain associated with inflammatory conditions can be challenging. Acupuncture can be a great alternative to aspirin or painkillers. This traditional healing method has been used for centuries to reduce pain associated with inflammation. Clinical studies regarding acupuncture for inflammatory pain have yielded mixed results, and more research is needed in this area. However, the World Health Organization recommends it for more than 40 different health conditions, including chronic pain. More than 15 million Americans have tried acupuncture for a variety of conditions, and some insurance companies cover acupuncture treatments.

If you want to try acupuncture, here are some tips from an article by Judith Horstman featured in *Arthritis Today*:

- Choose a licensed practitioner.

- Get a diagnosis before going.

- Don't stop medications without first discussing this with your doctor.

- Inform the acupuncturist about your health conditions and any medications you're taking, including herbs and over-the-counter medications.

- Be sure the acupuncturist uses sterilized or disposable needles.

- Tell the practitioner if you experience pain after the initial sting of the needle, or if you bleed more than a few drops of blood.

- Keep notes about your response to treatment to track your progress.

You may also want to ask your practitioner about using acupressure techniques, in which pressure is applied to the meridian points, and no needles are used.

● Vitamin C helps protect against oxidative damage. Though usually taken orally, it may be used intravenously to treat certain diseases.

● Vitamin D deficiency is associated with chronic inflammatory conditions including cancer.

● Vitamin E has been demonstrated to be effective in reducing inflammation and preventing cancer development in cellular and epidemiological studies; however, human studies have produced conflicting and inconclusive results.

The Anti-inflammation Plan

Antioxidants play an important role in preventing and treating chronic inflammation. But that's just the beginning. An anti-inflammatory diet combined with anti-inflammatory herbs and nutrients can help prevent and potentially reverse chronic inflammation. Homeopathic formulas may also be helpful. Because of the interrelationship between chronic inflammation and cancer, the anti-inflammatory plan that follows can be used as part of an overall cancer support plan.

Diet can play a huge role in controlling inflammation. The opposite is also true: A poor diet can contribute to internal inflammation. Insulin resistance is also a dangerous outcome of chronic inflammation. (Chapter 11 covers insulin resistance in depth.) Increased levels of the inflammatory compounds NF-kB and IL-6 have been linked to insulin resistance, so controlling chronic inflammation will help control insulin resistance. The reverse is true as well. Overweight individuals with insulin resistance have higher levels of NF-kB, IL-8, and IL-6. When these individuals lose weight, their NF-kB levels decrease. Specifically, reducing intake of simple carbohydrate-laden meals lowers inflammatory markers.

Dietary Recommendations

"Increase consumption of fruits and vegetables." That advice can start to sound like a broken record. But the fact is, fruits and vegetables are a key part of the anti-inflammatory diet. A diet high in fruits and vegetables will provide natural sources of the nutrients, including plenty of antioxidants, that are needed to help curb chronic inflammation. Anthocyanidins from berries are particularly effective at reducing NF-kB levels. For more dietary and lifestyle advice, refer to the "Foundational Health Plan" sidebar on page 84 in chapter 4.

Results from 206 human epidemiological studies and 22 animal studies demonstrated consistently that, because of their anti-inflammatory properties, increased vegetable and fruit consumption protects against cancers of the stomach, esophagus, lung, endometrium, pancreas, and colon. The most beneficial vegetables are carrots, any green vegetable, and cruciferous vegetables such as cabbage, broccoli, and cauliflower—all preferably raw.

"Good" fats will also help protect against chronic inflammation. There has been much debate regarding the benefits of a low-fat diet. Researchers at the Harvard School of Public Health and many others have confirmed that the type of fat you eat is often more important than the amount. This has special relevance in regard to inflammation. Polyunsaturated and mono-unsaturated fats reduce inflammation, whereas saturated fats and trans fats promote inflammation.

Because arachidonic acid is a polyunsaturated omega-6 fatty acid, you might assume that it's good for you. But when you eat excessive amounts of this fat, it enhances inflammation by metabolizing into harmful leukotrienes and proinflammatory prostaglandins. By reducing your intake of arachidonic acid, you can minimize the chronic inflammatory cycle. The primary source of arachidonic acid is animal foods: meat, poultry, dairy products, and so on. Trans fats also have damaging effects in terms of inflammation. When these synthetically transformed fats are incorporated into cell membranes, their altered structure interferes with the function of certain anti-inflammatory substances.

The essential fatty acids eicosapentaenoic acid (EPA) and docosahexaenoic acid (DHA), as well as conjugated linoleic acid (CLA), have direct anti-inflammatory effects and can help manage the inflammatory process. Most of the scientific data on essential fatty acids for inflammation is on EPA, an omega-3 fatty acid. Cold-water fish such as mackerel, herring, halibut, and salmon and shellfish such as shrimp are great dietary sources of EPA and DHA. There is growing scientific evidence regarding the anti-inflammatory and anticancer actions of CLA, which is found in dairy products. However, dairy products also contain the proinflammatory arachidonic acid, so if you consume dairy regularly, it is important to reduce consumption of other sources of arachidonic acid, such as meat and poultry. If it is difficult to get enough EFAs in your diet, they are available in supplement form. (Fish oil or sea algae capsules are the best source of EPA and DHA.)

Anti-inflammatory Supplements

In addition to antioxidant nutrients from diet, specific anti-inflammatory supplements can also help reverse chronic inflammation. However, if you are on chemotherapy or have concerns regarding safety and contraindications for your specific cancer, refer to the "Integrative Cancer Care Supplement Guide" starting on page 161 and the chart "Chemotherapy Drugs and Their Nutrient and Herb Interactions" starting on page 141. See the appendix for dosages.

- *Antioxidants*: Some antioxidant nutrients also have anti-inflammatory properties, particularly green tea, curcumin, CoQ10, alpha-lipoic acid, selenium, and vitamins C and E. (For more information, refer to the section "Antioxidants as Anti-inflammatories" starting on page 196.)

- *Enzymes (primarily bromelain)*: Dietary enzymes that break down proteins not only aid with digestion, they can also help reduce both acute and chronic inflammation. The most researched enzyme in this regard is bromelain, from pineapple. According to the National Institutes of Health website, "Several preliminary studies suggest that when taken by mouth, bromelain can reduce inflammation or pain caused by inflammation."

- *Curcumin (from turmeric)*: In a small pilot trial involving 21 patients with advanced pancreatic cancer, daily curcumin resulted in slowed disease progress in 14 percent (3 patients). In these patients, NF-kB was down-regulated.

- *Ginger*: Typically considered an antinausea herb, ginger also has anti-inflammatory properties; recent research from South Africa demonstrated that ginger has analgesic and hypoglycemic properties as well.

- *Probiotics*: Although we usually think of using probiotics to maintain healthy intestinal flora (which we'll discuss in chapter 12), several studies have demonstrated that they can also help control inflammation, specifically lowering IL-8 and NF-kB.

Though more clinical research is needed, homeopathic formulas have been shown to be beneficial for inflammatory symptoms. Arnica is perhaps the most popular anti-inflammatory homeopathic ingredient; others include Apis, Ruta, and Bryonia. Animal studies using a homeopathic formula known as Traumeel demonstrated effectiveness against swelling. The researchers concluded that the product did not block the development of swelling but did speed up the healing process.

A Call to Action

Inflammation is the body's call to action. Universities, researchers, and medical practitioners are recognizing the need to find answers for the chronic inflammatory alarm that is constantly ringing in so many of us. Hundreds of studies have concluded that chronic inflammation is linked to a number of serious illnesses, including Alzheimer's, diabetes, multiple sclerosis, heart disease, and cancer. According to a report in the journal *Oncology*, "A substantial body of evidence supports the conclusion that chronic inflammation can predispose individuals to cancer. The longer the inflammation persists, the higher the risk." Continued research in this area has recognized the link between inflammation and cancer progression. Increased inflammation is correlated with worsened prognosis in most cancers. "Today, some of the underlying cellular and molecular events linking inflammation and cancer have been unraveled," according to a recent report by Swiss researchers in the *Journal of Leukocyte Biology*. "Tumor cells exploit mechanisms that occur physiologically during inflammation to invade and metastasize."

Acute inflammation associated with an injury or infection may resolve quickly. However, in its cunning and resilient way, cancer can opportunistically turn a healing process into a deadly game of survival. To treat cancer and prevent a recurrence, we must reverse the process of chronic inflammation. This requires a comprehensive plan. Infection, injury, and oxidation fuel the inflammatory fire. Diet and supplements can douse the flame.

In the next chapter we will explore the role that endocrine function, specifically hormonal balance, plays in the body's response to cancer.

ten

Hormonal Influences

The human body is amazing. If you were asked which system of the body is the most significant, how would you respond? It is a difficult choice. Many would say it is the cardiovascular system, with its spectacular pump nestled in the chest. Or maybe you would choose the reproductive system because it can deliver the miracle of human life. Still others may identify the nervous system, which features a complex computer housed in the skull. And for those interested in cancer prevention and treatment, the immune system may be at the top of their mind.

In all likelihood, few people would rate the endocrine system as being the most amazing or important of all the body's systems. It is true that there is no headlining star in the endocrine system. However, even though the organs in this system are small and seemingly unimpressive, their collaboration can certainly steal the show when it comes to health. Strategically placed throughout the body, the organs and glands of the endocrine system work in concert to stimulate growth and development, control metabolism, and influence the performance of all other systems in the body.

The physiology of the endocrine system is quite complex, but because hormones can have such a huge impact on prevention, development, and treatment of cancer, a general overview is important. The primary glands of the endocrine system are as follows:

● Pituitary and pineal (in the brain)

● Thyroid and parathyroid (in front of the upper part of the trachea, in the neck)

- Thymus (in the chest—in front of and above the heart)

- Pancreas (behind the stomach and connected to the duodenum)

- Adrenals (one nestled atop each kidney)

- Ovaries in women and testes in men

These glands secrete messenger molecules that are carried throughout the body via the blood supply. On cue, these powerful messengers, known as hormones, help regulate and influence other body systems and important internal activities such as

- Calcium uptake by cells for strong, healthy bones

- Heart rate and blood pressure

- Lymphocyte development and other immune responses

- Breathing and various functions relating to respiration

- Secretion of digestive enzymes

- Blood sugar regulation

- Influence on brain function

- Development and function of the reproductive organs, including menstruation, pregnancy, and lactation

- Metabolic rate and energy level

As you can see, hormones significantly affect physiological function. (For a list of some of the most important hormones in the endocrine system and their actions, see the chart on page 206.) Hormones can influence cancers in both men and women, but before we discuss this, an overview of the endocrine system is in order.

To ensure and protect the body's internal harmony, hormone secretion is carefully regulated by a complex system of feedback loops among the various endocrine glands. Because each gland and its corresponding hormonal activity affect so many body functions, the hormonal activity of any one gland can have far-reaching effects within the body. Endocrine activity can be compared to threads in the garment of the body. When disruptive forces pull at these threads, they can unravel a large portion of the garment. The endocrine system is in constant response to both the internal and external environment. The interconnectedness of the endocrine system to the rest of the body allows for constant resetting and rebalancing, but it also means that any perpetual stress on a given endocrine gland will impact other bodily functions, such as immunity, digestion, and the nervous system.

Hormones in Action

Endocrinologist and mind-body expert Deepak Chopra, MD, has said that the endocrine system is like a web; if you touch one strand, the whole web trembles. Our endocrine glands diligently and synergistically work to maintain the dynamic internal equilibrium known as homeostasis. The endocrine system is comprised of glands communicating with each other. Within the endocrine system, there are glands that respond to signals from the nervous system. These master glands then send messages in the form of hormones to downstream glands, which respond to these messages by secreting their hormones. In order to maintain internal hormonal stability and responsiveness, each endocrine gland also has receptors for the hormones that its downstream glands secrete. When these receptors are filled by these downstream hormones, a signal is created within that gland to stop producing the hormone that it has been sending as a message. This process, known as negative feedback, allows for hormone production to be continually adjusted to the changing environment of the body. Nutrients, neurons, environmental factors, and other hormones influence hormonal production. This innate rhythmic flow of action, reaction, and interaction creates a dynamically adjusting system.

When the elements of the endocrine system are in step, we are likely to sail through our days without symptoms, sickness, or stress. However, when our hormones and our integrated feedback system are out of sync and unresponsive, so are we. When the finely orchestrated hormonal flow is out of rhythm, it's as if one gland is moving to a waltz while its partner is doing the tango. Being out of sync like this for too long can result in cancer, which capitalizes on the opportunity to cut in, becoming an unwanted dance partner incessantly tapping on your shoulder.

The connection between hormones and cancer goes beyond the commonly identified hormone-dependent cancers: breast, ovarian, and prostate. Beyond influencing many bodily functions, our hormonal milieu also affects malignant cells and can influence the growth of many cancers. This is because all cells have hormone receptors, and no matter where a cell is located, when the matching hormone attaches to a cell's receptor, it may set any number of processes into motion.

Hormones communicate with cells via hormone receptors on cell surfaces and within cells. Hormone receptors have sophisticated antennae waiting patiently for signals. Hormones and hormone receptors can also be compared to a key and a lock. As a hormone (the key) circulates, it looks for a receptor (a lock) on a corresponding cell to open. If the hormone's key fits the lock, the cell "opens," initiating a cascade of activity that ultimately alters the behavior of the cell in a specific way. Hormones are very potent chemicals, and when a hormone enters a cell it causes a chain of events that lead to various actions on the part of the cell and its nucleus. When the lock is held open or opened frequently, this intracellular chain of events happens repeatedly. This may result in an overamplified sequence of events and altered cellular behavior.

This overexpression can become problematic—especially if the cell receiving the hormonal messages is a cancerous cell. One of the key functions of hormones is to stimulate growth. In response to a hormonal signal, the cancerous cell may start to divide; it may send out other chemical messengers to increase its supply of blood or oxygen; or it may secrete hormones of its own that, in turn, stimulate various actions in neighboring cells. This is why, for example, the estrogen receptor status of breast cancer cells is so important. If they do have estrogen receptors, when estrogen binds to those receptors, the cell is encouraged to grow and divide. While there is a strong association between testosterone and androgens and prostate cancer in men, we've chosen to discuss the estrogen-cancer link in women in depth, because that's the most common hormone-cancer link. Nonetheless, the principles discussed in this chapter apply to other hormone-dependent cancers in both men and women.

The interactions between hormones and various physiological systems can also influence cancer development and progression. For example, hormones also activate or inhibit immune function and control the stress response; and to make things more complicated, those two systems interact with each other. When the stress hormone cortisol is present in high concentrations, it compromises the cancer-fighting ability of immune cells. Deficient immunity decreases our tissue defenses, resulting in tissue damage. This damage triggers a hormonal response that leads to more cortisol secretion. Elevated cortisol then suppresses immune function further. A vicious cycle ensues, with elevated cortisol causing impaired immunity, which in and of itself perpetuates elevated cortisol. Ultimately, this cycle can contribute to cancer growth via chronic immune suppression. This is not to say that stress causes cancer. However, the hormonal response to chronic stress, while necessary to manage the stress, can create collateral damage to immunity and this can create an environment that favors cancer development or impedes cancer treatment.

Hormones can also negatively impact health by causing excessive production of cytokines, immune system messenger chemicals that are critical to inflammation, infection, and allergies. You could almost think of cytokines as the "hormones" of the immune system, as they are secreted by one cell and exert their actions by binding to receptors on other cells, sometimes nearby and sometimes in distant areas of the body. They have pronounced effects on the cells they bind to, influencing the cell's function, viability,

Endocrine Glands and Their Hormones

Gland	Primary hormones	Actions
Pineal *(located in brain)*	Melatonin	Regulates daily rhythms such as sleep and wakefulness
Pituitary *(located in brain)*	Growth hormone	Stimulates growth
	ACTH (adrenocorticotropic hormone)	Increases cortisol production
	Luteinizing hormone	Causes ovulation and stimulates production of progesterone and testosterone
	TSH (thyroid-stimulating hormone)	Increases production of thyroxine (T4)
	Prolactin	Induces milk production
Thyroid and parathyroid *(located in front aspect of lower neck)*	Thyroxine and triiodothyronine	Stimulates metabolism and normal growth and development
	Calcitonin	Decreases blood levels of calcium and increases calcium uptake by bone
	Parathyroid hormone	Increases blood level of calcium and stimulates release of calcium from bone
Thymus *(located in the midchest region)*	Thymosin	Involved in immune system development and stimulation
Pancreas, specifically the islets of Langerhans *(located in the right upper quadrant of the abdomen)*	Glucagon	Increases blood glucose levels
	Insulin	Decreases blood glucose, increases cellular glucose utilization, and stimulates glucose storage
Adrenals *(atop the kidneys)*	Cortisol	Suppresses inflammatory reactions, raises blood sugar levels, stimulates mental alertness, suppresses immune activity
Ovaries *(located on each side of the pelvis)*	Estrogens	Involved in menstruation and maintenance of female reproduction
	Progesterone	Involved in menstruation, pregnancy, and lactation
Testes *(located in the scrotum)*	Testosterone	Maintains secondary sex characteristics

and growth. Hormone secretion is intimately connected with cytokine levels. If, for instance, growth hormone levels are elevated, this will result in increased levels of cytokines (such as interleukin-6 and tumor necrosis factor alpha [TNF-a]) that can impair immune surveillance and may hamper cancer treatment. High levels of cytokines are frequently observed in critically ill cancer patients.

One way we maintain healthy hormone balance and endocrine function is through detoxification of excess hormones, and the body has an efficient system for doing this. Most hormones are chemically altered in the liver, then packaged up and eliminated via the stool or urine. This is a critical body function that allows us to maintain hormonal homeostasis in the face of an ever-changing internal and external environment, both of which are under near-constant assault by foreign hormonal compounds. For instance, a wide variety of synthetic chemicals exhibit estrogenic activity, and these chemicals, known as xenoestrogens, are present in the air we breathe, the foods we eat, and food and drink containers. Our internal detoxification system identifies these foreign estrogen-like chemicals and attempts to eliminate them from the body by the usual hormone detoxification pathways. However, too many estrogens can overwhelm the detoxification system. These estrogens are then free to circulate and may find cell receptors to lock onto before they are eliminated. If many of these estrogenic compounds find estrogen receptors on breast cancer cells, for instance, this will stimulate growth of the cancer. Thus, one potential cause of cancer is the dangerous combination of too many estrogenic hormones and a sluggish hormonal detoxification system. (Chapter 12 will give detailed information about detoxification.)

"Estrogens can become carcinogenic only when natural mechanisms of protection [hormonal detoxification] do not work properly in our body," explains researcher Ercole Cavalieri, D.Sc., in an *Ascribe Newswire* article featured on www.mycancercompass.com. Cavalieri and associates published their findings regarding estrogens and increased risk of breast cancer in the journal *Carcinogenesis*. "In fact, if these protections go away due to genetic, lifestyle, or environmental influences, then metabolism of estrogen can get out of balance and cancer can be triggered." The link between hormones and cancer is clear. The most direct connection occurs in cancers that have a higher likelihood of being hormone-dependent, such as breast, ovarian, prostate, and some cases of lung cancer. However, the hormone-cancer connection is deeper and more significant than previously thought. Clinical trials have shown that prescription hormones can increase a woman's risk of developing breast and endometrial cancer, further illustrating the power that hormones can have. Correcting hormonal imbalances is of critical importance in comprehensive treatment of hormone-dependent cancers.

Hormonal Harmony

Just like other important body systems, the endocrine system relies on comprehensive support from a healthy diet, positive lifestyle choices, and dietary supplements (refer to the "Foundational Health Plan" in chapter 4). Beyond the general advice offered in our foundation plan, there are certain considerations specific to hormonal balance.

- Phytoestrogens are naturally occurring compounds present in a wide variety of plants, including some foods. There are more than 500 different phytoestrogenic compounds present in nature. The estrogenic activity of phytoestrogens present in alfalfa, red clover, and soy can help alleviate symptoms of estrogen deficiency, specifically menopause. However, people with a previous or existing diagnosis of an estrogen-dependent cancer or a strong family history of these cancers should avoid high intake of these herbs and foods, especially in concentrated form, such as standardized extracts.

- Soy products are rich in phytoestrogens. The phytoestrogens in soy are its isoflavones, namely, genistein and daidzein. Both of these compounds bind to and stimulate estrogen receptors. As a result, in someone who is estrogen deficient, the inclusion of soy in the diet, whether as tofu, tempeh, soy milk, or miso, will help alleviate some symptoms associated with estrogen deficiency. However, for this same reason, regular consumption of soy foods by those with estrogen-dependent cancers or at high risk for those cancers may cause increased proliferation of those tumors. It is important to understand that the information regarding soy and cancer is not definitive. A recently published prospective cohort trial of postmenopausal women with a history of breast cancer found that those who consumed the highest amount of soy *who were also taking tamoxifen* had a lower risk of recurrence. However, postmenopausal women with a history of estrogen receptor positive breast cancer who were not on tamoxifen and who consumed the highest amount of soy experienced an increased risk of recurrence. Interestingly, regular consumption of soy foods throughout adolescence and early adulthood lowers the risk of premenopausal cancers. This may be due to the fact that soy isoflavones, while stimulating to estrogen receptors, are more weakly stimulating than the estrogens that our bodies produce. Thus, over a lifetime, soy consumption could compete with our own stronger estrogens and in doing so lessen the overall estrogenic activity on breast cells. This may also be due to the fact that soy isoflavones have other anticancer actions including being antioxidant, antiproliferative, and anti-inflammatory. Until we know conclusively about whether soy contributes to the development of estrogen-positive breast cancer, our recommendation is that women should limit their consumption of soy-based foods to one serving daily. Individuals with a diagnosis of an estrogen-dependent cancer or a family history of these cancers should consult with a qualified health-care practitioner before taking soy isoflavones or any other concentrated phytoestrogen extracts.

- Green leafy vegetables and fruits should be included in the diet every day, as these foods contain trace minerals and vitamins that facilitate the health and function of endocrine glands. For instance, vegetables and grains, as well as lean meats, are excellent sources of selenium, which is necessary to activate the thyroid hormone. Kale, collards, okra, and chard are examples of vegetables rich in minerals. Eating fruits and vegetables in a rainbow of colors helps to ensure a wide spectrum of vitamins and minerals.

- Eat organic foods whenever possible to avoid exposure to strongly estrogenic compounds found in pesticides and herbicides. Select meat and dairy products that are guaranteed to be hormone free to avoid additional estrogen exposure. Choosing organic meat and dairy products is also important in terms of reducing your exposure to antibiotics and other chemicals, which can overwhelm the detoxification system.

- Avoid triggers and irritants, such as excessive caffeine, spicy foods, lack of sleep, and alcohol, which can aggravate the symptoms of estrogen deficiency in women and testosterone deficiency in men. Presumably, these various stimulants alter the tone of blood vessels, thereby altering blood flow and contributing to hot flashes (most commonly experienced by menopausal women, women on antiestrogen therapy, and men on androgen therapy).

Regarding dietary supplements, a comprehensive multivitamin-mineral supplement is always a good starting point, but beyond that, the following nutrients and herbs have demonstrated positive effects on hormonal balance and symptoms of hormonal imbalances:

- Antioxidant nutrients, such as vitamins C and E, can help reduce oxidative stress, which can reduce inflammatory triggers for excessive secretion of certain hormones (cortisol, insulin, growth factor), ultimately reducing the number of influences that can encourage cancer cell growth.

- Flavonoids, specifically hesperidin from the inner rind of citrus fruits, strengthen capillary integrity and help reduce hot flashes associated with estrogen deficiency.

- Calcium D-glucarate and indole-3-carbinol (I3C) as found in cruciferous vegetables or as supplemental 3,3'-diindolylmethane (DIM) play a role in metabolizing and thus detoxifying hormones. According to some very preliminary research, these supplements may be helpful in reducing the risk of developing estrogen-dependent cancers. Despite this research, in epidemiological studies the relationship between I3C or DIM and cancer risk is not evident. More data are needed to understand the influence of these compounds on modifying cancer risk.

- Chasteberry extract (*Vitex agnus*) is sometimes used by herbalists for its ability to inhibit prolactin secretion from the pituitary gland. Decreased prolactin appears to lessen menopausal symptoms, namely, hot flashes.

- Melatonin is a hormone secreted by the pineal gland. Melatonin can also be taken as a supplement. It has been shown to reduce estrogen influence by decreasing the synthesis of estrogen by the ovaries, blocking estrogen receptors, and inhibiting the aromatase enzyme (converts adrenal steroids into estrogen and testosterone).

- Mushrooms are natural aromatase inhibitors. Aromatase converts adrenal steroid hormones in fat tissue and in tumor tissue into estrogen or testosterone.

- Probiotics play an important role in hormonal balance. Excess hormones are broken down and then conjugated (bound to a protein) in the liver in order to be secreted into the intestines for elimination. An intestinal overgrowth of certain bacteria, such as *Bacteroides*, *Klebsiella*, and *Proteus* seen, for instance, in meat eaters, can deconjugate hormones, such as estrogen. The free estrogens are then reabsorbed into the blood. Beneficial bacteria such as *Lactobacillus* spp. and *Bifidobacterium* spp. can restore optimal bacterial balance and decrease the deconjugation of estrogen in the intestines.

In addition to diet and supplements, hormonal harmony can be achieved by focusing on the mind-body connection. Exercise, stress reduction, and acupuncture have all been shown to help maintain hormonal balance.

- Exercise helps reduce production of stress hormones (such as cortisol) and releases feel-good endorphins to enhance self-image and improve

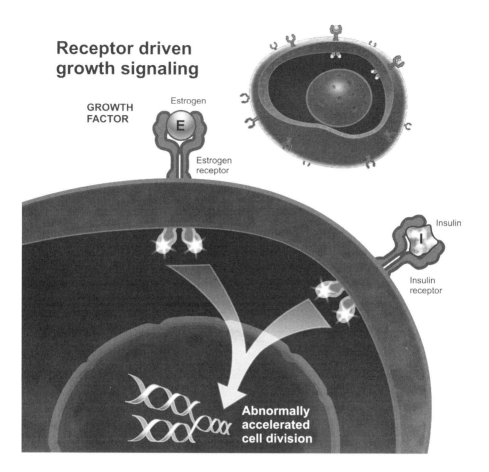

Receptor driven growth signaling

GROWTH FACTOR

Estrogen

E

Estrogen receptor

Insulin

Insulin receptor

Abnormally accelerated cell division

mood. Consistent physical activity also encourages proper digestion and elimination, which supports liver detoxification of hormones, such as estrogen, progesterone, and testosterone. And, as we all know, exercise can help maintain a healthy weight; and since being overweight can lead to excessive production of estrogen, this is extremely important.

- Relaxation and stress reduction techniques (such as meditation, reading, or walking) not only calm the mind, they calm the body, too, helping reduce levels of norepinephrine. Norepinephrine causes the adrenal glands to release cortisol, and as discussed previously, prolonged release of cortisol can disrupt immune function. Chronic stress can also be disruptive to our hormonal balance.

- Acupuncture has been shown to alleviate symptoms of estrogen deficiency, testosterone deficiency, elevated cortisol levels, and ovarian and thyroid disorders.

Hormonal Cancer Treatments in Conventional Medicine

Hormone replacement therapy (HRT) to manage menopause is different from hormonal blockades used to treat cancer. HRT consists of taking supplemental hormones such as estrogen and progesterone (usually synthetic) to increase levels of these hormones in the body. Hormonal therapy for cancer involves blocking the body's production of hormones, such as estrogen, testosterone, or androgens, or preventing hormones from binding to receptors on cancer cells. Hormone therapy for cancer is typically accomplished with the use of medications, although in some cases surgical removal of hormone-producing organs is necessary. Many new hormone drugs have been developed to treat cancer or prevent a recurrence.

Tumors, especially in breast cancer, express high quantities of estrogen and progesterone receptors on their cell surfaces. When estrogen binds to the estrogen receptor, the cell is stimulated to divide and the tumor grows (see the illustration on page 211). Estrogen- and progesterone-positive cancers are usually denoted as ER+ and PR+, while estrogen- and progesterone-negative cancers are denoted as ER- and PR-. Therapies for ER+ cancers include drugs that block the body's production of estrogen, thus preventing estrogen from binding to and activating estrogen receptor positive cancer cells or drugs that decrease the body's production of estrogen. Cancers that are most likely to respond to estrogen blockade include breast, ovarian, and endometrial cancers.

Several basic types of hormonal drugs are currently being used for ER+ cancer treatment: antiestrogens, aromatase inhibitors, luteinizing hormone–releasing hormone agents, and antiandrogens.

Antiestrogens

The first category, antiestrogens, or selective estrogen receptor modulators (SERMs), block estrogen receptors, thereby preventing estrogen from entering the cell and stimulating growth. Tamoxifen is the most well known and commonly used drug in this category and has led to significantly enhanced survival statistics for women with estrogen receptor positive (ER+) breast cancer. Tamoxifen is typically recommended to premenopausal women with a history of early-stage breast cancer in order to reduce the risk of recurrence. Tamoxifen is taken for five years and reduces the risk of breast cancer recurrence for an additional five years after it is discontinued. Tamoxifen reduces the risk of recurrence of invasive breast cancer, primarily estrogen receptor positive tumors, by 50 percent in most women, with women under 40 gaining even greater risk reduction up to 90 percent. Tamoxifen use increases the risk of fractures of the hip, forearm, and spine (due to osteoporosis as a result of estrogen deficiency), but it has no effect on the rate of heart disease (another risk elevated by estrogen deficiency). Other serious risks of tamoxifen include increased incidence of uterine and endometrial cancer, stroke, cataracts, and blood clots. Women taking tamoxifen may also experience symptoms similar to menopause, specifically, decreased libido, vaginal dryness, hot flashes, leg cramps, urinary tract infections, and incontinence. Raloxifene is a newer drug that can be used in place of tamoxifen. It has generally fewer side effects than tamoxifen, although it can cause muscle cramps, vaginal dryness, and weight gain. A five-year study ("Study of Tamoxifen and Raloxifene," or STAR) compared the two and found raloxifene to be as effective as tamoxifen in reducing the risk of invasive breast cancer, while also carrying a lower risk of stroke and cataracts. However, with raloxifene, there was a nonstatistically significant higher risk of noninvasive breast cancer. The risk of other cancers, fractures, ischemic heart disease, and stroke is similar for both drugs. No significant differences exist between tamoxifen and raloxifene in terms of quality-of-life issues. At this point, there is no consensus among medical practitioners about the superiority of tamoxifen or raloxifene. Another choice is toremifene, a synthetic analog of tamoxifen, which binds to and inactivates estrogen receptors. Toremifene binds to estrogen receptors four to five times more effectively than tamoxifen; however, toremifene can cause blood clots and liver inflammation. Toremifene is used in advanced cases of breast cancer in postmenopausal women.

Aromatase Inhibitors

The second category of hormonal drugs for ER+ cancer treatment is aromatase inhibitors. These drugs reduce the body's production of estrogen. In postmenopausal women, once the ovaries are no longer functioning, estrogen is produced in the fat cells. Adrenal androgens stored in fat cells are converted to estrogen with the help of an enzyme called aromatase. Currently, the Food and Drug Administration has approved three aromatase inhibitors: anastrozole, exemestane, and letrozole. These drugs cannot block ovarian estrogen production, so they are not as effective in premenopausal women who still have functioning ovaries.

Aromatase inhibitors have contributed significantly to the survival of postmenopausal women with breast cancer. Disease-free survival is significantly improved with anastrozole versus tamoxifen, an effect that is even more pronounced in women with ER+ and/or PR+ breast cancer. Anastrozole is one of the better-tolerated hormonal therapies, with reduced incidence of hot flashes, strokes, and vaginal bleeding or discharge, and it also carries the lowest risk for endometrial cancer. However, women taking anastrozole tend to have more musculoskeletal disorders and fractures (other than hip fractures) than women taking tamoxifen. Additional side effects of anastrozole and other aromatase inhibitors can include fatigue and dizziness.

Menopausal Management

Until recently, conventional hormone replacement therapy was almost universally recommended as a way to relieve menopausal symptoms. However, results from the Women's Health Initiative (WHI) in the United States and other large studies, such as the Million Women Study in the United Kingdom, have confirmed that conventional hormone replacement therapy (HRT) increases a woman's risk of developing endometrial and breast cancer. For this reason, many women are choosing a more natural approach to help ease their menopausal symptoms.

For some time, many women with a family history or previous diagnosis of breast cancer have been interested in natural alternatives to HRT. However, the WHI has changed the landscape. Now many other women, including those who were previously taking hormone replacement drugs, are also interested in natural alternatives. These women face quite a dilemma. How do they manage their symptoms, which can have significant impacts on quality of life, without increasing their chances of developing cancer or heart disease?

The answer may be found in a natural approach, including certain dietary modifications, lifestyle changes, and dietary supplements of natural hormonal agents, usually phytoestrogens. Many phytoestrogens (compounds from plant sources that have estrogenic effects) have a weaker effect than pharmaceutical agents and do not seem to confer an increased risk of developing cancer, yet they can still provide some symptom relief because of their estrogenic effects. Can phytoestrogens be used by women with a strong family history or personal history of breast, uterine, or ovarian cancers? The answer is likely no. Women in the high-risk category should avoid estrogenic compounds, whether synthetic, conjugated, bioidentical, or plant based. This includes prescription HRT drugs, estriol from a compounding pharmacist, soy isoflavones, and extracts of phytoestrogenic herbs such as alfalfa, red clover, gingko, and Panax ginseng.

Fear not, however; there are safe and effective alternatives. The following menopause management protocol is recommended for women who have a strong family history or personal history of estrogen-dependent cancer.

A wholesome diet featuring fresh fruits and vegetables, whole grains, and organic foods and minimizing or avoiding spicy or salty foods, alcohol, and caffeine can help alleviate many symptoms. Regular and sufficient sleep,

Ovarian tumors, infertility, and decreased bone mineral density have also been observed.

Luteinizing Hormone–Releasing Hormone Agents

Another category of hormonal drugs is luteinizing hormone–releasing hormone (LHRH) agents. These drugs signal the pituitary to release luteinizing hormone, which shuts down the production of estrogen and progesterone by the ovaries and testosterone by the testes. Drugs in this category include leuprolide for prostate cancer, goserelin for breast and prostate cancer, and triptorelin for ovarian and prostate cancer. These drugs are a mainstay of conventional management of advanced prostate cancer.

In men with prostate cancer, survival after treatment with LHRH drugs is equivalent to survival after removal of a testicle. The available LHRH drugs are equally effective, and no LHRH drug is superior to the others when adverse effects are considered. These drugs are not without side effects. Osteoporosis, unfavorable body composition (including breast enlargement),

although elusive for some women, is an important component of a symptom reduction plan. Here is a list of common symptoms and the nutrients and herbs that may help (for dosages, see the appendix):

- **Hot flashes and night sweats:** vitamin E, hesperidin, gamma oryzanol, (rice bran oil extract), and sage; black cohosh is also helpful.

- **Vaginal dryness:** vitamin E topically or via vaginal suppositories.

- **Anxiety and other mood swings:** gamma oryzanol and herbal sedatives such as chamomile, valerian, and St. John's wort (caution should be exercised when taking St. John's wort with other medications).

- **Insomnia:** melatonin, valerian, hops, or passionflower.

- **Lack of energy:** Siberian ginseng, CoQ10.

Many over-the-counter homeopathic remedies can also provide relief for some of the key menopausal symptoms. Commonly indicated homeopathic remedies include Sepia, Pulsatilla, and Apis.

Oftentimes, more serious worries weigh heavily on women as they go through menopause, including heart disease and osteoporosis. Heart disease remains the number one killer of women, and most heart disease occurs after menopause. Adding CoQ10 to your daily supplement regimen may be helpful, as it provides support to the heart. Additionally, garlic, fish oil, and niacin can be used to reduce the risk of developing clots and forming arterial plaques. Osteoporosis increases the risk of hip, foot, and vertebral fractures. Women at high risk of developing osteoporosis should take a quality calcium-magnesium bone-building supplement that also contains vitamin D and boron. However, because boron increases the action of estrogen on estrogen receptors, it could theoretically increase stimulation of estrogen-dependent cancer cells. For this reason, those with estrogen receptor positive cancers should not take supplemental boron.

Managing perimenopause and menopause can be very difficult for some women. Fortunately, there are many excellent books available that describe comprehensive ways to naturally and safely navigate through these challenging life transitions.

sexual dysfunction, and reduced quality of life are experienced by men undergoing testosterone deprivation therapy. Women taking LHRH are likely to experience symptoms similar to menopause, which can include fatigue, hot flashes, night sweats, mood swings, nausea, osteoporosis, and weight gain.

Antiandrogen Hormone Therapy

The final category of hormone therapy is antiandrogens. Antiandrogens, such as bicalutamide and flutamide, bind to androgen receptors and inhibit androgen uptake in androgen-sensitive prostate cancer cells. These drugs can cause heart attacks and high blood pressure, aggravate asthma, and contribute to osteoporosis. Other common side effects include hot flashes, nausea, dizziness, constipation, and pain.

Hormonal Drugs and Side Effects

Most of the time, hormone therapy is given as part of a multimodality treatment after chemotherapy, radiation, or surgery. Unfortunately, most

Kathi Magee: Breast Cancer Diagnosed at Age 34

I was on top of the world. Not only was I blessed with two beautiful sons, I worked with my mom and my sister. Life was great. Then one day it all fell apart.

It was just before my thirty-fifth birthday. I felt irritated that I had to take time off to go to my annual physical. I felt fine and was sure that nothing was wrong. During the breast exam, my doctor felt a lump. I recall that he had me feel it. My first thought was "How could I have missed that?" The doctor didn't say the C word, it was the B word—biopsy.

I was devastated. I went to work to tell my sister, Karolyn, and our mom, and just sobbed. We tried to be optimistic, but we have an extensive family history of cancer, specifically breast cancer. I think we all knew that it had finally hit home—our home. I pulled myself together and waited for the results.

After the biopsy, the C word came and I was diagnosed with cancer. It was like being forever branded. Once you have cancer, you can't go back.

I remember the week between the biopsy and the lumpectomy. I spent most nights sitting alone in my room crying, wondering why this was happening to me. I was so scared. I couldn't leave my boys, not yet. They were only nine and ten and they still needed me. I tried to be strong at work in front of my mom and sister. At night I would let down my guard and just cry—and pray.

Then it hit me. It was like a switch I could turn on—I found my inner strength. I had heard that term *inner strength* before but never thought much about it. I don't know if I just cried so much that there was nothing left to do but be strong. But I knew I was going to fight. I would do whatever I had to do to get through the surgery and treatment. I was simply not ready to leave!

My cancer was caught early. The tumor size was 1 inch, and the treatment called for a lumpectomy with seven weeks of radiation to follow. The type of cancer was very rare, but it happened to be a "good" rare, with a low rate of recurrence. I breezed through the treatment. With the support of my mom and sister, and all of my family and friends, I felt stronger than I ever thought possible.

advanced hormone-sensitive cancers will eventually become resistant to hormone treatment. According to the accumulated results of clinical trials, this is why women should not take tamoxifen for more than five years; after that, it is typically no longer effective.

While conventional hormonal cancer treatments show promise and have demonstrated effectiveness in certain populations, their use is not always without adverse effects. Quality-of-life issues associated with side effects should always be carefully considered. Complementary therapies can help manage some of the adverse effects of hormone therapy and therefore can be an important part of this treatment. Though certain supplements also have powerful effects on the endocrine system, they have not been well studied, so currently they cannot take the place of conventional hormone therapy for cancer. However, some nutrients and supplements can help offset the side effects and potentially enhance the anticancer effects of these drugs. Conversely, some nutrients and supplements should be avoided while undergoing hormone therapy. (For more information, refer to the chart "Hormone Drugs and Their Nutrient and Herb Interactions" on pages 156 and 157.)

Unfortunately, three years later a mammogram showed a small lump. It turned out to be the same type of rare cancer cells in the same area. While I could have chosen to wait and watch the area, I instead decided to go through with a mastectomy. Some might say I had a recurrence. I prefer to think those cells were left over from the first time.

I thought I was done with cancer and then when I was 48 years old, cancer paid still another visit. This time it was in my other breast and this time it was a more aggressive cancer. I would have to undergo surgery, reconstruction, and chemotherapy. I consulted with Dr. Lise Alschuler and my sister throughout my entire treatment process and used an integrative approach thanks to this book. I even gave a copy of the book to my oncologist. Today, I am doing better than ever. I met a wonderful man to share my life with and my sons continue to be the joys of my life.

One of the most important things you can do if you have been diagnosed with cancer is find out everything you can about the type of cancer you have and treatment options. Ask questions. Don't assume anything. If you are informed, you will feel more in control. If you have several options to consider, make an informed decision and then embrace that decision and don't look back. I chose an integrative approach that included dietary and lifestyle changes, nutritional supplements, and conventional treatment.

Surround yourself with friends, family, and positive people. There's nothing better than hearing about people who have survived cancer. I am living proof that cancer is not a death sentence. There is hope.

I mentioned earlier that once you have cancer, you can never go back. I'm not so sure that's a bad thing. While I wish cancer didn't exist and people didn't have to suffer, having cancer has made me stronger inside. I don't take things for granted anymore, and I have learned to really appreciate every day of my life.

I couldn't have traveled this journey alone. I would not have managed without the support of my family and friends. It has also helped to know that I have a purpose and my life has meaning. My two young boys are now fine young men. I am proud of them—I am proud of us.

In addition, it is important to support your body by using the comprehensive mind-body-spirit suggestions outlined in chapter 4.

The Endocrine Web of Life

The endocrine system embodies both strength and vulnerability. It controls the growth and development of the human body and, when balanced, its activity can positively impact health in powerful ways. Yet it is susceptible to imbalance, and the results of that imbalance are so profound as to potentially be a form of physiological chaos.

The silk strand of a spider's web is as strong as a steel thread the same size. In addition to being strong, it is flexible, sometimes stretching to double its length. The web of the endocrine system stretches throughout the human body, touching and influencing all other significant body functions. It is resilient and rhythmic as it adapts to our internally changing environment or merely holds on during the windstorms of our lives. But despite this strength, the endocrine system needs our support. Through healthy diet, lifestyle factors, and appropriate nutritional supplements, we can help create internal harmony, prevent illness, manage side effects, and even treat cancer.

Among the myriad of organs and tissues involved in the endocrine system is the pancreas. In addition to secreting enzymes essential for effective digestion, the pancreas produces insulin and glucagons, substances that help manage blood sugar levels and glucose metabolism. Though you may find it surprising, insulin is in fact a hormone, so the next chapter on insulin resistance and glucose metabolism and how they relate to cancer is really a continuation of this chapter's theme.

eleven

Insulin Resistance

According to the U.S. Department of Agriculture, the average American consumes between 150 and 170 pounds of simple sugars a year. Sugar consumption has increased dramatically since the introduction of high-fructose corn syrup just 30 years ago. High-fructose corn syrup, a form of sugar, is a key ingredient in numerous products. High sugar consumption has been linked to obesity and many illnesses, including cancer.

To fully understand the connection between insulin resistance and cancer, you must first understand blood glucose, which refers to the sugar that is circulating in your bloodstream, and how it gets there. What does it mean to have normal blood glucose or blood sugar levels? What happens when there is an increase or decrease of blood glucose? And how does insulin resistance potentially lead to cancer?

According to researchers from the Johns Hopkins Bloomberg School of Public Health, published in the *American Journal of Epidemiology*, "in the United States, impaired glucose tolerance [insulin resistance] is an independent predictor for cancer mortality." The results of their study demonstrated that people with insulin resistance were four times more likely to die from colon cancer and nearly twice as likely to die from any other type of cancer. In a large study of postmenopausal nondiabetic women, breast cancer incidence rates were 2.4-fold greater among those with the highest fasting insulin levels compared with the lowest fasting insulin level. Breast cancer and other estrogen receptor positive cancers are particularly susceptible to the growth influence of insulin because insulin and estradiol act in concert to promote cell cycle progression. Insulin resistance has been linked to the incidence and progression of several cancers, which has led many to examine the role of sugar in cancer development.

The insulin resistance story isn't just about sugar, though it plays a central role. We have to take a step back and look at carbohydrates as a whole. There are two different types of carbohydrates. Simple carbohydrates are made up of single sugar molecules or two sugar molecules joined together. Complex carbohydrates are also made up of sugars, but the sugar molecules are strung together to form longer, more complex chains. Complex carbohydrates include starches and fiber, and they are abundant in most plant foods, especially grains, legumes, and vegetables. In the body, complex carbohydrates are ultimately broken down into usable energy units—glucose molecules.

The simple carbohydrates, which are included in the 150+ pounds of added sugar consumed by the average American each year, are easy to recognize. They show up in the form of table sugar and sugar in sodas and other snacks. In fact, a key ingredient in fat-free foods is often sugar. So, you may think you are making a healthy choice, but it is possible that you are not.

The situation with complex carbohydrates is a bit more complicated. The body needs glucose for energy, and most complex carbohydrates in their natural form do a good job of supplying energy to the body in a slow, steady stream, which is better for us. But once complex carbohydrates are refined—stripped of fiber and other essential nutrients during milling and other processes—they behave much more like simple carbohydrates.

In truth, processing also plays an important role where simple carbohydrates are concerned. For example, fruits are fairly high in simple carbohydrates, yet they are a healthful food. Why? Because in their whole form they come packaged with complex carbohydrates, vitamins, minerals, enzymes, phytochemicals, and more—a veritable cornucopia of healthy nutrients. Plus, the fiber that they contain helps moderate the release of sugars into the bloodstream.

The insulin resistance story takes many twists and turns beyond what you eat. It includes when you eat, how much you eat, and many other factors, such as skipping meals, snacking habits, stress, and exercise. In this chapter, we'll explore how insulin resistance develops and how you can avoid or reverse it. When it comes to cancer, the body is better able to protect healthy cells and kill cancerous cells when blood glucose metabolism is normal. Conversely, blood sugar imbalances and insulin dysregulation can contribute to cancer growth and development and may impede successful cancer treatment.

Initiation of Insulin Resistance

The pancreas is one of the key organs of the endocrine system. As with all the organs of the endocrine system, the pancreas releases powerful hormones that significantly impact health. In addition to producing enzymes that aid digestion, the pancreas also secretes insulin and glucagon. These two hormones work together to ensure that blood sugar levels are always balanced and in the normal range. This is critical for many physiological systems because glucose is the primary energy source for all the cells in the body. This includes the nervous system (brain, spinal cord, and nerves), which is responsible for a complex array of important functions, including autonomic muscle and organ function, thought, emotions, and memory. Glucose is also essential for the production of energy in all tissues of the body, including the heart, muscles, and immune system.

The speed at which glucose is released into the bloodstream depends on a variety of factors, including what, when, and how much you eat. The pancreas will secrete either insulin or glucagon in response to the blood glucose level. If you skip a meal and eat fewer carbohydrates, your blood sugar level will decrease, which causes the pancreas to release glucagon, which in turn stimulates the liver to convert glycogen to glucose. (Glycogen, which consists of a long chain of glucose molecules, is the principal form in which the body stores glucose for later use.) Glucose is then released into the blood to meet the body's energy needs.

On the other hand, if you eat a lot of sugar and refined carbohydrates, your blood sugar level will rise, causing the pancreas to release insulin. Insulin facilitates cellular uptake of glucose. So, glucagon increases the blood glucose level while insulin decreases it. (The blood glucose flowchart on page 222 depicts this dynamic.) These two hormones—glucagon and insulin—work together continuously to keep blood glucose in the normal range. Whether you eat a lot or a little, go on a sugar binge, or skip a meal, this hormonal process is always at work.

Typically, we eat too many refined carbohydrates and simple sugars, which rapidly flood the bloodstream with glucose. Over time, as blood sugar levels are repeatedly elevated, tissues become resistant to the effects of insulin. It's as if insulin is knocking on the cellular door. At first, that door opens to insulin's knock. However, after a while, the irritating knocking is not heard and the door no longer opens. This is insulin resistance, also known as metabolic syndrome or syndrome X. It is a precursor to pancreatic failure in response to persistently elevated blood glucose levels, and it can lead to diabetes. It can also give cancer cells an unfair advantage.

Blood Glucose Flowchart

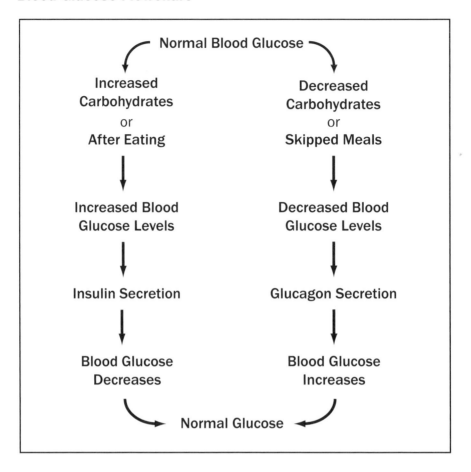

How Insulin Resistance Fuels Cancer

When the body's own cells and tissues stop opening the door to insulin, this doesn't mean the insulin goes away. It will keep knocking until it finds a door that still opens. Cells with the most doors (insulin receptors) are the ones that will likely still have doors that open. Cancer cells are loaded with insulin receptors, and they tend to retain their ability to accept insulin even once insulin resistance has developed. When insulin binds to the insulin receptors on a cancer cell, the cancer cell will be stimulated to divide. On a cancer cell, insulin acts as both a growth factor and a conveyor of glucose.

"As long as the pancreas can continue to produce large amounts of insulin in the face of insulin resistance, some individuals may avoid diabetes," explains Edward L. Giovannucci, MD, of the Harvard School of Public Health. "However, these individuals may be the ones most susceptible to cancer because they have the highest circulating insulin concentrations."

Like all cells in the body, cancer uses sugar as fuel. The primary method by which cells obtain sugar is through a process known as glucose uptake. Several studies have demonstrated that there is a high rate of glucose transfer from the blood into cancer cells. This is because cancer cells have more insulin receptors on their cell surfaces than do healthy cells. Insulin receptors facilitate the cellular uptake of glucose. It has been speculated that efficient glucose utilization gives cancer a competitive edge as it attempts to grow rapidly. It is believed that increased glucose uptake can also help protect cancer cells from apoptosis, or cell death.

It is true that cancer has a "sweet tooth." This may cause you to wonder whether you can eliminate cancer by avoiding sugar in your diet. Unfortunately, it is not that simple.

Cancer is extremely aggressive and adaptable. If you reduce your sugar and carbohydrate intake, cancer can adapt and thrive with less fuel. And because cancer cells are loaded with insulin receptors, they have a higher chance of obtaining glucose than healthy cells do. Therefore, it is nearly impossible to reduce glucose levels low enough to selectively kill the cancer. All cells require glucose to survive. The body needs glucose for energy, metabolism, and other important body functions. If you try to eliminate all sugar in an effort to starve cancer cells, you will starve your healthy cells first. In addition, avoiding sugar may lead some people to stop eating fruits and high-sugar vegetables like tomatoes and carrots. This is counterproductive because fruits and vegetables are valuable sources of anticancer agents such as antioxidants, flavonoids, and fiber, as well as vitamins the immune system needs to fight cancer.

Eliminating sugar and carbohydrates will not cure your cancer. However, a diet high in simple sugars and refined carbohydrates is dangerous and should be avoided because it "feeds" the cancer and because it leads to insulin resistance. Such a diet ultimately favors cancer growth, specifically, colon, pancreatic, kidney, breast, and endometrial cancers. On the other hand, a diet low in simple sugars and refined carbohydrates will prevent and help correct insulin resistance, thereby making the body a less hospitable host for cancer and more receptive to cancer treatment.

The Insulin Resistance–Diabetes-Cancer Connection

In addition to the strong link between obesity and cancer, a growing body of evidence makes a link between diabetes and cancer, as well. This is most likely due to the problems associated with insulin resistance; just as insulin resistance can fatigue the pancreas and ultimately develop into the insulin dysfunction known as diabetes, so too can the progression of insulin resistance heighten one's risk of cancer. In the *Journal of the National Cancer Institute*, Swedish researchers confirmed the association between diabetes and colon cancer. After their review of 15 clinical studies, they found a significant increase in the risk of colon cancer for people who also were diagnosed with diabetes.

Insulin is not just a hormone—it is a *growth* hormone that has powerful effects on cellular development and, ultimately, cell survival. In chapter 10, we discussed problems associated with excess estrogens in the bloodstream. A similar situation exists with insulin. There are insulin receptors on a variety of cells, and excess insulin molecules in the bloodstream are searching for homes, receptors they can lock on to. Once insulin connects to a receptor, one of three outcomes can occur:

1. The cell will divide.

2. Levels of other, more potent growth factors will be increased in the cell, causing cell division.

3. Cells will become more sensitive to other growth factors.

Growth factors are molecules that, when bound to a cell's receptors, stimulate division of that cell and subsequent growth of the tissue or tumor. Insulin-like growth factor (IGF) is a powerful growth factor, and although it is necessary for the regulation of normal physiology, it is also a very potent cancer-promoting agent. "A number of studies now show that individuals with higher levels of circulating IGFs are at increased risk for developing colon, premenopausal breast, and aggressive prostate cancers," according to Dr. Giovannucci. "Thus, in an insulin resistant state, such as induced by obesity, the higher circulating levels of insulin may have a cancer-promoting influence for at least some tissues."

Reversing Insulin Resistance

According to study results presented at the 2006 meeting of the American Diabetes Association, half of all Americans will develop insulin resistance, increasing their risk of developing diabetes, heart disease, and cancer. This is shocking, but luckily this condition can often be reversed. If you're concerned that insulin resistance may be an issue for you, your doctor can perform tests to assess the situation. One common test involves fasting, then drinking a standardized glucose solution. Blood is drawn before you drink the solution and then at regular intervals afterward to study how your glucose metabolism is functioning.

Diet and Exercise

Diet and exercise are the best ways to reverse insulin resistance. Although some studies have demonstrated that even people with a normal weight can have insulin resistance, weight reduction in overweight individuals has been shown to help reverse insulin resistance. A study featured in the *Journal of the American College of Nutrition* demonstrated that a moderate increase in physical activity along with a low-calorie, high-protein diet resulted in weight loss, as well as significant improvement in insulin sensitivity in premenopausal women.

A diet that emphasizes whole grains, fruits, and vegetables can help balance blood glucose levels. By reducing consumption of refined carbohydrates and sugars (any processed carbohydrates, such as white flour or high-fructose corn syrup), you can maintain a healthy weight and help reverse insulin resistance. This type of diet will also enhance your cancer treatment plan. Simple sugars and refined carbohydrates, such as added sweeteners, sugary drinks, candy, pastries, sugary snack foods, and anything made from refined flours—including bread and pasta—should be avoided.

At the same time, increasing fiber intake in the form of whole and unprocessed grains, as well as legumes, vegetables, and fruits, will improve your glucose metabolism. The body takes longer to break down these foods, thus avoiding releasing a rush of glucose into the blood. Refined carbohydrates, on the other hand, are processed similarly to simple sugars, sending a rush of sugar into the bloodstream and causing insulin levels to rise. As with managing a dam, it is usually much better to open the gate slowly so as not to flood the surrounding region. Unprocessed complex carbohydrates in the form of high-fiber foods allow the body to open the gate slowly, avoiding saturation of the bloodstream with insulin. For more information on sugar and fiber, refer to the sidebar on pages 226 and 227.

For more diet and lifestyle recommendations, refer to the "Foundational Health Plan" featured on page 84 of chapter 4. In addition to dietary changes, exercise has been scientifically demonstrated to prevent and improve insulin resistance. A recent study featured in *Circulation Journal* showed that exercise training improved insulin resistance in patients with chronic heart failure. Another recent study, from the University of California, Los Angeles, used a 16-week resistance-training program to increase insulin sensitivity among overweight Latino teenage boys. Researchers observed significant improvements in insulin resistance in this population. A combination of regular aerobic and anaerobic exercise is most beneficial.

Along with diet and exercise, a variety of herbs and nutrients can help curb or reverse insulin resistance. (For information about dosages, see the appendix.)

- *Alpha-lipoic acid*: Also known as thioctic acid, alpha-lipoic acid is an antioxidant and can also help regenerate other antioxidants. In vitro studies have shown that alpha-lipoic acid can increase cellular glucose

Hidden Sugars and Helpful Fiber

In order to prevent or reverse insulin resistance, you must become a proficient label reader. Pay careful attention to the first few ingredients listed. If the first ingredient is sugar, find out how much sugar has been added. Avoid drinks and snacks that have sugar listed as the first, second, or third ingredient. These foods typically have no nutritional value and instead simply load up the body with empty fuel. And remember, sugar appears in many guises, including the following: corn syrup, fructose, glucose, lactose, maltose, sucrose, and white grape juice concentrate.

The average soft drink has around 30 grams of sugar per 8 ounces, which is more than 6 teaspoons of sugar. That means that a 32-ounce soft drink has more than 25 teaspoons, or ½ cup, of sugar. Diet soda is not a good alternative because it contains aspartame and other harmful chemicals. Try natural soft drinks. They typically have less sugar and often have added beneficial ingredients like green tea and other nutrients.

Try to keep track of your daily sugar intake. According to the U.S. Department of Agriculture, a diet of 2,000 calories per day should not include more than 10 teaspoons of added sugar (meaning that just one supersized soft drink puts you way over the daily limit). Added sugar consumption can be hard to track because sugar, in so many forms, is added to so many processed foods. However, food supply data from the U.S. Department of Agriculture indicates that in 1996 each American consumed about 32 teaspoons, or ⅔ cup, of added sugar every day.

Because complex carbohydrates are converted to glucose in the body, carbohydrate consumption should be monitored as well. The healthiest carbohydrates are those closest to their natural state: whole grains and products made from whole grains. Because they have more fiber and break down more slowly, they are better for blood sugar control. Refined carbohydrates, on the other hand, which have been stripped of fiber and other important nutrients, are broken down more quickly, and as a result they can trigger a rush of insulin into the bloodstream, just like sugars do. As far as health is concerned, there's a world of difference between commercial white bread and a whole wheat kernel. There are gradations along the spectrum between the two, but to the extent possible,

uptake and help reverse insulin resistance. Clinical studies demonstrate that patients with diabetic neuropathy (nerve damage) show improvement with either intravenous or oral supplementation of alpha-lipoic acid. Neuropathy is also a common side effect of many chemotherapy drugs; however, alpha-lipoic acid is not typically helpful for this type of neuropathy.

- *B vitamins*: The B vitamins include thiamin (B_1), riboflavin (B_2), niacin (B_3), pantothenic acid (B_5), pyridoxine (B_6), folic acid (B_9), and cobalamin (B_{12}). Deficiencies of folic acid, B_6, and B_{12} have been linked to high homocysteine levels—a risk factor for both heart disease and cancer. Elevated homocysteine has also been linked with insulin resistance. Niacin has been shown to be beneficial in helping control blood glucose levels. Additionally, B_6 helps activate insulin receptors, thereby reducing insulin resistance.

opt for 100 percent whole grain products as often as you can.

Dietary fiber will help control blood sugar levels and assist with proper digestion, elimination, and detoxification, so look for foods that contain at least 2 grams of fiber per serving. The American Dietetic Association recommends that a diet of 2,000 calories per day should contain 25 grams of fiber and a diet of 2,500 or more calories should have 35 grams. Below is a list of some foods and their fiber content.

Food	Serving size	Grams of fiber per serving
Cooked garbanzo beans	1 cup	12
Cooked split peas	½ cup	8.1
Cooked lentils	½ cup	7.8
Raisin bran	1 cup	7.5
Cooked spinach	½ cup	7.0
Cooked fresh broccoli	¾ cup	7.0
Wheat bran flakes	¾ cup	4.6
Dried figs	2	4.6
Pears	1	4.0
Sliced strawberries	1 cup	3.8
Cooked brown rice	1 cup	3.5
Mixed dry-roasted nuts	1 ounce	2.6

- **Chromium**: This trace mineral is found in brewer's yeast, whole grain breads, fruits such as apples, bananas, and oranges, and vegetables such as green peppers, spinach, and carrots. According to the *Encyclopedia of Nutritional Supplements*, "The primary sign of chromium deficiency is glucose intolerance characterized by elevated blood sugar and insulin levels." Many studies have demonstrated that chromium can help control blood sugar levels.

- **Coenzyme Q10**: Animal models have shown that administration of this naturally occurring compound lowers circulating levels of insulin. A 12-week, randomized controlled trial involving 74 adults with type 2 diabetes and insulin resistance found that 200 mg of CoQ10 improved insulin sensitivity and blood sugar control.

- **Essential fatty acids**: Some studies have demonstrated that omega-3 fatty acids can help increase insulin sensitivity and control blood glucose levels. A diet high in cod protein and essential fatty acids has been demonstrated in a clinical trial to improve insulin sensitivity in obese, insulin-resistant men and women. Conjugated linoleic acid (CLA), a type of omega-6 fatty acid, may also help increase insulin sensitivity. Furthermore, insulin sensitivity progressively improves as the proportion of monounsaturated fats (olive oil) with respect to saturated fats increases.

- **Flax lignans**: Flaxseeds and flax oil are considered to be healthy sources of complex carbohydrates (lignans), phytoestrogens, and essential fatty acids such as ALA. In animal studies, the flaxseed lignan secoisolariciresinol diglucoside (SDG) has been shown to reduce levels of insulin growth factors in the blood. The reduction of insulin growth factors reduces tumor growth signals and can also decrease insulin resistance.

- **Green tea**: As discussed in earlier chapters, green tea and its active compounds have been studied extensively for cancer prevention and, more recently, cancer treatment. Preliminary animal studies have also demonstrated that green tea can improve insulin resistance.

- **Gymnema**: The Ayurvedic herb *Gymnema sylvestre* has been shown to help control blood sugar levels. Gymnema rejuvenates the function of the insulin-secreting cells in the pancreas. This is particularly important for diabetics. An animal study done by researchers at the University of Chicago Medical Center demonstrated that gymnema reduced body weight and improved glucose tolerance. Interestingly, liquid extracts of gymnema have the unique ability to selectively numb the sweet taste receptors on the tongue. After taking a swish of gymnema, a bite of chocolate tastes like bitter butterfat. Anecdotally, this property has been reported to be quite helpful for people trying to reduce their sugar intake.

- **Magnesium**: Magnesium is an important mineral for bone and heart health, but it also has many other benefits. There is a large concentration of magnesium in the body, and its primary role is to activate enzymes. It can increase insulin receptor sensitivity, and conversely, low levels of magnesium can result in a worsening of insulin resistance. Researchers from the University of Virginia have also shown that magnesium deficiency is associated with insulin resistance in obese children. They conclude in the journal *Diabetes Care* that "magnesium supplementation or increased intake of magnesium-rich foods may be an important tool in the prevention of type 2 diabetes in obese children." Magnesium-rich foods include wheat bran, nuts, tofu, brown rice, figs, apricots, dates, garlic, and fresh green peas.

- **Mushrooms**: Some mushroom extracts such as *Agaricus blazei* extract and maitake extract have each been shown in clinical trials to lower both insulin and blood sugar and to reduce insulin resistance.

- **Probiotics**: High-fat diets lead to insulin resistance. An animal study has found that oral probiotics treatment significantly reduces this insulin resistance induced by a high-fat diet.

- **Vitamin D**: A randomized six-week-long trial of 100 men over the age of 35 found that vitamin D_3 supplementation (three injected doses of vitamin D_3 of 120,000 IU each every 2 weeks) improved postprandial insulin sensitivity in men likely to have insulin resistance (obese but nondiabetic). Other trials that have utilized lower doses (400 IU) of orally supplemented vitamin D have not demonstrated this effect.

Breaking the Cycle

Preventing and reversing insulin resistance requires us to break the cycle of constant insulin secretion. To do so, we must do more than simply reduce or eliminate simple sugars; we need to avoid refined carbohydrates and eat more whole grains and complex carbohydrates in their natural forms. We also need to exercise to control blood sugar levels and maintain normal body weight. Specific nutrients and herbs may also help break the cycle that creates and maintains insulin resistance.

twelve

Digestion and Detoxification

Aside from your skin, your digestive system has the most contact with the outside world. From mouth to anus, this specialized canal accepts substances from the outside world, breaks them down, samples them for microbes, extracts nutrients, and discards the remainder. The digestive system, also known as the gastrointestinal system, is the ultimate food processor, security checkpoint, and garbage disposal. The goal is clear: turn food into fuel that is free of contaminants. From start to finish, it takes anywhere from one to three days for food to make it through the methodical, step-by-step process of the digestive system.

When everything is running smoothly, this process can easily be taken for granted. But when the digestive system is out of sync, you'll probably notice it immediately. Digestive dysfunction can be uncomfortable and painful, and can even result in serious illnesses such as cancer. In addition, digestive issues can arise during and after cancer treatment. Cancers directly connected to the digestive system include esophageal, stomach, colon, gallbladder, liver, and pancreatic. This is sufficient reason to support this key body system. But beyond that, unhealthy digestion, detoxification, and elimination can also indirectly contribute to other cancers.

Proper digestion has far-reaching health implications, as it influences all other body functions. A well-functioning digestive system is essential for efficient absorption of nutrients—nutrients that are essential for the function of every organ and cell in the body. Nutrients, and the energy derived from them, are essential for bone and muscle growth, neurological function, brain activity, blood formation, heart action, reproductive function, glucose metabolism, hormone synthesis, immune response, tissue repair, and a lengthy list of other physical functions.

The Digestive System in Action

The process of digestion may seem simple enough; after all, what goes in must come out. However, a lot can happen along the digestive path. The conversion of food to fuel requires both physical and chemical processing. Here are the basic steps of the digestive process:

1. In the mouth, chewing physically breaks down the food and saliva releases enzymes that start the chemical process of digestion.

2. The muscles of the esophagus narrow and expand in order to transport the food from the mouth to the stomach, where a valve opens to accept the food mass.

3. In the stomach, the food is showered with digestive chemicals, primarily consisting of stomach acid (hydrochloric acid, or HCl), for about three hours. The food is churned in the stomach as the acid breaks it down into smaller pieces before sending it on its way to the small intestine.

4. The gallbladder releases bile into the beginning of the small intestine—the duodenum and the jejunum. Bile, which is formed in the liver and stored in the gallbladder, dissolves fats into the watery food mass for easier absorption and elimination. (Bile also contains waste products that are secreted into the intestines for removal from the body.) The small intestine additionally receives digestive juices secreted by the pancreas, which help break down carbohydrates and proteins. Other enzymes, produced by the intestinal wall, also play a role in this phase. As the food makes its journey down the 25-foot-long, winding road of the small intestine, all of these processes are regulated by hormones and nerves.

5. While the food is still in the small intestine, islands of immune cells sample it for bacterial contaminants; any that are found are neutralized and passed into the large intestine. As the food progresses through the small intestine, it is broken down enough to be absorbed as nutrients. The small intestine consists of folds of tissue coated with villi—minute fingerlike projections that absorb nutrients into the bloodstream. One of the main activities that takes place in the small intestine is absorption. The partially digested food, known as chyme, is a thick, semifluid paste at this point. It passes across millions of

villi, which transport vitamins, minerals, proteins, carbohydrates, and fats across the intestinal lining and into the bloodstream. Following the flurry of activity in the small intestine, all that is left in the large intestine is a little water, some water-soluble vitamins, indigestible materials, and waste products. Only about one-tenth of the food and beverages we consume make it to the large intestine for elimination; the rest is absorbed through the villous lining of the small intestine. These nutrients absorbed through the small intestine are carried through the bloodstream and lymphatics directly to the liver.

6. The liver is considered part of the digestive system in that it screens all the compounds absorbed from the digestive system. Certain compounds are modified into less toxic forms, while others are altered into forms that other tissues of the body can use.

7. Food-derived material that is not absorbed, along with secreted waste products, moves into the large intestine, also known as the colon. The large intestine is not called large because of its length, but because of its diameter; in fact, it is only about one-fourth the length of the small intestine. The main function of the large intestine is to condense the remaining material into stool to be eliminated. During this process, excess water and certain water-soluble vitamins are absorbed into the blood from the large intestine. The resulting mass becomes drier and more formed; the material sits at the base of the colon for about 12 to 48 hours, until it is expelled via a bowel movement. The material loses about two-thirds of its size as it travels through the small intestine and large intestine. It is optimal to have a well-formed, easy-to-pass bowel movement one to three times daily.

Leaky Gut Syndrome

The absorptive process does not always work smoothly. There can be a number of causes, but one fairly common cause is leaky gut syndrome. In this syndrome, the intestinal wall becomes too permeable, allowing toxic particles that are normally contained within the intestines to instead pass through the intestinal barrier into the bloodstream. Larger food particles that are only partially digested also leak into the blood. Both of these—the toxic compounds and the larger molecules—require detoxification in the liver (see the illustration on page 235). This is problematic, because excessive detoxification can contribute to proliferation of free radicals and inflammation. Furthermore, the body considers the larger food particles that leak across the intestinal barrier to be foreign compounds. This triggers an immune response, which can ultimately lead to food allergies and autoimmune disease.

Leaky gut syndrome is caused by anything that inflames or damages the lining of the small intestine, including

- Inadequate digestion in the stomach

- Intolerance of specific foods

- Bacterial overgrowth

- Free radical stress

- Certain medications

- Impairment of normal intestinal movement (motility)

Leaky gut syndrome will often present itself as food intolerances or allergies to certain foods. Symptoms of leaky gut syndrome can be quite varied, and may include gas, diarrhea, headaches, fatigue, indigestion, and even mood swings and anxiety. Because leaky gut syndrome causes an increase in proinflammatory compounds in the blood, it can create a cycle of chronic inflammation. As we discussed in chapter 9, inflammation is a strong risk factor for cancer and can also impede treatment success.

You can avoid leaky gut syndrome, or help reverse it, by being alert to any food allergies or intolerances and avoiding those foods. Supporting beneficial intestinal bacteria by using probiotics is also helpful. And, as is so often the case, some surprisingly simple things can make a big difference, such as chewing well and taking sufficient time to eat in a relaxed manner. For some people, supplementation with digestive enzymes may be necessary to assist with digestion in the stomach so that there are fewer large food particles passing through to the small intestine.

Essential Bacteria

The intestinal lining is coated with "friendly" bacteria. These microorganisms aid in digestion, produce vitamins and energy for use by the body, support the immune cells in the digestive tract in recognizing and attacking disease-causing bacteria, and stimulate bowel contraction. Unfortunately, there are several factors that can destroy beneficial bacteria including antibiotic use and a diet high in meat and sugar and low in fruits, vegetables, and grains. A deficiency of friendly bacteria or imbalanced intestinal flora is known as dysbiosis, and a digestive tract thus afflicted is prone to becoming leaky, inflamed, constipated, and infected. Because dysbiosis unravels the immune process that occurs in the intestines, it can also contribute to problems in distant parts of the body, including infection, autoimmune disease, and inflammation.

There is another strong connection between digestion and immune activity. More than 70 percent of the cells of the immune system are housed in the digestive tract. This makes supporting healthy digestion and a healthy digestive lining even more critical to cancer treatment. This makes sense when you realize that the digestive tract is a tube that passes through the body, which means that its lining forms a semipermeable barrier between the outside world and the interior of the body. This barrier is challenged every time we eat. In addition to valuable nutrients, each meal also contains microorganisms, toxins, and harmful chemicals. A form of lymphatic tissue known as gut-associated lymphoid tissue (GALT) is located throughout the digestive tract in order to help protect us from these pathogens and harmful foreign compounds. When GALT is intact and fully functional, we are able to extract nutrients from food without being harmed by potentially damaging substances in the food. But when GALT is impaired, disease-causing microorganisms and other dangerous substances can escape the digestive system's immune defenses and invade the body. In addition, dysfunction and imbalances in GALT carry over to the immune system in the rest of the body, creating systemic immune imbalances that leave the body less defended against the development and progression of cancer. Probiotics, friendly bacteria in the form of dietary supplements, help support GALT.

Detoxification

Despite the digestive system's impressive defensive tactics—filtering out toxins and disabling pathogens—some harmful compounds inevitably make it into the bloodstream. And some toxic compounds are actually formed as a result of the body's process of digesting and metabolizing food. Fortunately, the body is well designed and backup systems exist. All of the immune processes described in chapter 8 play an important role, and detoxification is also crucial. The liver is the key organ of detoxification.

The liver is a hardworking organ. In addition to producing bile to aid in digestion, and storing glucose in the form of glycogen for later use, it works 24 hours a day to review all the nutrients, wastes, and toxins that are absorbed from the small intestine. Beneficial compounds may be stored, altered into more useful forms, or sent into the bloodstream for use by the body. When the liver detects toxic compounds, it breaks them down or otherwise alters them into less harmful forms, which are excreted into the bile and eventually eliminated during a bowel movement.

Though that may sound simple enough, the complex process of liver detoxification involves the activity of about 100 enzymes collectively known as cytochrome P450 (cP450). The main function of the cP450 enzyme system is to convert fat-soluble toxins into nontoxic water-soluble compounds

Detoxification

In the healthy liver, the toxins are converted by cytochrome P450 enzymes to intermediate substances (phase I detoxification) and then into water-soluble substances (phase II detoxification)

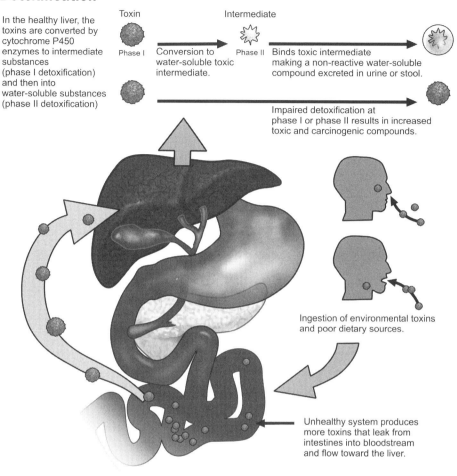

Toxin

Phase I Conversion to water-soluble toxic intermediate.

Intermediate

Phase II Binds toxic intermediate making a non-reactive water-soluble compound excreted in urine or stool.

Impaired detoxification at phase I or phase II results in increased toxic and carcinogenic compounds.

Ingestion of environmental toxins and poor dietary sources.

Unhealthy system produces more toxins that leak from intestines into bloodstream and flow toward the liver.

that can be excreted in the bile or urine. Detoxifying cP450 enzymes go through a two-step process to render the toxin harmless. An imbalance on either side of the process can be harmful.

Upon exposure to toxic substances, the activity of selected cP450 enzymes increases. This activity results in chemical alteration of the toxic substance into a reactive intermediate compound. This is referred to as phase I of detoxification. As a result of this phase of the detoxification process, chemicals are created that are even more reactive than the original compound. That's where phase II comes in. Phase II detoxification takes that intermediate, highly reactive, and often toxic chemical and renders it harmless, partially by binding it with proteins, sulfur, or methyl groups. The outcome of phase II detoxification is the creation of a conjugated compound that can be safely eliminated through urine or stool. It is important to note that medications and some supplements are also metabolized by the cP450 enzymes, and in some cases, these enzymes activate medications or compounds in supplements. So the activity of cP450 enzymes goes beyond detoxification and may determine how the body responds to medications, herbs, and supplements.

Health problems occur when there are imbalances between phase I and phase II detoxification. One scenario involves rapid phase I and slow phase II detoxification. This may occur as a result of chronic exposure to toxins, leading to chronic elevation of cP450 enzymes. The cP450 enzymes keep up their end of the job, eventually using up the conjugating compounds needed for phase II detoxification. But phase I doesn't stop just because phase II can't proceed. The result can be a buildup of toxic, highly reactive, intermediate compounds that cause tissue damage and inflammation, and can ultimately contribute to the development of cancer. Additionally, phase I enzymes generate free radicals as they metabolize compounds. An active phase I will generate significant free radicals, which can stimulate tumor growth, impair immunity, and aggravate adverse toxicity from drugs.

Factors that can increase cP450 activity include the following:

● Alcohol

● Nicotine

● Hydrocarbons formed during charcoal broiling or found in cigarette smoke

● Acetaminophen and phenobarbital (antiseizure medication)

● Iron deficiency

● A high-protein diet

Conversely, underactivity of cP450 enzymes slows down the initial phase of detoxification, leaving toxic compounds intact and free to circulate in the body. In addition to detoxifying foreign compounds, cP450 enzymes also break down compounds that naturally occur in the body, such as hormones and histamine. If cP450 activity is underactive, hormones and histamine are not adequately broken down. This leads to chronically elevated levels of hormones and histamine, which can lead to inflammation. And as discussed previously, inflammation and elevated hormone levels are linked to many health issues, including cancer.

Factors that can lead to decreased cP450 activity include the following:

● Nutritional deficiencies

● Fasting

● Protein deficiency

- A diet high in carbohydrates

- Phosphatidylcholine deficiency

- Benzodiazepines, such as triazolam, chlordiazepoxide, and diazepam (Halcion, Librium, Valium)

- Antihistamines

- Cimetidine (Tagamet)

- Naringenin (in grapefruit juice)

- Deficiency of vitamins A and C

- Bacterial toxins

- Aging

It is estimated that about 50 percent of the population has normal cP450 activity, about 30 percent are slow detoxifiers with depressed cP450 enzymatic activity, and about 20 percent are fast detoxifiers with elevated cP450 activity. The key is to promote balance between phase I and phase II detoxification. You can do this by being aware of the factors that increase and decrease cP450 enzymes, as listed above. There are also liver detoxification profile tests available that measure phase I and phase II activity. These tests must be ordered by a licensed health-care professional.

There are several natural substances that can help with both sides of the detoxification cP450 equation. For example, animal studies have demonstrated that curcumin neutralizes benzopyrenes from charcoal-broiled meat and also neutralizes toxic compounds in cigarette smoke (factors that decrease cP450 activity). For the 30 percent of the population who are slow detoxifiers, indoles from cruciferous vegetables and vitamin C may also help support phase I detoxification.

Other herbs, nutrients, and foods that can assist with effective detoxification by supporting or increasing phase I detoxifying enzyme activity are

- Carnosol (found in rosemary)

- Resveratrol (found in the skin of red grapes)

- Capsicum (found in cayenne)

- Eugenol (found in cloves)

- Quercetin (found in onions and apples)

- Garlic

- Green tea (especially EGCG)

The Liver Flush

The liver is the body's largest internal organ. It is also one of the most important, continuously undertaking countless tasks of metabolism and detoxification while also playing a role in digestion and elimination. Its role in detoxification is especially critical. As our world becomes ever more toxic, the liver can become overloaded. Supporting the liver with a healthy diet and lifestyle, appropriate herbs and supplements, and periodic gentle detoxification is an important part of any cancer treatment plan. But what about the liver flush, which is quite popular in some alternative medicine circles?

The liver's ability to detoxify can get bogged down by excessive environmental pollutants, an unhealthy diet, and unhealthful lifestyle choices, such as drinking and smoking. A liver flush is believed to support and enhance the release of bile from the liver while expediting the elimination of excess hormones, fats, parasites, and harmful food by-products and other toxins.

"A liver flush involves eating or drinking a combination of juices and oils, often with selected herbs, enzymes, and other components," according to the American Cancer Society. "The flush is usually done over the course of two or more days and results in several bowel movements." The American Cancer Society does not endorse the liver flush due to the lack of scientific evidence for this therapy.

Because a liver flush can include fasting, limited calorie intake, and other treatments such as coffee enemas, people with advanced cancers or those at risk of developing cachexia (a dangerous muscle-wasting condition) should be cautious about this questionable therapy. There is no clinical evidence that a liver flush will help treat cancer. In reality, a liver flush is most likely simply causing the gallbladder to contract and release its stored bile. Whether this action facilitates liver health is postulation; however, from a functional approach, supporting the liver before, during, and after cancer treatment makes sense. A gentle detoxification plan is recommended rather than the liver flush or any approach that incorporates extreme fasting combined with colonics. (For advice on gentle detoxification, see the sidebar "The Gentle Detoxification Plan" on page 136).

If you do opt to do a liver flush, be aware that some herbs in liver flush formulas may be contraindicated if you're taking certain chemotherapy agents. (Refer to the chart "Chemotherapy Drugs and Their Nutrient and Herb Interactions" starting on page 141 for more information on this.) In addition, some people doing a liver flush experience nausea, vomiting, and diarrhea. Before doing a liver flush, consult with an experienced integrative health practitioner who has worked with cancer patients.

There are nutrients that specifically support phase II detoxification. Glutathione is an important detoxifying antioxidant in phase II reactions. Researchers from the National Research Council of Canada and others have concluded that glutathione helps prevent cancer by alleviating oxidative stress and detoxifying mutagenic toxins. Additionally, sulfur and sulfur-containing foods such as eggs and cruciferous vegetables support phase II reactions.

High homocysteine levels can also be implicated in dysfunctional phase II detoxification. Normally, the body converts homocysteine into either glutathione or S-adenosylmethionine, both of which can serve as methyl donors as part of the conjugation process in phase II detoxification. However, deficiencies of vitamin B_6, vitamin B_{12}, and folic acid can interfere with the conversion of homocysteine into these beneficial compounds and thus interfere with phase II detoxification. Because of the importance of methylation in numerous metabolic processes, high homocysteine is actually indicative of much more than a deficiency in phase II detoxification; it's also a risk factor for cardiovascular disease, Alzheimer's disease, and certain cancers. High homocysteine is also correlated with worse prognosis in several cancers such as breast and prostate cancers.

Choline, which is also known as phosphatidylcholine, plays a critical role in detoxification and general liver function. Like B_{12}, folic acid, and S-adenosylmethionine (SAMe), choline can serve as a methyl donor and thus plays an important role in phase II detoxification.

For more information about gentle detoxification, refer to the sidebar on page 136.

Supporting Healthy Digestion

Just as there are natural ways to support effective detoxification, there are also methods to enhance healthy digestion, ease digestive disturbances, prevent digestive diseases, and in the process help treat cancer. Because digestion is directly related to what we eat and drink, the best way to support or create healthy digestion is with the diet. Dietary extremes that include excessive proteins, carbohydrates, or fats do not promote healthy digestion. In fact, simply eating too much—period—is hard on both the digestive system and detoxification. Your body must work to digest whatever you eat, and your liver must process the majority of the nutrients (and toxins) you take in. When you overeat, you overtax these systems. Conversely, undereating, while not particularly stressful on digestion, will deprive the body of required nutrients over time. Given enough time and sustained deficiencies, the tissues of the digestive system will be less able to perform the tasks of digestion.

The dietary advice in chapter 4 applies to healthy digestion, detoxification, and elimination. Review the advice in the "Foundational Health Plan" sidebar on page 84. Many compounds found in these fresh and nutritious foods can directly improve the efficiency of the digestion and detoxification systems. For example, enzymes and flavonoids found in some fruits can help with digestion, and indoles in cruciferous vegetables will help with a sluggish detoxification system. Fiber in fruits and vegetables is also critical to healthy digestion, detoxification, and elimination.

Avoiding high-calorie, low-nutrient "empty" foods is important. When you eat these foods, you're asking your body to do all the work of digestion for very little nutrient reward. Plus, these foods are often processed and laden with artificial ingredients, which increases the body's toxic burden and can damage the intestinal lining.

Eating sufficient fiber is especially important because it positively contributes to health on many levels, including digestion, detoxification, and elimination. "Sent to the intestines, the bile and its toxic load are absorbed by fiber and excreted," explain the authors of *How to Prevent and Treat Cancer with Natural Medicine*. "However, a diet low in fiber means that these toxins are not bound and are more likely to be reabsorbed." Oat fiber is a particularly good choice because it contains important water-soluble beta-glucans, which have been shown to be anticancer agents. Other good sources of dietary fiber include whole grains, legumes, and most fruits and vegetables.

Water is absolutely essential to healthy digestion—and to life. The average adult human body is made up of between 60 percent and 70 percent water. You can go without eating for several weeks, but without water, you would die in just a few days. Many people do not drink the recommended 64 ounces (2 quarts) of fresh water each day.

Just as important as what you eat is how you eat. Healthy digestion begins with chewing. Be sure to chew food thoroughly. Sit down, eat slowly, and take any steps necessary to have a stress-free dining experience. Reducing stress in all aspects of your life, not just while dining, will also promote optimal digestion.

Many lifestyle factors can positively or negatively affect digestive health. Chronic alcohol consumption greatly burdens the detoxification process, and it can also have a negative impact on digestion. A recent animal study featured in the *Journal of Acquired Immune Deficiency Syndromes* reported that long-term alcohol consumption affects turnover of immune system cells in the intestine and has an adverse effect on the intestinal mucosa.

Supplements for Healthy Digestion

A number of supplements can play a vital role in supporting healthy digestion and correcting underlying digestive problems, thereby helping to prevent and treat cancer. Among the most beneficial of these are bovine colostrums, L-glutamine, probiotics, and proteolytic enzymes. While many of these supplements have not been studied specifically as a cancer treatment, their ability to heal the digestive tract enhances the capacity to heal from cancer.

- *Bovine colostrum*: Colostrum is the name for milk given off during the first few days after giving birth, which has a different biochemical profile than the milk that follows. It is especially rich in growth factors, antibodies, and vitamins and minerals. For use in supplements, colostrum is collected from cows (don't worry, there is plenty left for the calves). A high-quality colostrum product should contain little or no lactose. It is believed that colostrum provides increased passive immunity in the digestive tract and can help prevent and treat diarrhea, allergies, infectious gastroenteritis, hepatitis C, obesity, peptic ulcers, *Heliobacter pylori* infection (a cause of ulcers and gastritis), and even cancer. The benefits attributed to colostrum are primarily anecdotal. More randomized, controlled trials are needed.

- **L-glutamine**: This is an important amino acid for many critical purposes, including proper intestinal cell function and regeneration, as glutamine is the preferred food source for intestinal cells. Scientific studies have shown that uptake of glutamine by the mucosal cells of the small intestine far exceeds the uptake of any other amino acid. In addition, studies have shown that L-glutamine protects the liver and acts as an antidepressant. In terms of cancer, it has been shown to reduce intestinal toxicity from chemotherapy drugs and increase concentrations of methotrexate (a chemotherapy drug) in tumors while selectively protecting normal tissues. And because fast-growing tumors can deplete the body's supply of glutamine, supplementing with this amino acid can help support muscle metabolism, in which glutamine is a key player.

- **Melatonin**: Melatonin is secreted in vast quantities by intestinal cells. Melatonin regulates intestinal motility and supplements can reduce constipation and irritable bowel syndrome. Melatonin also supports the immune system in the intestinal tract.

- **Probiotics**: There are more than 400 different species of "friendly" bacteria living in the gastrointestinal system. And as you've learned, the balance of "good" and "bad" bacteria in the gastrointestinal system has far-reaching health ramifications, including aiding absorption of nutrients from foods, maintaining healthy immune responses, and processing toxins. The most studied friendly bacteria are *Lactobacillus acidophilus* and *Bifidobacterium bifidum*. These "good" bacteria also help balance the "bad" bacteria that can accumulate in the digestive system. You can support a balanced internal ecosystem by using probiotics, substances that contain friendly bacteria in the form of supplements or cultured foods such as yogurt or sauerkraut. Several studies have demonstrated that probiotics can improve bowel health and the intestinal immune response. Probiotics also have systemic benefits, helping to reduce inflammation and infection throughout the body. Early research suggests that probiotics may reduce the risk of colon and other cancers.

- **Proteolytic enzymes**: Proteolytic enzymes, which help the body digest protein, are an often used and well-researched way to support healthy digestion. These enzymes include bromelain from pineapple, papain from papaya, and the pancreatic enzymes chymotrypsin and trypsin.

When these enzymes are taken with a meal, they support the body's own enzymes in breaking down food into smaller, digestible components. Proteolytic enzymes have also been studied and used as anticancer agents. If they are used to prevent or treat cancer, they are typically taken on an empty stomach.

Other nutrients and herbs that can assist with healthy digestion, detoxification, and elimination include the following:

- Deglycyrrhizinated licorice (DGL) supports repair of the mucosal lining of the stomach.

- Folic acid is necessary for tissue regeneration. People with inflammatory bowel disease are usually deficient in this B vitamin.

- Gamma oryzanol supports relief of stress-induced gastrointestinal disorders.

- Peppermint oil supplements relieve symptoms associated with dyspepsia and irritable bowel syndrome, including pain, pressure, bloating, and intestinal spasms.

- Vitamins C and E and beta-carotene are all powerful antioxidants that protect the gastrointestinal mucosa from free radical damage.

The Cancer Connection

Chronic digestive disorders may indicate a more serious problem, even cancer. In addition, correcting digestive disorders will complement any cancer treatment plan by reducing inflammation, improving detoxification, and increasing absorption of beneficial nutrients. This will likely enhance the success of the overall cancer treatment plan.

Effective digestion, detoxification, and elimination are critical to cancer prevention and treatment. Gastrointestinal health is important not just because of the direct functions it performs but also because of the influence it has on all other body systems.

As you learned in chapter 2, cancer is caused by many contributing factors collaborating in some cases over a long period of time—internal and external events that combine to create the dangerous internal domino effect we know as cancer. "A carcinogen may be present at a very low dose or for a brief time, but in combination with other chemicals and risk factors, it can start a chain reaction that leads to cancer," writes Mitchell Gaynor, MD, in his book *Nurture Nature, Nurture Health*. "Given what we know today about how cancer cells come to be, no single substance, genetic predisposition, or lifestyle would be sufficient to be called the sole cause of cancer."

Body Function Nutrient Chart

This chart represents natural agents with broad spectrum benefit to the five key body systems. These important substances influence more than one body system, making them useful for many individuals.

Body system	CoQ10	Curcumin	Botanical flavonoids	Garlic	Green tea	Omega-3 fatty acids	Melatonin	Mushrooms	Probiotics	Vitamins and minerals
Immune	•	•	•	•	•	•	•	•	•	A, C, D, E, and selenium
Inflammation	•	•	•	•	•	•			•	C, D, E, folic acid, and selenium
Hormonal			•				•	•	•	C, E
Insulin resistance	•	•			•	•		•	•	D, magnesium
Digestion and detoxification			•	•	•		•		•	C, E, beta carotene, and folic acid

Refer to Appendix: Dosage Ranges on pages 387–394 for dosages

The systems approach to cancer treatment considers all body functions, how they function individually, and how they interact as a whole. When the body is in harmonious homeostasis, key physiological systems support one another in ways that help us treat cancer. A variety of factors can disrupt any of these systems, and imbalance in any system can disrupt the harmony. The first domino can tip from any direction—immune function, inflammation, hormonal influences, insulin resistance, or digestion. As more and more dominoes fall, cancer can become firmly established. A cornerstone of cancer treatment is to do everything we can to improve or enhance the health of all of these important body functions.

Part IV
Addressing Specific Cancers

thirteen

Specific Cancer Overviews

Cancer is complex and multifaceted and can be extremely challenging to treat. You can develop cancer in virtually any place or organ in the body. Because each of us has a unique and dynamic genetic makeup, one could argue that there are as many different types of cancer as there are different types of people: because there are no two individuals with exactly the same genetic makeup, there are no two cancers that are exactly alike. For this reason, individualized cancer care is critical.

One potential "side effect" of a cancer diagnosis is the development of a voracious appetite for information. There is a desperate need to know. As cancer pushes its way into our homes, our relationships, and our lives, we push back with facts and data.

We understand the panic, desperation, and desire to gather as much information as possible. We've been there. Over time, our own personal experiences with cancer have taught us how to be methodical in the search for information—probing yet patient. This section features important details concerning 21 different cancers. Remember, however, new information becomes available every day, and important discoveries will undoubtedly be made while this book is in print.

We've done our best to sift through what's currently known to provide you with solid, straightforward information. The following chapters are not intended to provide comprehensive information about each type of cancer and its treatment. Rather, they present a synopsis of each with attention to the following aspects:

- General information

- Potential causes, symptoms, and diagnosis

- Basic information about conventional treatment

- Recommendations in regard to diet, lifestyle, and nutritional supplements

We want to emphasize that the information in these chapters is not meant to replace your doctor's advice. Self-diagnosis and self-treatment can be dangerous. Discuss all of your treatment options with your doctor and don't be afraid to get a second (or third) opinion.

Rather than repeating dosage recommendations for specific nutrients and herbs in each of the following chapters, we've compiled that information in the appendix. We have noted in brackets whether the recommended natural substances are preventive, anticancer, or supportive after each individual natural substance. *Anticancer* means there have been studies showing that the specific nutrient or herb kills cancer cells. *Preventive* means that the only studies done have shown that the nutrient or herb decreases the risk of develoopng cancer or a cancer recurrence. *Supportive* means the nutrient or herb has been shown to complement conventional cancer therapy by decreasing side effects and/or increasing the effectiveness of the conventional therapy in destroying cancer.

The scientific literature on cancer encompasses an overwhelming number of studies involving numerous nutrients, herbs, and other natural substances. We have focused on the most recent studies, along with a few compelling older studies, to help illustrate the promise associated with these powerful foods, nutrients, and herbs. However, it is important to emphasize that research in this area is still in its infancy. More human clinical trials are needed for nearly every natural substance we studied.

While the effectiveness of many of these substances hasn't been proven by the gold standard of research (randomized controlled trials), they are typically safer than conventional drugs, which makes them appealing. We are not suggesting that natural substances replace conventional treatment when there is expected benefit from that conventional treatment. We are, however, strongly advocating that the best medicine be used at all times. When used appropriately, natural substances work synergistically with conventional treatments to maximize benefit and minimize harm. They can also help offset the side effects of conventional treatments. In some cases, natural therapies comprise the best option. We believe the best medicine combines effective complementary medicine with conventional interventions. (For detailed information on the research supporting use of various nutrients and herbs and any concerns and contraindications, see the "Integrative

Cancer Care Supplement Guide" starting on page 161; for information on their interactions with chemotherapy drugs—whether they're supportive or contraindicated—see the chart "Chemotherapy Drugs and Their Nutrient and Herb Interactions," beginning on page 141.)

Cancer is an extremely individualized disease. The most effective approach to successfully treating your cancer and preventing a recurrence must be comprehensive, targeted to your specific cancer, and tailored to meet your individual needs. And just in case we haven't made ourselves clear, to achieve true healing, that comprehensive plan must include a healthy diet, positive lifestyle choices, and appropriate supplements.

fourteen

Bladder Cancer

The bladder is a flexible, balloon-shaped organ. The bladder expands when urine travels to it from the kidneys through tubes called ureters. It shrinks when the urine is emptied through a tube called the urethra. By contracting, the bladder muscle forces the urine out during urination. According to the American Urological Association, "more than 90 percent of all bladder cancers originate in the urothelium," the thin inside lining of the bladder. Most bladder tumors are contained within the bladder and do not penetrate the outermost bladder muscle. Bladder cancer is the sixth most common cancer in the United States.

Causes, Symptoms, and Diagnosis

Bladder cancer is 2.5 times more common in men than in women and is most common in the sixth and seventh decades of life. While not one of the most well-known types of cancer, bladder cancer illustrates the enormous impact of lifestyle and environmental changes. At least half of all incidences of bladder cancer could be avoided by healthy lifestyle and environmental changes. It is estimated that cigarette smoking causes 50 percent of all bladder cancers in the United States. Another 20 percent to 25 percent of bladder cancers are caused by long-term workplace exposure to chemical compounds. Specific chemicals linked to bladder cancer include aromatic amines used in the rubber, aluminum, and textile industries. Risk also increases with exposure to solvents and other chemicals used in dry cleaning, commercial painting, plumbing, heating, air conditioning, and the transportation industry. Arsenic in drinking water and other sources has also been linked to bladder cancer.

The most common symptom of bladder cancer is hematuria, a painless condition in which blood is present in the urine; however, hematuria by itself does not confirm bladder cancer. The blood can be visible in the urine, or it may only be detectable with a microscope. Pain during urination, known as dysuria, or frequent urination can also be signs of bladder cancer.

Upon receiving specific information about a patient's medical history, cigarette use, and symptoms, a physician will have a urinalysis done and may recommend cystoscopy, which allows direct viewing of the inside of the bladder. This simple procedure is done using local anesthesia or light sedation and involves insertion of a flexible fiber-optic scope (cystoscope) into the bladder, allowing the physician to examine the bladder and take tissue samples. If a tumor is discovered, further investigation to determine its stage is recommended. This usually involves a CT scan of the abdomen and pelvis and may also require an MRI of the abdomen. If at all possible, surgery to remove the tumor will be scheduled. The surgeon often will also remove small tissue samples from the area surrounding the tumor to be examined by a pathologist. This examination determines the cellular type of the cancer and the extent of cancer in the bladder—both of which give valuable information about whether follow-up therapy is needed and what type would be most helpful.

Conventional Treatment

Conventional treatment for bladder cancer relies heavily on surgery. Radiation and chemotherapy are used when cancer is more advanced and when it has spread.

Surgery

Surgery is used in almost all cases of bladder cancer. Approximately 70 to 80 percent of patients with newly diagnosed bladder cancer have superficial tumors, in which case surgery can usually cure the cancer. The goal of surgery is to remove all cancerous tissue and obtain a clean surgical margin. The margin size depends on the size and location of the tumor. Minimally invasive lesions may be completely removed by transurethral resection (TUR), which removes the cancer with minimal damage to the bladder. TUR is often performed during the initial biopsy surgery.

More advanced cancers may require a partial cystectomy (removal of part of the bladder and perhaps parts of nearby organs) or radical cystectomy. Radical cystectomy involves removal of the entire bladder, the pelvic lymph nodes, and the prostate in men, or the uterus and part of the vaginal wall in women. During or after a cystectomy, the surgeon may construct a new bladder made of the patient's own tissue, which in many cases preserves continence (the ability to control urination).

Surgery is an important first step following a diagnosis of bladder cancer. A recent study featured in the *Journal of Urology* found that patients who delayed bladder cancer surgery for more than three months experienced decreased survival rates compared to those who were operated on within three months of their diagnosis.

Radiation and Chemotherapy

While surgery leads to prolonged survival in the majority of patients with superficial cancers, those whose tumors have spread to tissues outside of the bladder require more than surgery. Additionally, in patients with tumors confined to the bladder but with invasion into the muscular layer, even successful surgical removal leaves an 80 percent chance of recurrence. Those with large tumors and tumors with a number of genetic mutations (determined from the biopsied tissue) or those who, in addition to having the primary tumor, also have carcinoma in situ (early-stage cancer) in other areas of the bladder are at the greatest risk of recurrence.

Radiation may be used with TUR, especially in more advanced cases. Preoperative radiation has received mixed reviews. More research is needed to confirm radiation's effectiveness in halting disease progression and preserving quality of life.

Chemotherapy can be targeted to the bladder using an intravesical approach in which chemotherapy drugs are pumped into the bladder through a catheter for about two hours, then drained. This has relatively mild side effects but can cause severe bladder irritation, depending on the dose used as well as the individual tolerance of the person receiving the treatment. Systemic chemotherapy, in which the drugs travel throughout the body via the bloodstream, may also be used in cases of advanced bladder cancer; however, side effects of the treatment are more serious. Typical chemotherapy agents used to treat bladder cancer include methotrexate, vinblastine, doxorubicin, cisplatin (M-VAC), mitomycin C, and cyclophosphamide. For information about how to counteract typical side effects of these medications, consult the conventional treatment chart "Chemotherapy Drugs and Their Nutrient and Herb Interactions" on page 141.

Other Conventional Treatments

An intravesical bacillus Calmette-Guérin (BCG) vaccine may be used to treat more advanced cases of bladder cancer. BCG is indicated in patients with multiple tumors within the bladder or recurrent tumors, or as a preventive measure against recurrence in people with high-risk cancer (determined by cellular classifications and genetic characteristics) after TUR. BCG is administered directly into the bladder or injected into the skin overlying the bladder. Treatment with BCG decreases and delays tumor recurrence and can prevent the need for more extensive surgery with recurrent disease.

Photodynamic therapy can be very effective in eliminating bladder cancer tumors. This therapy involves administering photosensitive substances that are taken up by the bladder cancer cells. These drugs are then locally activated by light to generate toxic free radical compounds that cause the death of the cancer cells. Interferon alfa-2a, delivered directly into the bladder, is also a viable treatment option for papillary tumors (a type of tumor that resembles enlarged fingerlike projections, or papillae, that grow into the hollow center of the bladder). This may be recommended as an initial treatment, and it may also be used if other therapies have failed to produce results.

People with advanced bladder cancer should always investigate clinical trials. The development of new and effective agents to treat bladder cancer is ongoing. Given the mixed response to radiation and current chemotherapy agents, exploring new conventional agents is important, as is an aggressive integrative approach.

Complementary Approaches

Refer to part II of this book regarding useful complementary approaches for all cancers. The following information is specific to bladder cancer.

Research has demonstrated that the more inflammation that exists with bladder cancer, the greater the likelihood of metastasis. There are specific inflammatory markers in the urine that can be tested to determine this. When these markers are elevated in patients with bladder cancer, an anti-inflammatory complementary approach is indicated.

Lifestyle and Diet

Avoiding the toxins mentioned previously, as well as cigarette smoke, is the most important lifestyle change people with bladder cancer can make. If you smoke, it is important that you quit. If you are regularly exposed to someone else's smoke (secondhand smoke), it is important to avoid this exposure. Antioxidant nutrients are particularly helpful to prevent the oxidative damage to bladder cells caused by the toxins mentioned above. The role of therapeutic doses of vitamins and minerals is significant in the prevention and treatment of bladder cancer.

Some studies have made direct links between eating fruits and vegetables and bladder cancer prevention and treatment. Japanese researchers who studied more than 38,000 atomic bomb survivors found that high consumption of vegetables and fruits is protective against bladder cancer. Another study, published in the *International Journal of Urology*, focused on 124 hospital patients diagnosed with bladder cancer. They concluded that people with "an increased risk of bladder cancer, such as smokers, may benefit from increasing their consumption of green-yellow vegetables."

As for other foods, researchers have paid some attention to probiotics, soy, olive oil, and fermented brown rice. Although these are food-based nutrients, the research has focused on standardized extracts of these foods taken as dietary supplements.

Research on soy in relation to bladder cancer has been primarily test tube and animal studies. Recent research at Harvard Medical School demonstrated that soy may help prevent bladder cancer from spreading, cause cancer cell death, and shut off the blood supply to the tumor. More human trials are needed.

Nutrients and Herbs

The majority of the studies done on nutrients and herbs as bladder cancer treatments have been test tube and animal studies. Although more research, specifically human trials, is necessary to determine their effectiveness as bladder cancer treatments, results thus far are promising. For information on dosages for the supplements listed below, as well as any potential contraindications, see the appendix.

- *Aloe vera*: This herb is believed to have some antitumor properties. New in vitro research has shown that a purified form of aloe vera leaves helps induce apoptosis in a human bladder cancer cell line. [anticancer]

- *Astragalus*: Mice exposed to a chemical that normally causes bladder cancer have a lower incidence of bladder cancer when given astragalus root extract. Astragalus has been shown to stimulate the immune system in a way that triggers bladder cancer cell death. [preventive, anticancer]

- *Cranberry*: We aren't aware of any studies linking cranberry extract to bladder cancer prevention or treatment; however, cranberries have been shown to help prevent urinary tract infections, which people with bladder cancer are susceptible to. [supportive]

- *Curcumin*: Test tube studies on bladder cancer cell lines demonstrated that the anti-inflammatory properties of curcumin, a main active ingredient in turmeric, help halt the progression of bladder cancer. Other in vitro studies have found that curcumin can suppress bladder cancer cell growth and induce apoptosis. Use caution with this herb, as it may interact with some drugs. [preventive, anticancer]

- **Ginger**: Animal studies have shown that orally administered powdered ginger significantly slowed the growth of bladder cancer. [anticancer]

- **Green tea**: Animal studies involving green tea and bladder cancer are very positive. In humans, green tea has been shown to reduce the cellular genetic damage that is caused by cigarette smoke. With more than 50 percent of all bladder cancer caused by cigarette smoke, it makes sense to utilize the preventive effects of green tea—especially if you smoke or are exposed to secondhand smoke. [preventive]

- **Kava**: It has been reported that there are lower cancer rates in three kava-drinking countries, namely, Fiji, Vanuatu, and Western Samoa. Researchers at the University of California, Irvine, found that kava kills bladder cancer cells in vivo. Kava may have some drug interactions and there have been a few cases of liver toxicity, so only use this herb under the guidance of a qualified health-care professional. [preventive]

- **Mistletoe**: Small human trials have yielded mixed results, with some showing benefit and others demonstrating no effect: a study of 45 patients featured in the *Journal of Urology* showed no effect, while a later study of 30 patients, featured in *Anticancer Research*, demonstrated effectiveness of a standardized extract applied intravesically following BCG treatment of noninvasive bladder cancer. [anticancer]

- **Probiotics**: In a 2005 review paper featured in the journal *European Urology*, German researchers conclude that "The potential of *L. casei Shirota* [a probiotic strain] to reduce the recurrence rate of bladder cancer is one of the most intriguing examples for the use of probiotics in medical practice. Clinical trials increasingly provide a profound scientific basis for the use of probiotics in medicinal practice including urology." A 2008 randomized control trial demonstrated that the addition of *Lactobacillus casei* (3 grams per day) to epirubicin therapy for superficial bladder cancer significantly improved recurrence-free survival versus epirubicin alone over a three-year period. [preventive]

- **St. John's wort**: Preliminary in vitro studies involving St. John's wort as an agent against bladder cancer cells show promise. St. John's wort has been shown to stop bladder cancer cells from growing and to cause cancer cell death. Caution should be exercised with this herb as it interacts with numerous drugs; it should only be used under medical supervision. [preventive, anticancer]

- **Vitamin A**: Several studies have indicated a preventive effect with oral consumption of vitamin A supplements. Additional small human trials also suggest that vitamin A may reduce the risk of recurrence of bladder cancer. Vitamin A enhances the antitumor effect of other treatments, such as interferon alfa-2a therapy. [preventive, supportive]

● *Vitamin B$_6$*: In some human trials, vitamin B$_6$ appears to be an effective way to reduce the risk of bladder cancer recurrence. However, other trials have failed to find this benefit. Taken as a whole, research indicates a favorable role for vitamin B$_6$ in the prevention and treatment of bladder cancer. [preventive, anticancer]

● *Vitamins C and E*: A combination of vitamins C and E and zinc was shown to decrease recurrence in patients with a previous diagnosis of bladder cancer. [preventive]

Summary

Prevention and early detection are important with bladder cancer, as there is significant opportunity to detour carcinogenic tissue changes back to normally functioning tissue through lifestyle changes. Additionally, early diagnosis dramatically increases the potential for cure. Eliminating or reducing exposure to cigarette smoke and the other toxins mentioned previously will help prevent bladder cancer. For those diagnosed with bladder cancer, a high-antioxidant diet with abundant fruits and vegetables is indicated. Additionally, flushing the bladder of mutagenic substances is of critical importance, hence the oft-repeated good advice to drink eight glasses of fresh water daily (about 2 quarts). Municipal water that is not filtered in the home should be avoided whenever possible. Herbal and nutrition-based therapies may help prevent recurrence.

fifteen

Bone Cancer

Bones, the support structure of our bodies, are made up of a variety of tissues: a hard, mineral-dense matrix; a fibrous outer covering called the periosteum; osteoblasts (cells that produce bone); osteoclasts (cells that break down bone); and a soft, internal tissue called marrow (consisting of fat cells and blood-forming cells). Any of the many cell varieties in bone can become cancerous.

Sarcomas start in bone tissue and are considered the main type of "true" bone cancer. Osteosarcoma is the most common type of bone cancer. Cancers of the bones and joints are some of the rarest forms of cancer, constituting only about 2,500 cases of the estimated 1.6 million cancers diagnosed in 2009 in the United States. Most cancerous tumors in bones are the result of cancers that originated elsewhere and have metastasized to the bones. Breast cancer, prostate cancer, and lung cancers are examples of cancers that tend to metastasize to the bones. Leukemia, multiple myeloma, and lymphoma, discussed in chapter 24, start in the cells of the bone marrow, but they're considered blood cancers rather than bone cancer.

Causes, Symptoms, and Diagnosis

The precise causes of bone cancer remain unknown, but risk factors include exposure to radiation or chemotherapy, preexisting Paget's disease, and age. Children and young adults are more likely to develop bone cancer than older adults; for example, osteosarcoma is a bone tumor that occurs primarily in adolescents, accounting for 5 percent of childhood tumors. Over 50 percent of all osteosarcomas begin in the femur near the knee, but they may occur in any bone, with the tibia, humerus, pelvis, jaw, fibula, and ribs being the next most common sites. Osteosarcoma tumors are bony growths formed by malignant cells. The majority of people diagnosed with osteosarcoma do not have metastatic disease at the time of diagnosis. However, for the 10 percent to 20 percent who do have metastatic disease, it is usually in the lungs and can be in other bones.

The most common symptoms of osteosarcoma are breakage of the affected bone or pain at the site of the tumor. Other symptoms may include tenderness in the bone, swelling, stiffness in surrounding tissue, fatigue, or fever.

To diagnose bone cancer, a doctor will typically take a medical history and perform an examination. Blood tests may reveal an increase of the enzyme alkaline phosphatase, which is a possible indicator of tumor activity, though not a definitive test for bone cancer. Doctors may look for bone tumors with imaging tests such as X-rays, bone scans, CAT scans, MRIs, and angiograms. Any suspected bone cancer must be evaluated by an orthopedic oncologist so a proper biopsy can be performed.

Conventional Treatment

Conventional treatment for bone cancer typically involves a combination of surgery, radiation, and chemotherapy.

Surgery

Surgery is used in most cases, with the goal of removing all cancerous tissue and obtaining a clean surgical margin. The margin size depends on the size of the tumor, and if the tumor is large, surgery may involve removal of pieces of bone or, less commonly, amputation of an entire limb. This may be followed by reconstructive surgery. Complete surgical removal of the primary tumor and all distant metastatic tumors improves the prognosis for long-term survival. However, more than two-thirds of patients will experience a recurrence at some point. If the cancer can be surgically removed upon recurrence, chances for long-term survival are greatly improved.

Radiation and Chemotherapy

Radiation may be used both preoperatively and postoperatively, or it may be used as an alternative method of controlling an inoperable tumor prior to chemotherapy. It is most often used for Ewing's sarcoma (a type of malignant bone tumor that affects children and young adults) and is not generally very effective for osteosarcomas.

Chemotherapy has an important therapeutic role in bone cancer. Osteosarcomas are considered to be micrometastasized at the time of diagnosis—even in the absence of detectable metastatic tumors. As such, systemic therapy, namely, chemotherapy, is considered essential for long-term survival. A combination of chemotherapy drugs is often used, and chemotherapy may be given prior to or following surgery. Prior to surgery, chemotherapy is used to reduce the size of the tumor to increase the chances that the limb, or more of it, may be spared. After surgery, chemotherapy is aimed at destroying any distant cancerous cells. Common chemotherapy agents used include methotrexate, doxorubicin, cyclophosphamide, cisplatin, ifosfamide, etoposide, and carboplatin. Refer to the chart "Chemotherapy Drugs and Their Nutrient and Herb Interactions" on page 141 for more information on supplements that can support your body during chemotherapy.

Complementary Approaches

Refer to part II of this book regarding useful complementary approaches for all cancers. The following information is specific to bone cancer.

Lifestyle and Diet

Because the specific causes of bone cancer are unknown, the best lifestyle advice is more general, using a basic approach. Although there are no dietary guidelines specific to bone cancer, a diet that promotes overall health and strong immunity is certainly a good idea. An interesting published case report involving a man with metastatic osteosarcoma underscored the importance of eating a healthy diet and doing intensive meditation in his long-term survival. Emphasize whole foods such as fruits, vegetables, whole grains, lean meats, and fish, and avoid or minimize consumption of processed foods and refined sugars. Eating more soy products may be beneficial, as one of the active ingredients in soy, the isoflavone genistein, has been shown to stimulate apoptosis of osteosarcoma cells in animals. In addition, there is some interesting research associated with sesame oil. In vitro studies have shown that sesamin, a lignan found in sesame oil, inhibits the growth of osteosarcoma cells.

Although physical activity is typically an essential component of a healthy lifestyle, this may not be the case in osteosarcoma. Exercise may be con-traindicated due to the fragility of bones with osteosarcoma, especially in children with tumors in the femur.

Nutrients and Herbs

For information on dosages for these supplements, as well as any potential contraindications, see the appendix.

- **Antioxidants and branched-chain amino acids**: Test tube and animal studies using a formula with a combination of vitamin C, lysine, proline, arginine, and green tea demonstrated a reduction in tumor size and cancer progression in cases of fibrosarcoma. Fibrosarcomas can be considered cousins to osteosarcomas, and the nutrients helpful in controlling fibrosarcoma growth may also be helpful in controlling osteosarcoma growth. [anticancer]

- **Genistein**: An animal study performed by researchers in Beijing found that genistein induced apoptosis of osteosarcoma cells. However, because of its estrogenic activity, genistein is contraindicated in cases where breast, prostate, or ovarian hormone-dependent cancers have spread to the bone. [anticancer]

- **Selenium**: In vivo and in vitro studies demonstrated that the essential trace mineral selenium, found in oats, whole wheat, and bran, inhibited osteosarcoma tumor growth and induced apoptosis. [anticancer]

Summary

Although they are rare, primary bone cancers can be difficult to treat if not discovered early. Additionally, osteosarcomas predominantly affect children and young adults. Many young people who are otherwise in peak health do not appreciate the significant risk for recurrence of this disease. As a result, an unusually high number of young people decline conventional therapy, opting instead for alternative treatment alone. Osteosarcoma is a cancer for which we recommend an integrative treatment plan with heavy emphasis on conventional treatment, given that there are few evidence-based alternative treatments for this cancer, the likelihood of recurrence, and the moderate success rate of conventional treatments for early-stage osteosarcoma.

In addition to the specific nutrients mentioned in this section, the recommendations in parts II and III of this book will support all key body functions and may improve the response to conventional therapy and further reduce the chance of recurrence. Although certain nutrients have shown promise in treating bone cancer in early trials, at this point little is known about the role of natural substances in the prevention or treatment of osteosarcoma.

sixteen

Brain Cancer

Primary brain cancers are relatively rare. Primary brain tumors, meaning cancer tumors originating in the brain, account for about 20 percent of all brain cancers. The other tumors in the brain are tumors that have spread from cancerous tumors originating in other organs of the body. Metastatic brain tumors occur in 10 to 15 percent of cancer patients. The most common cancers that metastasize to the brain are melanoma and cancers of the lung, breast, kidney, and head and neck. Primary brain tumors rarely spread to other areas of the body, but they can spread within the brain. Because there are more than 120 different varieties of brain tumors, effective treatment can be difficult.

The most common form of brain tumor is a glioma or glioblastoma. Gliomas are tumors of the glial cells; these are cells located in the brain and spinal cord that protect and support nerve cells. Of the glioma tumors, the most prevalent type are astrocytomas, which develop from star-shaped cells called astrocytes. There are several different subtypes of astrocytomas, ranging from relatively slow-growing, minimally invasive, and highly curable to fast-growing and invasive tumors with a poor prognosis. According to the National Cancer Institute, more than 22,000 new cases of primary brain cancer were diagnosed in the United States in 2009.

Causes, Symptoms, and Diagnosis

The causes of brain tumors are not known, but certain factors can increase risk. The most common environmental risk factor is exposure to radiation—

most frequently, radiation treatment given for already existing tumors. Exposure to industrial chemicals is another known risk factor. It has been suggested that artificial sweeteners and cell phone use may increase risk, but these claims are controversial. Immune system disorders are another risk factor, and in rare cases brain cancers may be hereditary.

According to the National Cancer Institute, common symptoms of brain cancer include frequent or worsening headaches, vomiting, loss of appetite, changes in mood and personality, changes in ability to think and learn, and seizures. Brain tumors are usually identified with an imaging test, such as a CT scan or MRI. If a suspected tumor is located, a tissue sample can be removed for biopsy by inserting a needle through the skull and into the tumor.

Conventional Treatment

Surgery and radiation are commonly used conventional treatments for brain cancer, with chemotherapy used occasionally.

Surgery

Surgery is used in many cases, with the goal being safe removal of the maximum amount of cancerous tissue possible. Superficial tumors are more easily accessed and removed. Deep-seated tumors are usually difficult to reach and often cannot be surgically removed without causing too much damage to other brain tissue. Oftentimes, the goal of surgery is to reduce the size of the tumor to improve neurologic function and increase the effectiveness of other therapies.

Radiation and Chemotherapy

Radiation is commonly used for brain cancer. It may be used preoperatively, postoperatively, or in cases where surgery is undesirable or impossible. Because of the surgical challenges, cutting-edge radiation technologies are often employed, such as stereotactic radiation, intensity-modulated radiation therapy (IMRT), tomotherapy, intraoperative radiation therapy, and proton beam therapy. Radiation plays a major role in the treatment of brain tumors and contributes substantially to both cure and disease-free survival.

Chemotherapy is occasionally used to treat primary brain tumors, depending upon the type of tumor, the presence of brain edema, and whether the tumor is amenable to surgery. If used, chemotherapy may lengthen the disease-free survival time. A significant challenge regarding brain tumor chemotherapy is delivery of drugs across the blood-brain barrier, that is, the blood vessels in the brain that only allow certain substances to leave the blood and come into contact with brain tissue. This selective barrier prevents potentially harmful substances from entering the brain, but it also makes it difficult for most chemotherapy agents to penetrate into the brain, significantly limiting the usefulness of chemotherapy for brain tumors. Brain swelling, which is common with brain tumors, can also impede the effectiveness of chemotherapy, as the fluid causing the swelling prevents the chemotherapy from finding and saturating the tumor tissue. For these reasons, chemotherapy is not typically considered a primary treatment, but it may be used preoperatively or postoperatively to treat certain types of tumors. Common chemotherapy agents used include surgical implantation of nitrosourea-based drugs and carmustine (BCNU). The direct implantation bypasses the blood-brain barrier and puts the chemotherapy agent in direct contact with the tumor tissue. Temozolomide can cross the blood-brain barrier and is utilized for certain types of brain cancer, such as glioblastoma and certain astrocytomas.

People with brain tumors that cannot be removed or people who have a poor prognosis should consider clinical trials with hyperthermia, interstitial brachytherapy, newly developed drugs, and biological response modifiers—agents that boost the body's immune system to fight cancer or other diseases.

Complementary Approaches

Refer to part II of this book regarding useful complementary approaches for all cancers. The following information is specific to brain cancer.

Lifestyle and Diet

While data are inconclusive, those concerned about developing brain cancer may want to reduce their exposure to possible contributing factors, such as regular use of cell phones and consumption of aspartame (a synthetic sweetener sold under the brand names NutraSweet and Equal, and added to many sugar-free foods and beverages). Preliminary reports have indicated exposure to pesticides may increase risk of brain cancer, but these reports are not conclusive. There have also been reports of higher incidences of brain cancer in children with high exposure to electromagnetic fields (EMFs), for instance, those living near high-voltage power lines. However, more recent research discounts the link between electromagnetic fields and childhood brain cancer.

A whole foods diet that minimizes processed foods and artificial ingredients is recommended. Eating organic foods will support overall health and may provide food-based nutrients that will support apoptosis of brain cancer cells. Aside from the data showing a potential link between pesticides and brain cancer as well as aspartame and brain cancer, no conclusive relationships between diet and brain cancer have been found. For now, avoiding consumption of pesticides and aspartame by keeping to an organic whole foods diet seems to be the best dietary advice.

Nutrients and Herbs

Some herbs and nutrients are showing promise as potential complementary treatments for brain cancer. For information on dosages for these supplements, as well as any potential contraindications, see the appendix.

- *Aloe vera*: A human trial of patients with solid tumors, including glioblastoma, for whom no standard anticancer therapies were available evaluated whether administration of aloe could enhance the therapeutic effects of melatonin (see below). These patients were treated with oral melatonin alone at a dose of 20 mg at bedtime or melatonin plus aloe vera tincture. This preliminary study found that melatonin plus aloe vera extract produced some therapeutic benefits, at least in terms of stabilization of disease and survival. [anticancer]

- *Curcumin*: Several cellular studies have found that curcumin significantly repressed invasion of glioma and other brain tumor cells in vitro. [anticancer]

- *Dong quai*: Early research on this herb commonly used in traditional Chinese medicine indicates promise for primary brain tumor treatment. Research in Taiwan demonstrated that dong quai had anticancer effects on glioblastoma cells. [anticancer]

- *Ginseng*: A recent report in the *International Journal of Cancer* indicates that a component in Panax ginseng (which the researchers call compound K) may help control the growth and invasiveness of brain tumors. [anticancer]

- *Green tea*: Canadian researchers found that epigallocatechin gallate (EGCG), an active ingredient in green tea, may help halt the progression of glioma cells in vitro. [anticancer]

- *Melatonin*: Brain tumor growth is at least in part stimulated by various growth hormones and inhibited by other hormones, such as melatonin. It makes sense, then, that a trial of patients with glioblastoma who received radiation therapy showed that those patients who also used the hormone melatonin at a dose of 20 mg at bedtime had better outcomes than those who received the radiation only. Both the survival curve and the percentage of survival at one year were significantly higher in patients treated with radiation plus melatonin than in those receiving radiation alone. Melatonin also reduced toxicity due to radiation and steroid therapy. [anticancer, supportive]

- *Phosphatidylserine and ginkgo biloba*: Other supplements to consider for primary brain tumors include phosphatidylserine and ginkgo biloba, which are known to enhance brain function. These nutrients may reduce treatment-related side effects such as cognitive dysfunction and memory loss. Additionally, they may exert some preventive effects by stimulating apoptosis and reducing genetic damage to brain cells. [preventive, supportive]

Other Complementary Approaches

Although there are some case reports of success using magnetic therapy, there are no studies confirming its effectiveness against brain cancer. Antineoplaston therapy as performed at the Burzynski Research Institute in Houston, Texas, shows some promise. In 1970, Dr. Stanislaw Burzynski isolated a group of compounds that he called antineoplastons from human blood and urine. A 1991 National Cancer Institute review of seven brain tumor patients treated by Dr. Burzynski found that the antineoplastons had antitumor activity. A phase II study of antineoplastons in children with incurable glioma was conducted in 2004 and found that at the time of the publication, 10 out of the 12 patients were alive and well with either stable disease, reduced tumor, or complete remission. The study continues to recruit patients. In a 2006 report published in *Integrative Cancer Therapies*, 18 patients with inoperable brain tumors who received the antineoplaston therapy demonstrated a 22 percent overall five-year survival rate. This is in contrast to a typical five-year survival rate of 5 percent.

Summary

Brain cancers are difficult to treat because doing so requires penetration of the blood-brain barrier. In addition, operating on some portions of the brain or radiating the brain can be challenging and quite possibly damaging to the patient. Success using chemotherapy as a sole treatment is limited, but chemotherapy may be a helpful adjunct treatment in some cases. Substances such as melatonin and phosphatidylserine, along with herbs such as curcumin and green tea, may provide some additional benefits by stimulating apoptosis of brain tumor cells. Dr. Burzynski's research using antineoplastons may yield some innovative therapies for certain brain cancers.

seventeen

Breast Cancer

American Cancer Society statistics indicate that breast cancer is the second most frequently diagnosed cancer in the United States and the most common cancer among women. In 2009, more than 192,000 women were diagnosed with breast cancer—that represents one out of every eight adult women in the United States. Of all breast cancers diagnosed in women, 74 percent are diagnosed in postmenopausal women and 26 percent in premenopausal women. Only 6 percent of those diagnosed with breast cancer have metastatic disease, whereas the others have localized cancer.

Among the structures of the breast are lobes, subdivided into smaller sections called lobules, and tiny bulbs capable of producing milk. These structures are interconnected by tubes called ducts. Breast cancer most commonly originates in the duct tissue (ductal carcinoma) but can also begin in the lobes or lobules (lobular carcinoma). Inflammatory breast cancer is a less common type of cancer in which the breast swells and becomes red.

Causes, Symptoms, and Diagnosis

Factors contributing to the likelihood of contracting breast cancer are numerous. Women are at 100 times greater risk than men. The chance of getting breast cancer increases with age, with 80 percent of breast cancer cases occurring in women over 50. Heredity plays a part in about 5 to 10 percent of breast cancer cases. Women with a mother, daughter, or sister with breast cancer are twice as likely to contract the disease as women with no close relatives with breast cancer. Gene mutations, specifically of the genes

BRCA1, BRCA2, and p53, are associated with a 40 to 85 percent lifetime risk of developing breast cancer.

Other factors that increase the risk include exposure to radiation and early onset of menstruation. Women who have taken birth control pills any time during the previous ten years are thought to have a slightly higher risk of breast cancer than those who have not. Previous pregnancy and having breast-fed are both thought to lower breast cancer risk slightly. Using hormone replacement therapy (HRT) to treat symptoms of menopause increases the risk of breast cancer (and other diseases). Alcohol use, obesity, and a sedentary lifestyle also increase risk. Other potential risk factors include smoking, eating charred red meat regularly, and exposure to pesticides, PCBs, and other pollutants.

In its early stages, breast cancer is typically not painful; the first symptom may be an obvious lump in the breast tissue. The presence of a lump is typically noticed before any additional symptoms occur; however, some breast tumors develop in areas of the breast that cannot be felt. As breast tumors grow, symptoms can include breast discharge, nipple inversion, changes in the skin of the breast, and fatigue. In later stages, possible symptoms include changes in the size, shape, or color of the breast, nipple, or skin surrounding the nipple, as well as discharge or bleeding. Breast tumors are typically detected by screening mammograms, breast self-examination, or an examination by a health-care practitioner. Mammography increases the likelihood of early detection, and despite public concern, it has not been found to increase the risk of developing breast cancer. In fact, mammography has been associated with an overall decreased risk of death due to breast cancer. Any new or suspicious breast lump should be immediately investigated with a follow-up diagnostic mammogram. There is much debate regarding when women should start getting regular mammograms. For the American Cancer Society Recommendations, see page 29. Recently proposed guidelines based upon comprehensive research indicates that unless you are a woman at high risk (family history or past diagnosis) or have a suspicious breast lump, you should not start getting mammograms until age 50. Regular mammogram screenings should continue at least every two years (every year if you are at high risk). We emphasize, however, that the decision about when to begin mammogram screening is one that needs to be made by both you and your doctor based on your individual total risk factors and index of concern.

If cancer is suspected after mammography or palpation, more imaging tests, such as an ultrasound or breast MRI, will be done. Of note, it is of critical importance to obtain mammograms and other imaging studies of both breasts, as the presence of disease in one breast increases the chances of cancer in the other. If the imaging is not conclusive, a patient may be a candidate for breast-specific gamma imaging (BSGI), which is a molecular breast imaging technique that can detect very small breast lesions. BSGI is particularly useful in detecting ductal carcinoma in situ and lobular carcinoma. If cancer is still a concern after these imaging studies, the person should undergo a biopsy, the only definitive diagnostic method for breast cancer.

Suspicious areas need to be biopsied. Most patients will undergo a fine-needle biopsy to extract cells for analysis. Some patients will undergo a core needle biopsy, which removes more of the tissue. Pathologists then review tumor tissue to determine whether the tumor is ductal or lobular carcinoma. Infiltrating or invasive ductal cancer is the most common type of breast cancer, comprising 70 to 80 percent of all breast cancers. Additionally, the tumor will be evaluated for its grade of differentiation, proliferative activity, and status in regard to estrogen receptors (ER), progesterone receptors (PR), and human epidermal growth factor receptors. All of these factors have significant implications in terms of prognosis and treatment options.

Oncotype DX Test

The FDA recently approved the use of a multi-gene diagnostic assay test in cases of breast cancer. This test, known as the oncotype DX test, is designed to help oncologists tailor the treatment to the individual. Used in conjunction with the standard staging, grading, and tumor marker analyses, this assay can give insight into the chances of recurrence and may help determine the most appropriate treatment strategy. This test looks for the presence of mutations in a set of genes in breast tumor cells. These mutations are associated with response to treatment and also with the likelihood of recurrence. Presently, studies indicate that this test is most appropriate for those with newly diagnosed stage I or II node-negative, estrogen receptor positive breast cancer who will be treated with tamoxifen. According to the developers of this assay, clinical studies in other breast cancer populations are under way. This test is promising and is likely to become an accepted part of a diagnostic workup for early-stage breast cancers. The test is performed by using part of the tumor tissue removed with lumpectomy or mastectomy surgery.

Conventional Treatment

Conventional treatment for breast cancer relies heavily on surgery, often followed by radiation therapy. Chemotherapy and hormone therapy are used in cases of metastatic or advanced breast cancer.

Surgery

Surgery is used in almost all cases, with the goal of removing all cancerous tissue and obtaining a clean surgical margin. The margin size depends on the size and location of the tumor. There are several surgical options, depending on the stage and aggressiveness of the cancer, including

- Lumpectomy (removal of the tumor and a clean margin)
- Lumpectomy with removal of sentinel nodes (removal of the tumor and one or a small number of lymph nodes that are the first to receive

Lymphedema

Lumpectomy or mastectomy with removal of the axillary nodes can produce arm and hand swelling (edema), which can, in turn, cause numbness, tingling, and occasionally pain. Women will need to take precautions to minimize this complication. Massage, physical therapy, and acupuncture may help. Discuss edema prevention and treatment options with your doctor.

drainage from the tumor and that are most likely to harbor metastatic disease)

● Mastectomy (removal of the breast)

● Modified radical mastectomy (removal of the breast and axillary lymph nodes, located in the armpit)

● Radical mastectomy (removal of the breast, axillary lymph nodes, and chest wall muscles)

Mastectomy surgery may include immediate breast reconstruction, but reconstructive surgery may also be delayed to a later time, and some women may elect not to have reconstructive surgery at all. As with any major surgery, there are always risks that should be discussed with your surgeon prior to the procedure.

With advances in detection technology, more breast cancers are being found early. As a result, breast-conserving surgery is often a safe and effective option. Several studies indicate that better disease-free survival is achieved for premenopausal women with breast cancer and positive axillary lymph nodes if breast surgery is performed during the second half of the menstrual cycle (days 15–36; the luteal phase) rather than in the first half (the follicular phase). Other studies have not confirmed this finding, so the optimal timing of surgery remains controversial and should be evaluated on a case-by-case basis.

Radiation and Chemotherapy

In cases of early-stage breast cancer (carcinoma in situ and tumors less than 1 centimeter in diameter), lumpectomy and close follow-up is one treatment choice. However, even in these early-stage breast cancers, local radiation treatment will typically be recommended in order to prevent local recurrence. In a study with 818 women, disease-free survival at eight years was 75 percent for those who underwent lumpectomy plus radiation therapy, versus 62 percent for those who underwent lumpectomy alone. With types of breast cancer that are more invasive or have the potential to be more invasive, radiation, chemotherapy, or a combination of both will be recommended in addition to surgery.

Lobular cancer in situ is typically managed by lumpectomy. For those tumors that are ER+, hormonal therapy such as tamoxifen is used. Ductal carcinoma in situ is typically managed with breast-conserving surgery

Prophylactic Surgery

Some women at high risk who have not been diagnosed with breast cancer consider prophylactic (preventive) surgeries. This includes mastectomy (removal of the breasts) and can sometimes include a complete hysterectomy (removal of the uterus and ovaries). While many studies have confirmed there is less breast and ovarian cancer among women who have had these organs removed, subsequent studies have questioned the use of such radical preventive measures because of quality-of-life issues and long-term side effects.

Since the introduction of prophylactic surgery, the medical community has failed to focus on issues of surgical complications and communicating risk-to-benefit information. A database search of studies on prophylactic mastectomy for the prevention of breast cancer uncovered research bias, poorly designed studies, and inappropriately prequalified participants. Researchers who evaluated 23 studies involving more than 4,000 patients concluded in a report featured in the *Cochrane Database System Review* that more rigorous prospective studies are needed, because "the state of the science is far from exact in predicting who will get or who will die from breast cancer. By one estimate, most of the women deemed high risk by family history (but not necessarily BRCA1 or 2 mutation carriers) who underwent these procedures would not have died from breast cancer." The researchers reported that body image and feelings of femininity were adversely affected.

Another study, which evaluated 269 women who underwent bilateral (both breasts) prophylactic mastectomy, found that two-thirds experienced at least one complication following the surgery (such as infection or excess bleeding).

While many genetic counseling centers and research facilities continue to encourage these surgeries, women are advised to evaluate this decision carefully. Genetic testing is not designed to be a diagnostic tool. While research has confirmed that mutations of the BRCA1 and BRCA2 genes cause a predisposition to breast and ovarian cancer, many other genes have been identified that also can increase a woman's risk. Until more research is done, genetic testing should not be the sole tool used to recommend serious surgeries.

High-risk women with a family history of breast cancer or who have tested positive for mutation of the BRCA1 or BRCA2 gene are advised to undertake an aggressive integrative prevention plan that incorporates the guidelines outlined in chapter 4. In addition, those who are not taking tamoxifen can derive additional protection from indole-3-carbinol (abundant in cruciferous vegetables) or supplemental diindolylmethane (DIM). Aggressive screening is also recommended for these women. This may include the combination of mammogram with ultrasound and, for those with risk for ovarian cancer, an annual pelvic ultrasound. If your risk level is high, ask your doctor how you can step up your screening program.

followed by radiation. For tumors that are ER+, tamoxifen or aromatase inhibitor hormonal therapy is used. Radiation therapy often entails side effects such as local skin irritation and fatigue, and in some cases delayed complications from radiation therapy—including radiation pneumonitis, heart damage, arm edema, and increased risk of subsequent malignancies—can occur months or years after radiation. (See the sidebar "What's New with Radiation?" on page 90 for information about current advances in radiation therapy that better localize the radiation and minimize these toxic effects.) Despite some of the adverse effects of radiation therapy, it can lower the risk of local recurrence. However, radiation therapy does not lower the risk of recurrence in the opposite breast or elsewhere in the body. In an effort to lower the risk of recurrence at distant sites, conventional treatment includes tamoxifen after radiation. Tamoxifen blocks estrogen receptors on cancer tumor cells. This is significant because the estrogen receptor is used by the cancer cell to stimulate growth. Studies indicate that for ER+ tumors, tamoxifen (premenopausal women) or aromatase inhibitors (postmenopausal women) can be effective at reducing recurrence. This recommendation is based on data from clinical trials. For more information about tamoxifen, refer to the section "Other Conventional Treatments" in this chapter.

Despite the early stage of the disease, patients with stage I (local, not in the lymph nodes) through stage III (has spread to the lymph nodes) breast cancer require a multimodality approach to treatment. The treatment strategy is determined based on tumor characteristics, oncotype DX results (refer to the sidebar on page 267), and patient characteristics. The goal is to lower the risk of occurrence while weighing the pros and cons of the treatment. Keep in mind that most breast cancers are considered curable at an early stage but highly incurable once metastatic. Surgical treatments include (1) lumpectomy plus radiation to the affected breast or (2) mastectomy of the affected breast with or without prophylactic removal of the opposite breast. Women who carry the BRCA1 or BRCA2 genetic mutation who are diagnosed with breast cancer are statistically more likely to develop disease in the other breast and therefore are often encouraged to have a mastectomy of the affected breast and a prophylactic mastectomy of the other breast (for more information on prophylactic mastectomy, see the sidebar on page 269). Mastectomies may include immediate reconstruction. Following surgery, additional treatments are likely indicated:

- Radiation therapy to the affected breast

- Radiation therapy to the affected breast plus the lymph nodes and/or chest wall

- Chemotherapy (typically includes adriamycin, cytoxan, and/or paclitaxel) (Note: Women with HER-2/neu-positive tumors will benefit from adriamcyin, whereas women with HER-2/neu-negative tumors will not)

- Hormonal therapy (typically tamoxifen for premenopausal women or an aromatase inhibitor for postmenopausal women)

Women with metastatic breast cancer will usually receive chemotherapy along with hormonal therapy and trastuzumab (for an explanation of Herceptin see page 95) if their tumor is HER-2/neu-positive (about 25 percent of breast cancers). Most people do not experience side effects while on Herceptin; however, for women with underlying heart conditions, there is a risk of serious heart damage. Radiation is used as a pain control measure in metastatic disease, as it can help shrink tumors. This is especially indicated when these tumors are large enough to be causing tissue and nerve compression and associated tissue dysfunction and pain. In these instances, the symptom relief provided by radiation-induced tumor shrinkage typically outweighs any adverse reactions to the radiation itself. There are several chemotherapy agents used for metastatic breast cancer, including doxorubicin, cyclophosphamide, fluorouracil, methotrexate, epirubicin, carboplatin, paclitaxel, and docetaxel. Women with node-positive, ER-positive, PR-positive, and HER-2/neu-positive tumors tend to respond most favorably to chemotherapy. Adverse toxicity from chemotherapy is expected, and integrative management of these symptoms is important. For information about how to counteract typical side effects, consult the chart "Chemotherapy Drugs and Their Nutrient and Herb Interactions" that begins on page 141.

Chemotherapy Considerations

A recent meta-analysis by the Early Breast Cancer Trialists' Collaborative Group has uncovered survival benefit from chemotherapy even in women with early-stage breast cancer. Among these women, six months of an adjuvant anthracycline-based chemotherapy regimen reduced the annual mortality rate from the disease by 38 percent in women younger than 50 and by 20 percent in women 50 to 69 years old. In more advanced cancers (stages II through IV), chemotherapy provides the most benefit in women under the age of 50, with 10-year survival rates increasing from 71 to 78 percent in node-negative disease and from 42 to 53 percent in node-positive disease. In women 50 or more years of age, on the other hand, the 10-year survival rate only improved from 67 to 69 percent for node-negative disease and from 46 to 49 percent for node-positive disease. These data suggest that chemotherapy is most advantageous for women under the age of 50 with early-stage cancer.

Other Conventional Treatments

Hormone-blocking treatments may be beneficial in women with ER-positive or ER-unknown breast tumors. In women with estrogen receptor positive disease, five years of adjuvant tamoxifen reduced the annual death rate by 31 percent, regardless of age. Survival advantages and decrease of risk of recurrence conferred by tamoxifen increased with length of use up until five years; after that point continued use did not provide additional benefit.

Tamoxifen is not without adverse effects, however. Tamoxifen increases the risk of deep vein thrombosis, pulmonary emboli, and endometrial cancer. Women taking tamoxifen need routine follow-up annual gynecological exams and may be candidates for raloxifene (Evista) instead. (See chapter 10 for further discussion of hormone involvement in cancer, and the "Hormone

Drugs and Their Nutrient and Herb Interactions" chart on pages 156 and 157 for nutrients and herbs that may help with side effects from hormone therapy.)

Studies have demonstrated that aromatase inhibitors (for example, anastrozole) are more effective than other hormone-blocking treatments in postmenopausal women. A recent study from the University of Athens, Greece, demonstrated that aromatase inhibitor treatment was well tolerated and helped extend life among 60 postmenopausal women with advanced stage IV breast cancer. For more information on conventional hormone cancer treatments, refer to the chart "Hormone Drugs and Their Nutrient and Herb Interactions" on page 156.

Women with HER-2/neu-positive tumors will likely receive a recommendation to take Herceptin, which has been shown in clinical studies to provide benefit.

Zoledronic acid (Zometa) is used to treat breast cancer bone metastasis. Recent data indicate it may also help prevent breast cancer metastasis to bone and elsewhere in premenopausal women with breast cancer.

Complementary Approaches

Refer to part II of this book regarding useful complementary approaches for all cancers. The following information is specific to breast cancer.

Lifestyle and Diet

As mentioned in previous chapters, many studies have indicated that exercise will help women with breast cancer, as it stimulates immune activity, enhances detoxification, encourages positive self-image, and helps prevent or reduce obesity. Exercise directly reduces risk factors for the development and progression of breast cancer, primarily via its effect on the body's metabolic process. A report in the *Journal of Clinical Oncology* demonstrated that a combination of exercise (30 minutes 6 days per week) and diet (5 servings of vegetables and fruits daily) actually cut the risk of dying of breast cancer in half among early-stage breast cancer patients.

Increasing consumption of colorful fruits and vegetables is especially important in regard to breast cancer prevention and treatment. Many studies have demonstrated a link between breast cancer prevention and increased consumption of cruciferous vegetables and antioxidant-rich foods. Researchers at the University of California, San Diego, reported in the journal *Nutrition and Cancer* that a low-fat, high-vegetable diet helped reduce the risk of recurrence among breast cancer survivors. Another study in the same journal in 2006 demonstrated that a low-fat, high-fiber diet rich in fruits and vegetables improved overall survival of postmenopausal women who had previously been diagnosed with breast cancer.

Reducing fat consumption is critical to the prevention and treatment of breast cancer and maintaining normal body weight. According to researchers from Uruguay, women with a strong family history of breast cancer were more susceptible to the cancer-promoting effects of the Western high-fat diet, in which increased dietary fat and decreased fiber consumption results in increased circulating free estrogens (growth factors for breast cancer) in the bloodstream. Obesity is an identified risk factor for the development of breast cancer. A 2009 *Journal of Clinical Oncology* study found that obesity was associated with increased oxidative stress and increased breast cancer risk. Another dietary consideration with regard to breast cancer is soy. Increased soy in the diet is controversial. Consumption of soy foods appears to reduce the risk of premenopausal breast cancer; however, women with breast cancer should minimize dietary soy, as it may act as a growth factor for the established breast cancer tumors.

A diet high in sugar should also be avoided. A 2009 study featured in *Cancer Causes and Control* found that frequent consumption of sweets, particularly desserts, specifically in premenopausal women, doubled the risk of breast cancer development. High-sugar diets increase insulin resistance, which promotes breast cancer growth. Several studies have demonstrated a direct link between insulin resistance associated with a high carbohydrate intake and diets with high glycemic index and ER+/PR- breast cancer risk.

Alcohol consumption has been clearly linked to an increased risk of breast cancer. The relationship between alcohol and breast cancer is linear, meaning that each additional serving of alcohol confers additional risk of breast cancer development. Additionally, new research published in the *Journal of the National Cancer Institute* shows that alcohol raises breast cancer risk among women who use hormone replacement therapy. An article featured in the *British Medical Journal* concludes that "an adequate dietary intake of folic acid may protect against the increased risk of breast cancer associated with alcohol consumption." Folic acid, also known as folate, is found in various beans, asparagus, and spinach.

Nutrients and Herbs

A wide variety of nutrients and herbs have been studied for preventing and treating breast cancer. Here are some of the more notable findings:

- **Ashwagandha (*Withania somnifera*)**: In vitro studies have shown that ashwagandha reduces cell proliferation and increases apoptosis in ER+ and ER- human breast cancer cells. [anticancer]

- **Black cohosh**: Two different observational studies involving breast cancer patients have demonstrated a significant protective effect on the rate of recurrence (one study was 27 percent and the other was 61 percent reduction). [preventive]

- **CoQ10**: Early studies demonstrated that CoQ10 is effective at improving the health of those with advanced breast cancer. [supportive]

- **Curcumin**: This phytochemical found in turmeric decreases oxidative damage to cells and inflammation, interferes with growth factor stimulation of breast cancer cells, and reduces tumor growth in animal and in vitro studies. Curcumin should not be taken if the chemotherapy drug doxorubicin is being used. [preventive, anticancer]

- **Diindolylmethane (DIM)**: DIM, which is a metabolite of indole-3-carbinol (I3C), influences metabolism of estrogen into safer end products. DIM has also been shown in vitro to stimulate the destruction and decrease the invasive potential of breast cancer cells. [preventive, anticancer]

- **Fermented wheat germ extract (Avemar)**: In vitro study indicated that Avemar enhances tumor destruction when combined with hormonal therapies. In an animal study Avemar also increased tumor inhibition in both ER+ and ER- breast cancer. [anticancer]

- **Flaxseed lignans**: Several cellular and animal studies have demonstrated that the lignan secoisolariciresinol diglucoside (SDG) can reduce tumor growth and help prevent metastasis. In addition, human trials have shown that high plant lignan intake is associated with reduced risk of postmenopausal breast cancer. [preventive, anticancer]

- **Green tea**: Several studies have demonstrated that green tea has a protective effect against breast cancer and can also inhibit cancer cell growth and invasion. In human studies, women with a history of stage I breast cancer who drank at least five cups of green tea daily had longer disease-free survival, a 57 percent lower recurrence rate, and decreased extent of recurrent disease. [preventive]

- **Indole-3-carbinol**: Recent research featured in the *British Journal of Cancer* found that indole-3-carbinol (I3C) can help prevent development of cancer in women with mutations of the BRCA1 and BRCA2 genes. I3C should not be taken with tamoxifen, as it may increase the speed at which tamoxifen is metabolized (thus reducing the time it is active). There is controversy about the safety of isolated I3C. Although it is purported to divert estrogen's metabolic breakdown products away from carcinogenic metabolites and toward noncarcinogenic metabolites, some studies have shown that I3C may actually stimulate metabolism of estrogen toward both carcinogenic and anticarcinogenic metabolites. This isn't a problem with dietary I3C, which is found in cruciferous vegetables; it is considered safe in food form and is highly encouraged as a part of an anticancer diet. But again, caution is recommended when taking I3C supplements. [preventive]

- *Iodine*: This mineral has been shown in several cellular studies to down-regulate estrogen receptor stimulated growth of breast cancer cells and increase apoptosis. Iodine also increases the enzyme activity that breaks down estrogen in the body. Note: Iodine should only be supplemented when there is confirmed deficiency. [preventive]

- *L-glutamine*: Recent animal studies demonstrated that oral glutamine could increase the effectiveness of chemotherapy drugs, such as methotrexate and paclitaxel, in cases of breast cancer. [supportive]

- *Melatonin*: After estrogen binds to an estrogen receptor on a breast cancer cell, melatonin inhibits that receptor's signaling for cell division. In vitro studies have demonstrated that melatonin induces apoptosis and reduces breast cancer invasiveness and metastasis. These mechanisms are further demonstrated in human trials. In a study in 2005, women in the highest quartile of melatonin metabolite levels had a 40 percent lower risk of invasive breast cancer than those in the lowest quartile. The researchers concluded that higher melatonin levels are associated with a lower risk of breast cancer. Melatonin inhibits the enzyme aromatase, which normally converts androgens in fat cells into estrogen. Androgens are the primary source of estrogen in menopausal women, so inhibition of aromatase is a significant way to lower breast cancer risk in menopausal women. [preventive, anticancer]

- *Mistletoe*: A five-year clinical trial involving breast cancer patients who have completed conventional therapy found that use of mistletoe extract resulted in significantly fewer disease- and therapy-related complaints including mouth sores, fatigue, pain, and headache. [supportive]

- *Mushrooms*: A component of medical mushroom known as PSK was shown in studies to significantly extend survival in stage II ER- breast cancer patients. The dosage used in the study was 3 grams per day. [anticancer]

- *Omega-3 fatty acids*: Omega-3 fatty acids, found in flax oil, algal oil, and fish oil, have been shown to reduce breast tumor growth in animal models. [anticancer]

- *Proanthocyanidins*: These phytochemicals found in grape skins (such as resveratrol), seeds, fruits, and vegetables specifically kill breast cancer cells in vitro. [anticancer]

- *Probiotics*: According to a paper featured in the journal *Medical Hypothesis*, cancer recurrence could potentially be minimized when employing probiotics. [preventive]

- *Vitamin D*: Although this vitamin has been studied primarily for its role in preventing breast cancer, new research indicates that prognosis may also be improved with vitamin D therapy. Studies indicate that women with low levels of vitamin D tend to have more advanced breast cancers while women with higher levels of vitamin D tend to have less advanced cancers. [preventive]

- *Vitamin E*: A cellular study from the University of California at Los Angeles found that vitamin E inhibited estrogen receptor positive cancer cell growth by altering cellular response to estrogen. [anticancer]

Summary

It is estimated that one in eight women in the United States will develop breast cancer. Some progress has been made in lowering the incidence of breast cancer among menopausal women, an effect attributed to the dramatic reduction of hormone replacement therapy in use by these women since 2003. At that time, the Women's Health Initiative demonstrated that there is an increased risk of heart disease and breast cancer in women taking a combination of premarin and progesterone (Prempro). This led to a decline in hormone replacement prescriptions and a reduction in breast cancer. Slight improvements have also been made in the prognosis for all women, primarily due to early detection followed by comprehensive treatment. Screening and early detection are critical. Surgery to remove the cancer is prudent and recommended. Follow-up radiation, chemotherapy, and hormonal therapy are part of the standard of conventional care for this cancer. Additionally, many natural substances offer promise as adjunctive treatment aids—especially in the earlier stages of breast cancer. Among the most promising are green tea, melatonin, curcumin, and vitamin D. All of these interventions rest upon a foundation of a healthy lifestyle that includes a balanced diet, exercise, stress management, and strong support systems.

eighteen

Cervical Cancer

The cervix is the narrow, lower end of the uterus that connects it to the top of the vagina. It is sometimes referred to as the neck of the uterus. About half of the cervix can be seen with appropriate medical equipment, and the other half lies above the vagina and cannot be seen. The tissue of the cervix changes during menstruation, stretching slightly to allow the endometrium to be shed. The cervix also dilates during the final phases of childbirth so the baby can pass through. According to the American Cancer Society, just over 11,000 new cases of cervical cancer were diagnosed in 2009.

Causes, Symptoms, and Diagnosis

The major risk factor for cervical cancer is infection of the cervix by human papillomavirus (HPV), a sexually transmitted virus. HPV causes more than two-thirds of cervical cancer cases. The Centers for Disease Control has estimated that each year more than six million Americans will become infected with genital HPV. In June 2006, the FDA approved the sale of a vaccine (trade name Gardasil) to prevent cervical cancer. The three-shot series contains weakened and non-disease-producing viruses of three types known to cause the majority of cervical cancers and has been demonstrated to be nearly 100 percent effective in protecting against the two primary strains of HPV, which cause most of the HPV-related cancers.

Other risk factors for cancer of the cervix include sexual intercourse at an early age, smoking, giving birth numerous times, sexual promiscuity, use of birth control pills, and compromised immune function.

Symptoms of cervical cancer include vaginal bleeding or discharge, heavier menstrual flow, pelvic pain, or pain during sexual intercourse. In its early stages, cervical cancer usually doesn't have noticeable symptoms. It is typically detected during a regular gynecological checkup. Early detection of cervical cancer greatly improves the outlook for recovery.

A Pap test is used to detect cervical cancer. The American College of Obstetricians and Gynecologists recommends that women who are 18 years old or older and sexually active receive an annual Pap test; once there are three consecutive normal Pap tests, less frequent screening is acceptable, but should be evaluated in the context of other risk factors (such as new sexual partners). Pap tests can identify both cancer cells and atypical cells that may be precancerous; the latter condition is known as cervical dysplasia. Cervical cancer typically develops gradually in the cervical tissue and progresses from dysplasia to cervical cancer in situ to invasive cancer over a 10- to 12-year period. However, it can progress from in situ to invasive cancer within a year in about 10 percent of women. Obtaining annual Pap tests is an essential screening measure to monitor any tissue changes. If Pap test results are suspicious, your doctor may remove a sample of tissue from the cervix for biopsy. Progressive cervical cancer invades the cervical tissue locally and can spread via regional lymph nodes or the bloodstream to distant sites.

Conventional Treatment

Conventional treatment for cervical cancer involves a variety of techniques in addition to surgery, radiation, and chemotherapy.

Surgery

Methods to remove precancerous or cancerous in situ cervical lesions include LEEP (loop electrosurgical excision procedure), laser therapy (the use of high-intensity light to destroy cancerous lesions), conization (surgical removal of the precancerous or cancerous tissue from the cervix), or cryotherapy (destruction of precancerous or cancerous tissue by freezing). (See the "Noninvasive Alternatives" sidebar on page 280 for alternative forms of treatment.)

If cancer is present, surgical removal of the cervix is usually the first line of treatment. The goal is to remove all cancerous tissue and obtain a clean surgical margin. The margin size depends on the size and location of the tumor. The surgery may remove as little as the tip of the cervix, or it may be necessary to remove the entire cervix and parts of the uterus; it may even entail a radical hysterectomy (removal of the cervix, uterus, ovaries, and fallopian tubes, and possibly surrounding tissue and lymph nodes).

Removal of the cervix can also be done with a laparoscope via a small abdominal incision. Even if the tumor appears to be well confined within the cervix, a full metastatic workup is advised; in some cases, an apparent locally invasive cervical cancer has actually given rise to distant metastatic lesions.

Radiation and Chemotherapy

Radiation may be used preoperatively or postoperatively, and is commonly used to treat recurrent cases. In nonmetastasized cases, it may be used instead of surgery. Several different types of radiation therapy are used, including the traditional external beam pelvic radiation and intracavitary brachytherapy, which places radioactive isotopes directly into the uterine cavity. Intracavitary brachytherapy may be the only treatment required after surgical removal of a cancer that has invaded less than 3 millimeters deep into the cervical tissue. For locally advanced lesions between 3 millimeters and 5 millimeters in size, survival rates of 85 to 90 percent can be achieved with either radical hysterectomy or radiation therapy. Radiation can be used in combination with chemotherapy in cases of advanced disease.

Chemotherapy may be used preoperatively or postoperatively. In recurrent cases, chemotherapy is often combined with radiation therapy as this decreases risk of death (reduction of 30 to 50 percent). Most chemotherapy regimens for cervical cancer include cisplatin with or without another agent, including fluorouracil, ifosfamide, irinotecan, paclitaxel, or gemcitabine. (For information about how to counteract typical side effects of these medications, consult the chart "Chemotherapy Drugs and Their Nutrient and Herb Interactions" starting on page 141.) According to *Cancer Management: A Multidisciplinary Approach*, "Chemotherapy [for cervical cancer] has traditionally been used for the palliative management of advanced or recurrent disease that can no longer be managed by surgery or radiation therapy." Because many chemotherapy drugs have not been successful in treating cervical cancer (other than in some recurrent cases), new biological agents are being tested, including the angiogenesis inhibitor TNP-470.

Complementary Approaches

Refer to part II of this book regarding useful complementary approaches for all cancers. The following information is specific to cervical cancer.

Lifestyle and Diet

Preventing cervical cancer or its recurrence requires the practice of safer sex with barrier methods to avoid contracting HPV. In addition, immune system support is critical. Reduce your exposure to secondhand smoke, and if you smoke, it is important to find a way to quit. Cigarette smoke is an

Noninvasive Alternatives

For precancerous cervical lesions, local herbal escharotic treatments may be a reasonable alternative to LEEP, laser therapy, conization, or cryotherapy. In herbal escharotic treatments, a naturopathic physician applies a treatment to the cervix that contains enzymes and herbs that digest the cervical tissue, thereby killing precancerous cells and encouraging regrowth of healthy cervical cells. Additional treatment includes vitamin E creams, and suppositories to reduce inflammation of the cervix. Any alternative treatment for precancerous conditions must be followed with regular pelvic examinations and Pap tests.

independent and significant risk factor for invasive cervical cancer, and quitting should be your highest priority. Genital hygiene is also important. If possible, use all-natural sanitary and body care products. Avoid using talc powder on the genital area; this is directly associated with an increased risk of ovarian cancer, and some speculate it may contribute to other health problems associated with female genitalia.

According to a report featured in the journal *Cancer*, women who are overweight have twice the risk of developing cervical cancer as women who are not overweight. Maintaining proper weight through diet and exercise will also likely help with treatment of cervical cancer. There is also an association between a compromised immune system and the development of cervical cancer. For this reason, all of the advice in chapter 8 may be helpful, especially the dietary tips. Eat plenty of fruits and vegetables, which are high in antioxidant nutrients. Several studies confirm that low levels of antioxidants are directly correlated with a higher incidence of cervical cancer. Often, a vegetarian diet or a diet emphasizing whole grains, vegetables, beans, nuts, and seeds will help women with cervical cancer.

Nutrients and Herbs

The following nutrients have been shown to help prevent and treat cervical cancer. For information on dosages for these supplements, as well as any potential contraindications, see the appendix.

- *CoQ10*: An interesting study from the Bronx-Lebanon Hospital Center in New York compared blood concentrations of CoQ10 and vitamin E between women with normal Pap tests and those with biopsy-confirmed cervical cancer. They found low blood levels of both antioxidants in the women with confirmed cervical cancer. [preventive]

- *Curcumin*: A study featured in the journal *Nutrition and Cancer* found that mice fed a diet with 5 percent cumin seed (*Cuminum cyminum*) had a much reduced incidence of cervical cancer development when exposed to known carcinogens. In this model, it appeared that cumin seeds alter the body's metabolism of carcinogens, thus preventing the onset of cervical dysplasia. [preventive]

- *Flavonoids*: Compounds found in berries, known as flavonoids, inhibited proliferation of human cervical cancer cells in vitro. [anticancer]

- *Folic acid*: Folic acid appears to help prevent dysplasia from progressing; however, it does not seem to have a significant role in preventing or delaying established cervical cancer. [preventive]

- *Mushroom extract*: A human study of 100 patients with cervical, ovarian, or endometrial cancer undergoing chemotherapy treatment demonstrated that a mushroom extract, *Agaricus blazei* Murill Kyowa (ABMK), reduced chemotherapy-associated side effects, including loss of appetite, hair loss, emotional instability, and general weakness. However, in this study, this particular mushroom extract did not appear to stimulate increased immune activity, as mushroom extracts usually do. [supportive]

- *Vitamins C and E*: Very few nutrients have been studied as cervical cancer treatments. However, researchers at the Albert Einstein College of Medicine in New York have determined that vitamins C and E may play a protective role in preventing development of cervical intraepithelial neoplasia (CIN), a precancerous condition. In their recent follow-up report featured in the journal *Nutrition and Cancer*, researchers concluded that HPV-infected cervical tissue with deficiencies of several antioxidants, specifically vitamins C and E, was more susceptible to free radical damage. High levels of vitamin C are associated with reduced risk of cervical cancer, and low intake of vitamin C from food sources is correlated with increased risk of cervical cancer. Vitamin C may be particularly helpful for lowering the risk of dysplasia in situ and invasive disease among smokers. Vitamin E and carotenoids appear to reduce the risk of all stages of cervical cancer. Dosage recommendations for these antioxidants are listed in the appendix. [preventive]

Summary

If cervical cancer or precancerous cervical conditions are caught early, there is a good chance for full recovery and remission. Practicing safe sex, quitting cigarette smoking, and losing weight (if overweight) are key lifestyle changes associated with lowering the risk of cervical cancer. With cervical cancer, a naturopathic component can be an especially helpful adjunct to the overall treatment approach. Immune support, particularly in the form of increased antioxidants, in the diet and in the form of herbs and supplements, is critical with cervical cancer.

nineteen

Colon Cancer

The colon, also known as the large intestine, is the last part of the digestive tract, connecting the small intestine to the anus. It consists of the ascending colon, transverse colon, descending colon, sigmoid colon, rectum, and anus. Most colorectal cancers begin as a polyp, a growth in the lining of the colon or rectum. According to the American Cancer Society, even though more people are diagnosed with breast cancer than colon cancer, each year more people die of colon cancer than breast cancer. Colon cancer, also referred to as colorectal cancer, occurs at almost equal rates among women and men. It is the second most deadly cancer, but it is actually highly curable, especially if detected and treated early.

Causes, Symptoms, and Diagnosis

Age is a strong risk factor for colorectal cancer—90 percent of those diagnosed with the disease are over 50. A personal or family history of conditions such as colonic polyps, ulcerative colitis, or Crohn's disease, or a family history of colorectal cancer, increases the risk of developing colorectal cancer. Smoking, heavy alcohol use, obesity, a high-fat diet, regular consumption of red meat, and lack of exercise all contribute to increased risk as well. Jews of eastern European descent are known to have a higher incidence of colon cancer.

Symptoms of colon cancer, which can be subtle, may include diarrhea, blood in the stool, abdominal pain, intestinal obstruction, changes in bowel habits, and weight loss. Colon cancer can also occur without symptoms, which is one of the reasons screening tests are so important. Tests used to screen for colorectal cancer include stool blood tests; sigmoidoscopy or colonoscopy (insertion of a fiber-optic tube through the rectum into the colon to examine the colon); and a barium enema with air contrast (a liquid suspension of barium sulfate administered as an enema into the colon to render it radiopaque for an abdominal X-ray). If you have a family history of colon cancer or are over age 50, ask your doctor about colon cancer screening. Being diligent about consistent screening is critical.

Diagnosis of colon cancer requires a biopsy of the lesion. Depending upon the size of the tumor, a metastatic workup may also be part of the diagnostic process and would include imaging tests of the abdomen, lungs, bone, and brain. Stage I and stage II colon cancer are tumors that are confined to the colon. Stage III includes tumors that have spread into the nearby lymphatic tissue. Stage IV includes spread of the cancer to any other organ or tissue. The five-year survival rate for stage I colon cancer is 85 to 95 percent; for stage II, 60 to 80 percent; for stage III, 30 to 50 percent; and for stage IV, 5 percent. Fortunately, these statistics are changing with advances in treatment options.

Conventional Treatment

Conventional treatment for colon cancer usually entails surgery, with chemotherapy used in some cases.

Surgery

Surgery is used as primary treatment in almost all cases of colon cancer, with the goal of removing all cancerous tissue and achieving a clean surgical margin. The margin size depends on the size of the tumor, but is usually much larger than in other cancers. The surgery includes removal of the affected part of the colon and the regional lymph nodes, and will also include removal of cancerous tissue from nearby organs. A colostomy may be performed in cases where the distal bowel (farthest from the small intestines and closest to the anus) has been removed or it is impossible for feces to pass through the colon. A colostomy involves surgically creating a small opening through the abdominal wall that connects the proximal colon (the part of the colon that follows the small intestines) to the outside surface. A catheter is secured to this opening and leads to a plastic bag (a colostomy bag) that is worn outside of the body to collect intestinal waste. A colostomy can be temporary in cases of inflammation or permanent in situations when a significant portion of the large intestine has been removed.

Radiation and Chemotherapy

Radiation is typically not indicated for most colon cancers, as it does not appear to grant significant survival advantage and causes significant damage to the intestines. However, localized radiation is indicated for early-stage rectal cancer to help prevent recurrence. Nonetheless, radiation does not improve survival in cases of stage II or III rectal cancer.

Chemotherapy may be used in metastatic and advanced cases of colon cancer or when the cancer is node-positive (cancerous cells are detected in the lymph nodes). Significant advances have been made in recent years in the chemotherapy offered for colon cancer. There are enough effective chemotherapy agents now available for colorectal cancer that should the initial chemotherapy combination be ineffective, oncologists are able to offer up to three or more chemotherapy combinations, each with a good measure of effectiveness. Chemotherapy delivery methods also enhance effectiveness. The most common site of metastasis is the liver. Chemotherapy can be delivered directly into the liver via a catheter fed through the femoral artery and into the hepatic artery.

Chemotherapy agents used for colon cancer are typically used in combination and include leucovorin, fluorouracil, floxuridine, capecitabine, irinotecan, and oxaliplatin, with cisplatin and mitomycin used intra-arterially directly into the liver. (For information about how to counteract typical side effects of these medications, consult the chart "Chemotherapy Drugs and Their Nutrient and Herb Interactions" beginning on page 141.) Additionally, drugs in other classes have been introduced in an attempt to improve patient outcomes. Some of these newer drugs bind to growth factors on cancer cells, thereby inhibiting their growth and slowing down angiogenesis. These new drugs have improved response to treatment and include bevacizumub and cetuximab. These newer drugs are generally better tolerated than conventional chemotherapy drugs, but they are intended to be used in combination with chemotherapy, not to replace those regimens.

NSAIDs and Colon Cancer Prevention

Some research indicates that NSAIDs or anti-inflammatory COX-2 inhibitors may help prevent colon cancer. However, researchers from the University of California, San Francisco, and the University of Michigan Health System concluded that colonoscopy, as a screening and early detection tool, is a far more cost-effective prevention strategy than using COX-2 inhibitors. Research featured in the *Journal of the American Medical Association* indicated that using NSAIDs to prevent colon cancer would require a higher dose than is recommended for cardiovascular disease prevention, and that the risks associated with gastrointestinal bleeding must be considered and may outweigh any cancer prevention benefits.

Complementary Approaches

Refer to part II of this book regarding useful complementary approaches for all cancers. The following information is specific to colon cancer.

Lifestyle and Diet

Recent research featured in the *Journal of Clinical Oncology* concluded that physical activity following a colon cancer diagnosis can substantially reduce the risk of death due to the cancer. This study evaluated 573 women diagnosed with stage I through stage III colorectal cancer, as well as 832 patients with advanced colon cancer. The researchers warn that patients who have received chemotherapy that can affect heart function should take extra precautions and talk to their doctor before embarking on a vigorous exercise program.

According to a study in the *Journal of the American Medical Association* that featured more than 3,000 asymptomatic people ages 50 to 73, smoking and consumption of more than seven alcoholic drinks per week was strongly associated with an increased risk of developing colon cancer. Another study, published in *Nutrition and Cancer*, demonstrated that alcohol consumption was associated with a significant risk of developing colon cancer.

Several studies have confirmed a connection between red meat and colon cancer. A study published in the *Journal of the National Cancer Institute* demonstrated that people who ate at least six ounces of red meat and processed meat daily had a 35 percent higher chance of developing colorectal cancer than those who ate very little red meat—less than ⅓ ounce. Additionally, the study showed that individuals who consumed at least three ounces of fish per day had a 30 percent reduced risk of developing colorectal cancer. Another study, featured in the *Archives of Internal Medicine*, had a broader conclusion, stating that those who eat the typical Western diet, featuring red meat, sweets, desserts, fried foods, and refined grains, had a 50 percent greater chance of developing colon cancer than those who consumed few of these foods. Interestingly, diets with a high glycemic index and glycemic load are associated with an increased risk of rectal cancer but not colon cancer.

A recent report in *Public Health Nutrition* explains that the initial findings of the European Prospective Investigation into Cancer and Nutrition (EPIC) study demonstrates that "one of the most important results is a protective effect of high fiber intake and fish consumption against colorectal cancer, while high red and processed meat intake increase the risk." Data from more than 452,000 participants in EPIC showed that consumption of fruits and vegetables significantly reduced the risk of colon cancer.

Nutrients and Herbs

Because colon cancer is the second most deadly cancer, much research is devoted to its treatment, and that includes research into nutrition, herbs, and supplements. Several nutrients and herbs have shown particular promise as complementary colon cancer treatments. For information on dosages for the supplements listed below, as well as any potential contraindications, see the appendix.

- *Aged garlic extract*: A recent cellular study featured in the *Journal of Nutrition* showed that aged garlic extract has potential in suppressing tumor formation and inhibiting angiogenesis of colorectal cancer cells. Previous studies have demonstrated that garlic consumption provides a protective effect against colon cancer. [anticancer]

- *Anthocyanidins*: Extracts from berries, particularly bilberry, chokeberry, and grapes, have shown multiple mechanisms of action in test tube and animal studies, including an ability to protect against colon cancer development. [preventive]

- *Arabinogalactans*: This polysaccharide derived from the larch tree may prevent the spread of colon cancer cells to the liver, thus preventing or reducing liver metastasis. [anticancer]

- *Curcumin*: This powerful phytochemical found in turmeric inhibits cell growth, has apoptotic effects, and reduces inflammation. [preventive, anticancer]

- *Flavonoids*: Flavonols (metabolite of flavonoids) from beans, onions, apples, and tea were studied in a randomized control trial. High intake of these flavonols significantly decreased the risk of colon cancer recurrence in patients who previously had colon cancer. [preventive]

- *Flaxseed and flax lignans*: Recent animal studies showed that flaxseed meal helped prevent colon cancer development; it also decreased levels of inflammatory COX-1 and COX-2. [preventive]

- *Folic acid*: The Cancer Prevention Study II showed a modest reduction in colon cancer mortality among people who took a multivitamin containing folic acid, specifically in cases of moderate to heavy alcohol use. [preventive]

- *Green tea*: Both in vitro and animal studies have demonstrated that green tea can help protect against colon cancer; however, a recent research review featured in *Carcinogenesis* concluded that the evidence to support its effectiveness in humans is inconclusive. But in human studies involving other cancers, green tea has been proven an effective anticancer agent. [preventive]

● *Indole-3-carbinol (I3C)*: This compound found in cruciferous vegetables can inhibit proliferation of colon cancer cells. [anticancer]

● *L-glutamine*: One study of 70 colon cancer patients receiving chemo-therapy demonstrated that L-glutamine reduced permeability and absorption issues associated with the drug and that this amino acid may be of benefit in preventing chemotherapy-induced diarrhea. [supportive]

● *Melatonin*: Many studies have demonstrated that melatonin shows promise as an agent against colon cancer. In cellular studies, melato-nin induced apoptosis of human colon cancer cells while stimulating a directed antitumor immune response. [anticancer]

● *Mistletoe*: A human clinical trial involving 62 patients demonstrated that when given prior to surgery, mistletoe extract prevented surgical-induced suppression of natural killer cells, important cells of the immune system. [supportive]

● *Mushroom extracts*: Extracts of various mushrooms (maitake, reishi, *Cordyceps*, and others) contain polysaccharides that stimulate cytotoxic aspects of the immune response and may hinder metastatic spread. [anticancer]

● *Omega-3 fatty acids*: EPA and DHA, abundant in cold-water fish, induce apoptosis of colon cancer cells. They can also delay the onset of cachexia (lean body mass wasting) associated with metastatic colon cancer and reduce its severity. [supportive]

● *Probiotics*: The beneficial bacterial strains of *Lactobacillus rhamnosus* and *Bifidobacterium lactis* combined with prebiotics improved immune function in patients with colon cancer. [supportive]

● *Quercetin*: This phytonutrient has been shown to modify genetic expression in colon cancer cells, resulting in reduced cell division and apoptosis of cancer cells. [preventive, anticancer]

● *Resveratrol*: A recent animal study showed that resveratrol inhibited colon cancer development. [anticancer]

● *Vitamin D and calcium*: According to the *Journal of the American Medical Association*, a study of more than 3,000 people (mentioned previously) showed a strong correlation between vitamin D and calcium intake and reduction of colon cancer. Several other studies have made the same connection. [preventive]

- *Vitamin E*: This specific form of vitamin E succinate has been shown to inhibit colon cancer cells in vitro and in vivo; it appears to suppress tumor growth through apoptosis and reducing cell proliferation. High doses of vitamin E have been shown to increase natural killer cell activity in patients with advanced colon cancer. [anticancer]

Summary

Lifestyle modifications can help prevent this deadly cancer. The key to successfully treating colon cancer is proper screening so it can be caught early, when it is very treatable. The American Cancer Society recommends that people over age 50 have a fecal occult blood test annually, a sigmoidoscopy every five years, and a colonoscopy every ten years. Individuals who have a family history of colon cancer are advised to discuss their testing program with their doctor. Reducing consumption of red meat and processed meats, simple sugars, and alcohol can make an enormous contribution to both prevention and treatment, as can eating more cold-water fish and fiber, and supplementing with specific nutrients.

twenty

Esophageal Cancer

The esophagus is the long hollow tube that runs from your throat to your stomach. After you eat, food travels down your esophagus to the stomach where it can be digested. Esophageal cancer can occur anywhere along that path; however, in the United States, the most common site is the lower portion of the esophagus. According to the American Cancer Society, for all groups combined, the lifetime risk of developing esophageal cancer in the United State is 1 in 200. It is 3 to 4 times more common in men than women with more than 16,000 new esophageal cancer cases diagnosed in 2009. There are two primary types of esophageal cancer: adenocarcinoma, the most common form in the United States, and squamous cell carcinoma, the most common form in other countries.

Causes, Symptoms, and Diagnosis

While the exact cause of esophageal cancer is unknown, there are several factors that can put you at risk for developing this type of cancer, including increased alcohol intake, chewing tobacco or smoking, poor diet, obesity, gastroesophageal reflux disease (GERD), and radiation treatment to the chest or upper abdomen.

In its early stages, esophageal cancer typically causes no symptoms. As it progresses, symptoms appear. Because esophageal cancer often creates obstruction in the esophagus, difficulty swallowing is a hallmark sign of the disease. Fatigue, losing weight without trying, and chest pain (e.g., pressure or burning) are also signs of esophageal cancer. Frequent hiccupping, hoarseness, and a feeling that there is food stuck in your throat or chest can be signs of esophageal cancer.

This type of cancer is diagnosed following an upper gastrointestinal series of X-rays, endoscopy (using a lighted, flexible endoscope to view the upper GI), and/or with a barium swallow test. With the barium swallow test, a special liquid is ingested, which coats the walls of the esophagus so X-rays can clearly outline the esophagus and any irregularities on its surface. Even small, early cancers can be seen using the barium swallow test. If there is concern that the cancer has spread beyond the esophagus, a CT scan may be required. The only way to get a definitive diagnosis of esophageal cancer is by analyzing a biopsy of tissue taken from the tumor site, typically during an endoscopy.

Conventional Treatment

Depending on the extent of the cancer, surgery, chemotherapy, radiation, or a combination of the three will be used to treat esophageal cancer.

Surgery

Removal of the cancerous part of the esophagus (esophagectomy) is meant to either cure the cancer or ease symptoms. Esophageal cancer surgery is very complex and a specialist should perform the operation. In some cases, a portion of the stomach may need to be removed as well. After the cancerous part of the esophagus is removed, the remaining ends of the esophagus are reattached to one another or a part of the small or large intestine may be used to replace the removed part of the esophagus. Some complications of this surgery can be very serious and even fatal. A second opinion is recommended prior to undergoing surgery for esophageal cancer.

Radiation and Chemotherapy

Radiation therapy alone will not cure this type of cancer, so it is often combined with surgery and/or chemotherapy. Radiation therapy can help shrink the tumor to relieve pain associated with difficulty swallowing but can also cause esophageal strictures or narrowing, which can contribute to ongoing difficulties with swallowing.

Chemotherapy as a sole treatment also cannot typically cure this type of cancer. Thus, it is used in combination with surgery and/or radiation therapy. Chemotherapy is often used to help relieve symptoms of advanced cancers and to shrink the cancerous tumor. Using chemotherapy to shrink tumors prior to surgery is still a novel approach and more research is required before this becomes widely recommended. According to a 2007 review featured in the *Annals of Thoracic Surgery*, chemotherapy and radiation prior to surgery only gleaned a modest improvement of 40 days in life expectancy. The researchers concluded that surgery alone was a preferred strategy when considering quality-of-life issues. Typical chemotherapy drugs used to treat esophageal cancer include cisplatin and 5-fluorouracil (5-FU).

Photodynamic Therapy (PDT)

PDT is the use of laser light through an endoscope (a flexible tube inserted through the mouth into the esophagus with a fiber-optic camera on the end). First a harmless light-sensitive chemical is injected into the bloodstream. This chemical then settles at the tumor site. Once this occurs, a special laser light is aimed at the tumor. The light changes that chemical into a new chemical that can actually kill the cancerous tumor. PDT is best used in cases of early diagnosis of cancers that are near the surface. This therapy does not work for cancers that are deeper or that have spread to other organs. Sometimes PDT is used to reduce tumor size in advanced cases to help relieve symptoms.

Complementary Approaches

Refer to part II of this book regarding useful complementary approaches for all cancers. The following information is specific to esophageal cancer.

Esophageal cancer can be very difficult to treat because it is often discovered at an advanced stage. As a result, most of the research involving complementary therapies has focused on pain management strategies including acupuncture, guided imagery, hypnosis, massage, and other relaxation techniques.

Lifestyle and Diet

Consumption of red meat, but not poultry, is significantly associated with increased esophageal cancer risk. Consumption of fruits and vegetables as well as olive oil and tea are significantly associated with reduced risk of esophageal cancer.

Obesity and increased weight even within normal weight range (as measured by the Body Mass Index) is associated with increased risk of esophageal cancer. Smoking, chewing tobacco, and alcohol use can also dramatically increase your risk of developing this type of cancer.

Nutrients and Herbs

Because individuals with esophageal cancer are often not eating normally or have a restricted diet due to uncomfortable swallowing, they may benefit from a comprehensive powdered multivitamin-multimineral supplement. Caution is warranted even with powdered supplements, as some supplements can be irritating to the esophageal tissue if they remain in contact with it for too long. This can occur if swallowing is inadequate. The challenges to swallowing can result in the need for a gastric feeding tube. If this tube is placed, nutritional needs will be met through the use of special enteric nutritional feeding products. Additional nutritional supplementation can be provided with intravenous therapies under the direction of qualified medical, osteopathic, or naturopathic physicians or dieticians.

Assuming that swallowing is adequate for supplementation, the following supplements may be of benefit for people with esophageal cancer.

- **Eicosapentaenoic acid (EPA)**: In a double-blind design, esophageal cancer patients undergoing esophagectomy (removal of a portion of the esophagus) were randomized to a standard enteric formula or a formula enriched with 2.2 grams EPA/d for 5 days preoperatively (orally) and 21 days postoperatively (j-tube feeding). The EPA group maintained all aspects of body composition postoperatively, whereas patients in the standard enteric nutrient group lost significant amounts of lean body mass. Thus, EPA supplementation preserved lean body mass in esophageal cancer patients after surgery. [supportive]

- **Vitamin E**: Alpha-tocopherol, a form of vitamin E, has been found to be inversely associated with the risk of developing esophageal cancer. This vitamin appears to protect and repair damaged esophageal tissue. [preventive]

- **Glutamine**: Thirteen patients with stage III or IV esophageal cancer were randomly assigned to two groups, a control group and a glutamine-supplemented group who received 1 gram three times daily for 28 days. All subjects underwent a 3-week course of radiation therapy and received chemotherapy of cisplatin and 5-FU for the first 10 days. The lymphocyte activity was depressed in the control patients compared with the patients receiving the oral glutamine supplement. Glutamine repletion was also beneficial in the maintenance of gut integrity compared to the control group. The results suggested that glutamine supplementation boosts cytotoxic T cell activity against tumor cells in patients with advanced esophageal cancer. [supportive]

Summary

When caught early, esophageal cancer is very treatable. Unfortunately, lack of symptoms can make diagnosis elusive until the cancer is more invasive. Conventional medicine offers some options. Scientific research regarding natural substances specifically for esophageal cancer is limited. More research is needed in this area.

twenty-one

Gastric Cancer

The stomach is a saclike muscular organ that is located in the upper left quadrant of the abdomen. The average human adult stomach can hold about 1.5 quarts of food or liquids, and in some cases as much as 4 quarts. Gastric cancer refers to those cancers occurring in the stomach. The incidence of gastric cancers has remained fairly stable over the past several years, with about 21,000 cases diagnosed in 2009. It occurs more frequently in men and is one of the less common digestive system cancers overall.

Causes, Symptoms, and Diagnosis

Many factors can contribute to increased risk for gastric cancer: a family history of gastric cancer; infection by *Helicobacter pylori* (a bacteria that is a common cause of ulcers and chronic gastritis); having type A blood; a diet with large quantities of dry salted meats and other foods containing nitrosamines; a personal history of pernicious anemia (a severe blood disease); chronic atrophic gastritis (stomach inflammation); or adenomous gastric polyps (glandular benign stomach tumors).

Symptoms of gastric cancer may be similar to those of less serious illnesses, such as ulcers, heartburn (gastric reflux), gallstones, and even irritable bowel syndrome. This overlap of symptomology may result in delayed diagnosis. These symptoms may include bloating, vague or premature abdominal fullness, abdominal discomfort, breath odor, and excessive belching or flatulence. More serious symptoms can include loss of appetite, difficulty swallowing, nausea and vomiting, abdominal pain, vomiting blood, and unintentional weight loss.

Diagnosis of gastric cancers involves a physical examination of the abdomen, an upper GI series (X-rays of the esophagus and stomach taken after ingestion of a barium solution), and endoscopy (insertion of a lighted fiberoptic tube into the stomach through the mouth and esophagus to examine the stomach and remove a sample of tissue for biopsy). As is usually the case, the best prognosis occurs when gastric cancer is diagnosed early, namely, before it extends beyond the stomach wall and before it involves lymph nodes; in such cases, a cure is expected in more than 50 percent of patients.

When the cancer is confined to the mucosa and treated by surgical removal of the stomach and regional lymph nodes, long-term survival rates are more than 90 percent. Once the cancer has spread outside of the stomach and into regional lymph nodes, only 10 to 15 percent of patients can expect to survive at least five years. This is a poor prognosis, but current treatment strategies offer much improvement in terms of quality of life and some prolongation of life.

Conventional Treatment

Conventional treatment for gastric cancers primarily involves surgery and sometimes radiation. Chermotherapy is used in some cases.

Surgery

Surgery is used in most cases, with the goal of removing all cancerous tissue. Achieving a clean margin is important, and the margin size depends on the size and location of the tumor. Surgery may involve resection (removal of the tumor and a clean surgical margin), partial gastrectomy (removal of part of the stomach and perhaps parts of nearby organs and tissues), or radical gastrectomy (removal of the entire stomach, plus other organs or parts of organs). Depending on the extent of the surgery, reconstructive surgery may be required.

Radiation and Chemotherapy

Radiation may be used preoperatively or postoperatively, especially in advanced cases. Certain types of gastric tumors are associated with localized recurrence. In these cases, radiation can be effective, particularly for symptom management. Bleeding, pain, and nausea are some of the symptoms that radiation therapy can alleviate.

Chemotherapy alone shows little value except when used to shrink inoperable tumors or slow the growth of advanced cancers. When combined with radiation, it shows some success in reducing advanced cancers. Radiation combined with chemotherapy (fluorouracil and leucovorin) after surgery for cancers of the upper stomach lends a significant five-year survival advantage (three-year survival of 50 percent) over surgery alone (three-year survival of 41 percent). Typical chemotherapy agents used to treat gastric cancer include fluorouracil (5-FU), doxorubicin, mitomycin C, cisplatin, epirubicin, etoposide, and methotrexate. (For information about how to counteract typical side effects of these medications, consult the chart "Chemotherapy Drugs and Their Nutrient and Herb Interactions" beginning on page 141.) According to *Cancer Management: A Multidisciplinary Approach*, "Numerous prospective, randomized trials have been conducted in the United States and Europe [involving various chemotherapeutic agents], with contradictory results." The decision as to whether to undergo chemotherapy should be based on your oncologist's thorough assessment of potential benefit, taking into account cancer type, stage, and location, as well as characteristics specific to you.

Complementary Approaches

Refer to part II of this book regarding useful complementary approaches for all cancers. The following information is specific to gastric cancer.

Lifestyle and Diet

Key lifestyle factors that can contribute to gastric cancers include smoking, alcohol consumption, and obesity. Smoking directly damages DNA in gastric epithelial and mucosal cells. Smoking also depletes the body of certain essential antioxidant nutrients that could otherwise help repair damage from ingested carcinogens. Alcohol directly damages the mucosa of the stomach, leaving the underlying cell layer exposed and susceptible to *H. pylori* infection, which is associated with an increased risk of stomach cancer. A link between obesity and increased rates of gastric cancer has been identified in some epidemiological studies. In a recent study published in the *International Journal of Cancer*, researchers conclude, "An increasing prevalence of obesity may be associated with the increasing incidence of gastro-esophageal cancer observed in many populations." In addition, physical activity is associated with a reduced risk of gastric cancer.

Diet can influence gastric cancer risk and may also contribute to successful treatment. Garlic and onions can protect the gastric epithelium and should be part of an overall prevention program. In fact, garlic is perhaps the most studied natural substance for gastric cancer. There is a much higher incidence of gastric cancer in Japan, and that is where much of the research on garlic originates. Human trials have shown that garlic offers protection against *H. pylori* infection, as well as gastric cancer. Research featured in the *European Journal of Cancer Prevention* found a reduction of stomach cancer development in animals fed a diet high in garlic and lycopene (from tomatoes).

Researchers from Loyola University Medical Center found that a high intake of cereal fiber significantly reduced the risk of gastric cancer. Japanese researchers have found that dietary soy intake reduces gastric cancer risk. Although the direct link between fruit and vegetable intake and the prevention and treatment of gastric cancer is controversial, given all of the other health benefits of fruits and vegetables, it certainly makes sense for the person with stomach cancer to eat more of these healthful fresh foods.

It's also important to avoid certain foods. Smoked and cured meats are carcinogenic to the stomach. Thus, minimizing ingestion of dried and salted meats, cured meats, and nitrosamine-containing foods can help prevent stomach cancer. There are several high-quality studies demonstrating that a variety of important nutrients can help prevent gastric cancer, including selenium, beta-carotene, and vitamin E.

Nutrients and Herbs

Research regarding herbs and nutrients for the prevention and treatment of gastric cancer is increasing. Following are a few that show promise. For information on dosages for the supplements listed below, as well as any potential contraindications, see the appendix.

- *Astragalus*: In a study involving 120 gastric cancer patients undergoing chemotherapy, the patients were given the herb astragalus via injection. The researchers found that astragalus helped inhibit tumor growth, decrease toxic effects of chemotherapy, increase immune activity, and improve quality of life. Previously, in vitro studies involving astragalus have shown that it specifically inhibits gastric cancer cell growth. Additional human trials are needed to determine the full potential of this herb for the treatment of gastric cancer. [anticancer, supportive]

- *Ginkgo biloba*: This antioxidant herb has been shown in vitro to inhibit the growth of gastric cancer cells. One study, which involved 86 patients, demonstrated that ginkgo biloba extract taken orally resulted in markedly improved clinical symptoms, although its effect on disease progression was not evident in this study. This herb should not be taken prior to surgery, as it can interfere with certain anesthetics used during surgery and may also contribute to increased risk of abnormal bleeding during surgery. [supportive]

- *Green tea*: Drinking green tea is also associated with a reduced risk of gastric cancer. In fact, in vitro studies have demonstrated that epigallocatechin gallate (EGCG), an active ingredient in green tea, induces apoptosis of human gastric cancer cells. Consumption of increasing quantities of green tea is inversely correlated with the incidence of gastric cancer. In addition, in vitro and in vivo studies have shown that green tea causes profound growth inhibition of *H. pylori*, which is a significant risk factor for gastric cancer. [preventive, anticancer]

- *Mushroom polysaccharides*: A trial featuring 262 gastric cancer patients demonstrated that the mushroom polysaccharide-K (PSK; an extract from the fungus *Coriolus versicolor*) enhanced survival time and produced a positive immune response. The PSK was combined with chemotherapy following surgery. [anticancer]

- *Panax ginseng*: A small study involving stage III gastric cancer patients demonstrated that Panax ginseng enhanced immune activity during postoperative chemotherapy. More research is needed to confirm ginseng's effects. [supportive]

- *Proanthocyanidins*: These phytochemicals from fruits such as cherries, grapes, and berries have antioxidant activity. An in vitro study demonstrated that proanthocyanidins from apples had an apoptotic effect on gastric cancer cells. Conjugated linoleic acid (CLA) has also been found to induce apoptosis of gastric cancer cells in vitro. [preventive, anticancer]

- *Probiotics*: A special beneficial bacterial strain, *Lactobacillus rhamnosus GG*, was shown to reduce the growth of gastric cancer cells in vitro. [anticancer]

- *Vitamins C and E*: Studies involving antioxidants to prevent gastric cancers have yielded conflicting results. Some human studies have found a protective effect with vitamins C and E, while others have found no association. According to a review of the Cochrane Central Register of Controlled Trials, selenium demonstrated a protective effect against gastric cancers. Vitamin E, specifically gamma tocotrienol, has also been shown to reduce metastasis of gastric cancer cells in vitro. [preventive, anticancer]

Summary

Preventing and treating *H. pylori* infections is critical to the prevention and treatment of gastric cancers. Historically, prospects for long-term survival of people with gastric cancer have not been favorable; however, this is changing significantly. Conventional medicine can offer lifesaving surgery, and combined radiation and chemotherapy does extend life expectancy. Minimizing alcohol, smoking, and red meat are important lifestyle changes both for prevention and to support treatment and prevent recurrence. Many nutrients and supplements show promise as potential complementary treatments for gastric cancer. Dietary interventions appear to be an essential foundation for any comprehensive treatment plan.

twenty-two

Head and Neck Cancer

According to the American Cancer Society, men are more frequently diagnosed with head and neck cancer than women. These cancers can occur in the mouth, nose, sinuses, salivary glands, throat, and lymph nodes of the neck. Because the thyroid gland is located at the lower part of the neck, it can sometimes be categorized as a head and neck cancer. In this book, chapter 33 deals specifically with thyroid cancer. Cancers of the throat (pharynx) and voice box (larynx) accounted for just over 12,000 new cancers in 2009. About 60 percent of cancers of the larynx start in the vocal cords themselves. Squamous cell carcinoma in the cells that line the inside of the nose, mouth, and throat is the most common type of head and neck cancer. If found early, head and neck cancers are often curable. Advanced head and neck cancers can have a less favorable prognosis.

Causes, Symptoms, and Diagnosis

According to the National Institutes of Health, 85 percent of head and neck cancers can be attributed to tobacco use, both smoking and smokeless tobacco. Alcohol use, sun exposure, the human papillomavirus (HPV), and airborne toxins—specifically asbestos—also increase the risk of developing head and neck cancers. Symptoms of head and neck cancers can include

- A lump in the neck that does not go away

- A mouth or throat sore that does not heal

- A sore throat that does not go away

- Difficulty swallowing or painful swallowing

- Change in the voice or hoarseness that lasts more than two weeks (hoarseness occurs when the vocal cords are involved or if the cancer is in a later stage)

- Ear pain that won't go away

- Difficulty breathing

- Unexplained weight loss

Head and neck cancers are diagnosed using a physical exam and other tests such as an endoscopy (using a lighted, flexible endoscope to view the upper GI). Confirmation of head and neck cancers is made via a biopsy of the suspicious tissue.

Conventional Treatment

Typically, early-stage head and neck cancers are cured with either radiation or surgery, which accounts for one-third of the patients. The remaining two-thirds of head and neck cancer patients have locally advanced disease and are usually treated with a combination of surgery and radiation, or surgery and radiation combined with chemotherapy. Approximately 65 percent of patients with locally advanced disease experience a recurrence within five years.

Surgery

If the cancer can be removed through surgery, this is the first-line treatment course. Surgery can be relatively minor or quite extensive, involving the removal of significant tissues in the neck region. It is important to receive surgery from a surgeon who specializes in the head and neck in order to achieve the most complete removal of cancerous tissue along with the best cosmetic results.

Radiation and Chemotherapy

In some cases, the tumor may be too large or inoperable, so radiation is used before surgery to shrink the tumor. Radiation can include external beam therapy (EBT) or intensity-modulated radiation therapy (IMRT). Both of these forms of radiation are designed to selectively target the tumor and spare the surrounding healthy tissue as much as possible. Radiation prior to surgery makes the surgery more difficult because the radiation creates scar tissue in the area, which compromises blood flow and can interfere with tissue healing. Therefore, radiation prior to surgery should be considered carefully and should involve consultation between the surgeon and the radiation oncologist.

Chemotherapy may be indicated if the cancer is stage III or stage IV. The most common chemotherapy agents used for head and neck cancers are cisplatin and 5-fluorouracil (5-FU). The targeted therapy, cetuximab, is also sometimes used in combination with radiation or chemotherapy and radiation.

Complementary Approaches

Refer to part II of this book regarding useful complementary approaches for all cancers. The following information is specific to head and neck cancer.

Lifestyle and Diet

Consumption of vegetables, fruit, and whole grain cereals has been inversely related to laryngeal cancer risk. A strong association between fiber intake and reduced risk of laryngeal cancer risk has been identified, so fiber may be one of the most beneficial components of vegetables and fruit. In addition, moderate to vigorous exercise improves quality of life, reduces fatigue, and lessens depression in people with head and neck cancer. Also, consumption of green tea reduces the risk of head and neck cancer and can prevent precancerous lesions of the mouth from developing into oral cancers. Smoking is a major risk factor for oral cancer.

Nutrients and Herbs

Several natural agents may provide significant anticancer actions against head and neck cancers.

- **Artemisinin**: Artemisinin is a compound isolated from the plant *Artemisia annua L.* (sweet wormwood). Preliminary in vitro data indicate that artemisinin has antitumor effects by inducing apoptosis in oral cancer cells. [anticancer]

- **Green tea**: Both in vitro and in vivo studies have demonstrated the ability of green tea, specifically EGCG, to inhibit head and neck cancer progression. Phase I clinical trials have also demonstrated green tea's safety in patients with head and neck cancer. [anticancer]

- **Honey**: This common sweetener has mild immune-stimulating properties, significant wound-healing actions, and pain-relieving effects. It also provides potent anti-inflammatory and soothing effects on the tissues of the mouth and throat. This is especially helpful during chemotherapy and radiation therapy. Several randomized clinical trials of patients with head and neck cancer have demonstrated that honey reduces mouth sores associated with radiation. In one such study, subjects who used 20 ml of honey 15 minutes before radiation therapy, then again at intervals of 15 minutes and six hours after radiation, had significantly reduced rates of severe mouth sores (mucositis) and yeast infections of the oral cavity (candidiasis). [supportive]

● *Lycopene*: A flavonoid compound known as lycopene, found in tomatoes, has been found in vitro to inhibit the growth of squamous cell cancers of the mouth. [preventive, anticancer]

Note: It is important for head and neck cancer patients who are current smokers or those who have smoked in the past not to take vitamin E during radiation therapy. One randomized clinical study showed that alpha-tocopherol (vitamin E) and beta-carotene taken during radiation therapy and for three years after completion of the therapy resulted in fewer side effects from the radiation, but also significantly increased the risk of disease recurrence and of dying from the cancer.

Summary

Early-stage head and neck cancer is highly curable by conventional treatments. Head and neck cancers can be difficult to treat in their advanced stage. Research into natural substances for head and neck cancer patients is expanding. More research is needed regarding targeted conventional therapies and complementary treatments.

twenty-three

Kidney Cancer

The kidneys are fist-sized, bean-shaped organs located on either side of the spine in the middle of the back just below the rib cage. The kidneys are responsible for filtering toxic substances from the blood and directing them into urine. The kidneys also help regulate blood pressure and mineral status, as well as maintain a constant volume of water in the body. The most common type of kidney cancer is called renal cell carcinoma; it begins in the cells lining the small tubes—proximal tubules—inside the kidneys. In 2009, the American Cancer Society reported that more than 57,000 new cases of kidney cancer were diagnosed, with men affected more often than women.

Causes, Symptoms, and Diagnosis

Risk of developing kidney cancer (also known as renal cancer) increases with age. Other risk factors include smoking, obesity, long-term use of phenacetin (a prescription painkiller), long-term dialysis, and exposure to asbestos or significant amounts of radiation, or prolonged proximity to steel industry facilities.

Symptoms often do not appear until later stages of the disease. These symptoms can include blood in the urine and unexpected weight loss or fatigue. Symptoms such as low back pain, unaccountable fever, or swelling in the ankles and legs can also indicate kidney cancer.

When renal cancer is suspected, patients typically undergo a physical examination and provide a complete medical history. Most cancers cannot be diagnosed without the removal of tissue for biopsy. Kidney cancer, however, can often be diagnosed using imaging tests such as CT scans, MRIs, intravenous pyelograms (an X-ray procedure that uses an injection of a dye to make the kidneys visible), or ultrasound due to the obvious prominence of a renal cell cancerous tumor on these imaging tests. If a positive diagnosis is made, chest X-rays or bone scans may be used to determine if the cancer has spread to other parts of the body. Lymph nodes, abdominal soft tissue, lung, and bones are common sites where renal cancer metastasizes. Fortunately, the majority of people with renal cancer are diagnosed when the disease is confined to the kidney, and it is highly curable if diagnosed at this stage.

Conventional Treatment

Conventional treatment for kidney cancer relies primarily on surgery, with radiation as a palliative treatment. In stage I disease, treatment is considered curative; however, advanced renal cancer is more difficult to treat. Patients with advanced renal cancer may wish to explore clinical trials.

Surgery

Surgery is used in most cases, with the goal of removing all cancerous tissue and obtaining a clean surgical margin. Radical nephrectomy (complete removal of the affected kidney and adrenal gland perirenal fat and may include regional lymph nodes) or laparoscopic radical nephrectomy (performed via laparoscopic guidance) are the most common surgical treatments. If permanent dialysis would result following radical surgery, partial nephrectomy may be considered in some patients.

Radiation and Chemotherapy

Radiation is indicated in cases of advanced disease as a pain control measure, not as a curative treatment. Metastatic renal cancer is not responsive to chemotherapy. The lack of sensitivity to chemotherapy is not well understood. It may be related to the fact that it is difficult for a chemotherapy agent to reach the kidneys intact or due to inherent chemoresistant characteristics of renal cancer cell tumors.

Other Conventional Treatments

Various nonchemotherapeutic biological agents provide good response rates in some individuals. Biological agents are naturally occurring substances that are administered in very large doses to create a powerful effect. These agents are usually chemicals secreted by immune cells to regulate the immune response. Commonly used biological agents include interferon and interleukin. Interferon alfa produces a response in approximately 15 percent of patients with metastatic renal cancer. Both high- and low-dose interleukin-2 therapies produce a response rate similar to interferon alfa and can produce long-term remissions in about 5 percent of patients. Combining interferon and IL-2 does not seem to improve overall response rates. In advanced cases, thalidomide may be given. Pregnant women may not use this drug, as it can cause severe birth defects.

Sunitinib and sorafenib are multitargeted receptor tyrosine kinase inhibitors that have antiangiogenic and antitumor activity in metastatic renal cell carcinoma. Tyrosine kinases are enzymes that are a key component of cellular signaling involved in cell proliferation, metabolism, survival, and apoptosis. Several protein tyrosine kinases are activated in cancer cells and thereby drive tumor growth and progression. Thus, these drugs bind to the tyrosine kinase receptors and inhibit the signaling pathways. Temodar is a chemotherapy drug that inhibits DNA synthesis and cell division and may be of some value in the treatment of renal cell cancer.

Complementary Approaches

Refer to part II of this book regarding useful complementary approaches for all cancers. The following information is specific to kidney cancer.

Lifestyle and Diet

Toxic environmental compounds are typically detoxified into nontoxic compounds in the liver by phase I and II detoxification enzymes and conjugating nutrients. However, some environmental toxins, along with heavy metals, are not detoxified prior to elimination. As the kidneys filter these toxic compounds into urine, the kidneys can be damaged. Repeated or severe damage to the kidneys can initiate cancer development. Thus, avoiding toxic environmental compounds that are eliminated via the kidneys is critical. The carcinogens in cigarette smoke should be avoided. The chemicals found in cigarette smoke are highly carcinogenic to the kidneys and bladder. Other toxins known to increase risk of kidney cancer that should be minimized include solvents, pesticides and herbicides, copper sulfates, benzene, benzidine, coal tar, soot, pitch, creosol, lubricating oil, mustard gas, vinyl chloride, and DNT (technical dinitrotoluene).

Hypertension, or high blood pressure, and diabetes also increase the risk of renal cancer. Both hypertension and diabetes damage the capillary network in the kidneys, which makes the kidney prone to abnormal cell growth. Additionally, diabetes is characterized by increased insulin and insulin-like growth factor, both of which are growth factors for cancer. For more information on diabetes, refer to chapter 11. If you are at high risk of developing hypertension, talk to your doctor about an integrated prevention plan.

A recent report featured in the *International Journal of Cancer* found that obesity increases kidney cancer risk in women. Obesity is linked to increased risk because of the corresponding increase in insulin and insulin-like growth factor in overweight individuals. Dr. Tobias Pischon of the German Institute of Human Nutrition concludes that the increasing prevalence of obesity may explain the increasing incidence of renal cancer. A study involving more than 482,000 patients demonstrated that physical activity, including physical activity during childhood, reduces the risk of developing kidney cancer.

Following the dietary advice in chapter 11 will help control insulin levels and maintain normal body weight. A diet high in protein or fat increases the risk of kidney cancer. Avoid specific foods that may damage the kidneys, especially foods that contain preservatives, artificial colorings, and hormones. Carcinogens formed during grilling and charring of red meat can also damage the kidneys and increase the risk of kidney cancer. Lowering blood pressure by eating less salt is also a good idea.

Nutrients and Herbs

While there is limited research showing a direct link between nutrients and herbs and treatment of kidney cancer, some key natural substances show promise in providing overall kidney health support. For information on dosages for the supplements listed below, as well as any potential contraindications, see the appendix.

- *Alpha-lipoic acid*: This antioxidant nutrient reduces oxidative stress in the kidneys, as well as the liver and nerves, which results in decreased inflammation and may improve response to treatment and survival. [preventive]

- *Green tea*: Green tea extracts may be especially beneficial. Epigallocatechin gallate (EGCG), an active ingredient in green tea, up-regulates the p53 tumor suppressor gene, which is the most frequently mutated gene in human cancers. Mutated p53 does not effectively suppress abnormal cell growth. EGCG increases apoptosis, or death of tumor cells, by up-regulating healthy, unmutated p53. [preventive, anticancer]

- *L-carnitine*: This amino acid is synthesized in the kidneys. Previous studies involving kidney disease and dialysis have demonstrated that L-carnitine supplements may benefit people who have experienced chronic kidney failure. Natural substances such as L-carnitine that improve kidney function may be beneficial to those with kidney cancer. [supportive]

- *Melatonin*: In a phase II study with 22 patients, melatonin was found to be synergistic with interferon in metastatic renal cell carcinoma. However, melatonin may exaggerate some of the adverse side effects of interleukin-2 (IL-2), so it should not be taken by those undergoing IL-2 treatment. [supportive]

● *Panax ginseng*: In vitro studies have demonstrated that Panax ginseng can inhibit renal cell carcinoma, specifically by inhibiting proliferation. While this is promising preliminary research, the human applicability of this finding is unknown. [preventive, anticancer]

● *Shark cartilage (Neovastat liquid extract)*: Neovastat, a liquid extract of shark cartilage, has been shown in multiple in vivo models to inhibit angiogenesis (new blood vessel growth) in various tumor tissues. A phase II survival analysis of 22 patients with advanced renal cell cancer found that a daily dose of 240 ml of Neovastat resulted in a median survival of 66.3 months compared to a median survival of 7.1 months for those patients who received 60 ml daily. A phase III trial was also completed in 2007 that confirmed significant increased survival advantage for renal cancer patients taking Neovastat. [anticancer]

● *Vitamin A*: People with kidney cancer have been found to have low levels of vitamin A and also of zinc. Both nutrients support apoptosis and, while the theory remains unproven, it stands to reason that supplementing these two nutrients would stimulate apoptosis in established tumors. [anticancer]

● *Vitamin D*: This vitamin inhibits proliferation of cancer cells by stopping their ability to divide and replicate, induces apoptosis, and reduces invasiveness and angiogenesis. Vitamin D also increases insulin sensitivity, thereby improving sugar metabolism and reducing production of insulin-like growth factor (IGF) and IGF receptor activity. A 2008 clinical trial demonstrated that vitamin D enhanced the effectiveness of interferon in renal cancer. [preventive, supportive]

● *Vitamin E*: This vitamin induces apoptosis in a variety of renal cancer cell lines in vitro. [preventive, anticancer]

Summary

Conventional medicine has limited offerings for people with kidney cancer, although new treatment options are continually being investigated. The kidneys are key organs of elimination, and supporting them with all the diet and lifestyle recommendations outlined earlier is critical. Careful detoxification may help people who have been exposed to kidney toxins and can be used as a preventive measure or as a component of an integrated treatment plan (for more information about detoxification, see chapter 12). Avoid exposure to cigarette smoke and environmental toxins. In addition, a low-protein, low-fat diet is recommended, and if adequate protein is maintained, a vegetarian diet may be most helpful. Supplementing the diet with key nutrients and herbs such as vitamin A, zinc, green tea, Panax ginseng, and vitamin D may interfere with disease progression.

twenty-four

Leukemia, Lymphoma, and Myeloma

Leukemia, lymphoma, and myeloma are names for cancers of the blood, lymphatic system, and bone marrow, respectively. Although the variations of these cancers are too disparate and numerous to describe here in detail, we'll take a look at the most common types. Let's begin by understanding the terminology. Leukemias are cancers that affect the body's immature leukocytes, or early white blood cells. Lymphomas are cancers that originate from lymphocytes that accumulate in the lymphatic tissues, producing swollen lymph nodes. And myelomas are cancers that involve bone marrow cells, also known as myelocytes, that result in a proliferation of plasma cells that, in turn, produce large quantities of abnormal antibodies.

The major types of leukemia are acute myelogenous, acute lymphocytic, chronic myelogenous, and chronic lymphocytic, but there are further subclassifications of these types. Leukemia is caused by a genetic mutation of progenitor cells in the bone marrow, leading to elevated white blood cell counts. A normal white blood count range is between 5,000 and 10,000; people with leukemia can have counts of 50,000 to 500,000, with most of those cells being abnormal white blood cells. The rapid growth of these abnormal white blood cells can crowd out normal healthy blood cells produced in the bone marrow. Acute leukemia is a rapidly progressive disease that affects most of the undifferentiated white blood cells in the body. These cells are not fully mature and cannot perform their immune-related functions. Acute lymphocytic leukemia is the most common type of leukemia among children. Chronic lymphocytic leukemia is the most common type of leukemia in the Western world; its incidence increases with age, occurring especially after the age of 60. In chronic leukemia, which progresses more slowly, some white blood cells fully mature and maintain some overall immune function. Eventually, the abnormal leukemic cells can outnumber the healthy immune cells, undermining immune function. Leukemia results in impaired immune function and increased infection.

Lymphoma refers to a cancer of the white blood cells, usually originating in the lymph nodes or in lymphatic tissue. More than half the cases of blood cancers diagnosed each year are lymphomas. Lymphomas are divided into Hodgkin's lymphoma and non-Hodgkin's lymphoma. Non-Hodgkin's lymphoma, which is associated with a specific cell type, is more common in young adults, and unlike Hodgkin's lymphoma, it can spread beyond the lymphatic system. Lymphomas are the result of mutated lymphocytes that develop into tumors within the lymphatic system—usually in lymph nodes or in the lymphatic tissue of the stomach or intestines. Unlike leukemia, lymphomas present as solid tumors.

Myeloma is a type of cancer originating in the cells of the bone marrow that produce plasma cells, or B lymphocytes. This results in damaged B lymphocytes, or B cells, that aren't able to produce a full range of effective antibodies. These B cells proliferate, crowding out healthy B cells and their antibodies. Most cases of myeloma affect many locations in the body simultaneously and are referred to as multiple myeloma. Myeloma occurring as a single tumor outside the bone marrow is known as extramedullary plasmacytoma. Myeloma tumors (plasmacytomas) can form in any of the body's tissues. Smoldering myeloma is a type of myeloma that progresses slowly.

According to estimates from the National Cancer Institute, in 2009 more than 140,000 people were diagnosed with lymphomas, leukemia, and myelomas. Non-Hodgkin's lymphoma is the most common of these (nearly 66,000 cases), with all leukemias next (nearly 45,000 cases), and multiple myelomas (nearly 21,000 cases) being fairly rare. Leukemia is the most common form of cancer among children.

Causes, Symptoms, and Diagnosis

The exact causes of leukemia are unknown. Genetic predisposition and exposure to benzene chemicals, excessive radiation, or viruses are believed to directly increase the risk of developing leukemia. Symptoms of leukemia can include weakness or chronic fatigue, anemia, fever, bone pain with no apparent cause, easy bruising, blood in urine or stools, unexplained weight loss, and enlarged lymph nodes or spleen. A blood test can suggest the possibility of leukemia, but a bone marrow biopsy is necessary to conclusively diagnose it. In order to biopsy the bone marrow, a lumbar puncture, also known as a spinal tap, is performed.

Infection with HIV increases the risk of contracting non-Hodgkin's lymphoma by as much as 100 times. Elevated rates of non-Hodgkin's lymphoma in agricultural communities suggest that exposure to herbicides and pesticides may also increase risk. Epstein-Barr virus may increase the risk of non-Hodgkin's lymphoma, too. Epstein-Barr is a common virus but remains dormant in most people. Hodgkin's lymphoma represents about 12 percent of all lymphomas. It is most common in adolescents and young adults. The five-year survival rate in children and young adults is more than 78 percent. Causes of Hodgkin's lymphoma are unknown.

Symptoms of both Hodgkin's and non-Hodgkin's lymphoma often include a painless swelling of the lymph nodes in the neck, chest, armpit, abdomen, or groin. Other symptoms include fatigue, night sweats, generalized itching, weight loss, and flulike symptoms. Those suffering from Hodgkin's lymphoma may feel pain in the lymph nodes after drinking alcohol. Those with non-Hodgkin's lymphoma may experience pain or pressure in the lower back, possibly extending into the legs; bone pain, coughing, and pressure in the face and upper chest are also possible. Any symptoms suggestive of lymphoma require further medical evaluation. Diagnosis relies upon imaging, usually radiographic (X-ray) imaging and biopsy of enlarged node(s).

The most common symptom of myeloma is bone pain, usually in the back or ribs. This is because myeloma cells secrete cytokines that stimulate other cells to dissolve bone. Fatigue, anemia, and repeated infections are also possible. Infections are often the first indication of myeloma. The process of diagnosing myeloma includes a complete medical history and physical exam; laboratory examination of the blood, urine, and bone marrow, including a biopsy of the bone marrow tissue; and imaging tests (X-rays, CT scans, MRIs, PET scans) of the bones. Characteristics that lead to a definitive diagnosis of myeloma are an increased number of malignant plasma cells in the bone marrow biopsy; the presence of a specific immunoglobulin (M protein) and protein (Bence-Jones protein) in the blood; and loss of bone mass or fractures in the bones.

Conventional Treatment

Conventional treatment for these cancers relies almost exclusively on radiation and chemotherapy.

Surgery

Surgery is not indicated for leukemia, lymphoma, or myeloma, because in these cancers there is not a primary site of the cancer to remove. These cancers result from genetic defects in bone marrow production rather than starting as an originating tumor. They are considered to be disseminated at the time of diagnosis. Non-Hodgkin's lymphoma sometimes creates tumors in the skin, lungs, stomach, or other organs, which cause pressure-related pain or are unsightly. These tumors can be removed surgically.

Radiation and Chemotherapy

Treatment for leukemia has resulted in a tripled five-year survival rate in the past 45 years. Acute lymphocytic leukemia has a five-year survival rate of 65 percent overall and 88 percent for children under the age of 4. Chronic lymphocytic leukemia has a 74 percent five-year survival rate. Acute myelogenous leukemia has a 20 percent five-year survival rate overall and a 52 percent survival rate for children under the age of 15. Chronic myelogenous leukemia has a 39 percent five-year survival rate.

Chemotherapy is the primary treatment for leukemia. Some types of leukemia progress slowly, and chemotherapy may be withheld during early stages until progression becomes evident. Radiation is used to supplement treatment to the brain, spine, and testes, which cannot receive chemotherapy through the bloodstream.

Treatment for lymphoma relies on both chemotherapy and radiation. Hodgkin's lymphoma is treated with chemotherapy or radiation, or a combination of the two. The 86 percent five-year survival rate for Hodgkin's lymphoma has made this one of the most curable types of cancer. Early or indolent non-Hodgkin's lymphoma may be treated with radiation alone. Relapses are treated with a combination of chemotherapy and radiation. More aggressive types of non-Hodgkin's lymphoma require intensive chemotherapy for treatment, which produces five-year survival rates between 50 and 60 percent. Chemotherapy drugs for both leukemia and lymphoma are used as combination chemotherapy regimens. Chemotherapy drugs used for both types of lymphoma include carboplatin, carmustine, chlorambucil, cisplatin, cyclophosphamide, dacarbazine, fludarabine, ifosfamide, bleomycin, doxorubicin, idarubicin, etoposide, vinblastine, vincristine, and paclitaxel. (For information about how to counteract typical side effects of these medications, consult the chart "Chemotherapy Drugs and Their Nutrient and Herb Interactions" beginning on page 141.) Steroidal agents, including dexamethasone and prednisone, are immunosuppressive, and therefore limit the proliferation of lymphocytes, including malignant ones. While effective in treating cancer, these agents do depress immune function in general.

Monoclonal antibodies (alemtuzumab, rituximab, tositumomab, ibritumomab, and tiuxetan), which are antibodies created in the laboratory from mouse cells, destroy malignant immune cells by targeting very specific antigenic molecules located on the surface of immune cells. These antigens are expressed in large numbers on the surface of malignant immune cells, making the malignant immune cells preferential targets for these therapies.

Myeloma treatment relies exclusively on chemotherapy, with radiation therapy not playing a role. Chemotherapy drugs used for myeloma include melphalan, vincristine, doxorubicin, carmustine, bortemozib, and cyclophosphamide. Thalidomide selectively suppresses plasma cell proliferation by altering tumor necrosis factor. Immunosuppressive steroidal agents, including prednisone and dexamethasone, are used to exert immunosuppressive effects.

Other Conventional Treatments

In advanced cases of leukemia and lymphoma that are resistant to chemotherapy, a stem cell transplant may be recommended. In an allogenic transplant, stem cells are harvested from a healthy donor who has been matched with the patient. The patient's bone marrow is destroyed with radiation or potent chemotherapy. The previously harvested stem cells are then infused into the patient. These stem cells migrate to the bone marrow and fill the void. If the transplant is successful, these new stem cells will take over the production of white blood cells in the bone marrow, effectively replacing the damaged cell line. Nonmyeloablative allogenic stem cell transplants use lower doses of chemotherapy that do not destroy all of the bone marrow. The infused stem cells will replace damaged white blood cells and will also seek out and destroy damaged cells.

In all allogenic transplants, graft-versus-host disease, in which the immune system rejects the transplanted material, is a constant concern. A type of transplant that avoids graft-versus-host disease is an autologous transplant. In an autologous transplant, the patient first receives growth factors to mobilize stem cells into the blood. These stem cells are then collected from the patient's blood. The patient then receives high-dose chemotherapy or radiation therapy to purge or partially purge diseased cells from their marrow. Next, the healthy stem cells are returned to the patient and stimulated to reproduce. This type of transplant is typically reserved for difficult-to-treat cases.

Complementary Approaches

Refer to part II of this book regarding useful complementary approaches for all cancers. The following information is specific to leukemia, lymphoma, and myeloma.

Lifestyle and Diet

Smoking, poor nutrition, and previous exposure to chemotherapy or radiation can increase the risk of developing cancers of the blood and lymph, such as leukemia, lymphoma, and myeloma. To help prevent the development of secondary cancers, it is prudent to restore immune function after chemotherapy or radiation, in addition to quitting cigarette smoking and improving nutrition.

The *American Journal of Epidemiology* featured a report by Canadian researchers demonstrating that physical inactivity and obesity were associated with an increased risk of developing non-Hodgkin's lymphoma. The researchers found that men with the highest level of physical activity had a 21 percent decreased chance of developing the cancer. In contrast, women who were considered obese had a 59 percent increased chance of developing the cancer. Maintaining healthy weight, exercising consistently, and eating foods that stimulate a positive immune response, such as fruits and vegetables, are all important for people with leukemia, lymphoma, or myeloma. Research from Harvard University in 2009 also showed that intake of cured or smoked meats and fish increased the risk of children of developing leukemia. They speculate it is because of the high nitrite and nitrosamine content. Conversely, they demonstrated that intake of vegetables had a protective effective.

Several studies have shown that exercise can be beneficial for children and adults with these cancers. One study demonstrated that a home-based exercise intervention program involving children receiving maintenance therapy for leukemia improved cardiovascular health. In another study, patients receiving myeloma treatment received many physiological benefits from a exercise program.

Nutrients and Herbs

Most of the studies involving natural substances for these cancers are small and preliminary. Using natural substances for cancers of the immune system is particularly challenging in that many natural anticancer substances stimulate immunity—both cell proliferation and function. Therefore, in some cases these therapies may stimulate proliferation of malignant immune cells. For this reason, it is especially important to employ a conservative approach to using natural substances for cancers of the immune system. For information on dosages for the supplements listed below, as well as any potential contraindications, see the appendix.

- **Astragalus**: In a small controlled trial involving two groups of children receiving chemotherapy for acute leukemia, one of the groups also received astragulus. The group receiving 90 grams of astragulus combined with chemotherapy showed an increase in the number and activity of dendritic cells (an important immune cell that stimulates other immune cells to destroy cancerous and infected cells). [supportive]

● *Flavonoids*: In separate in vitro studies, resveratrol from red grapes, curcumin from turmeric, quercetin from fruits, and lutein from vegetables were shown to inhibit proliferation of leukemia cells. A constituent of curcumin reduces growth of leukemia cell lines by inducing apoptosis. However, caution is advised with curcumin and quercetin, as they may interfere with common chemotherapy drugs used for cancers of the blood and lymph. Other cellular and animal studies have indicated that flavonoids induce apoptosis in human leukemia cells. [preventive, anticancer]

● *Genistein*: Researchers from the Henry Ford Health System in Michigan found that the soy isoflavone genistein was effective in vitro at inducing apoptosis of lymphomas. [preventive, anticancer]

● *Green tea*: Several cellular studies have demonstrated that green tea can contribute to leukemia cell death and antiangiogenesis (blocking the formation of new blood vessels to supply cancer cells). Abnormal angiogenesis has been observed in people with leukemia and myeloma. In a study featured in the journal *Blood*, researchers from the Mayo Clinic recommend that more studies be done on EGCG (epigallocatechin gallate) from green tea as a possible nontoxic treatment in early-stage leukemia or for individuals at high risk. [anticancer]

● *L-carnitine*: This amino acid involved in the biochemical pathways of white blood cell development is able to promote differentiation of a specific leukemic cell line into normal mature cells. This reduces the number of undifferentiated cells, which are incapable of carrying out the functions of fully mature cells. [preventive]

● *Melatonin*: Preliminary studies have shown that melatonin has potential as a complement to conventional therapy for cancers of the blood and lymph. A small clinical study of 12 patients (6 non-Hodgkin's, 2 Hodgkin's, 2 myeloma, and 2 leukemia) demonstrated that melatonin used in conjunction with low-dose interleukin-2 (IL-2) therapy helped halt disease progression in 8 of the 12 patients. Melatonin is, however, contraindicated with high-dose IL-2 therapy, as it can cause significant hypotension (drop in blood pressure). An animal study combining melatonin and the immune-stimulating herb echinacea enhanced survival in leukemic mice. However, melatonin should be used with caution by those with leukemia, lymphoma, and myeloma, as its immune-stimulating actions could cause growth of the mutated immune cells implicated in these cancers. In one study, melatonin increased proliferation of myeloma cells. This same concern applies to echinacea. [supportive]

- *Mistletoe*: There is conflicting evidence regarding mistletoe and lymphoma. A retrospective analysis involving more than 200 lymphoma patients in Germany who were treated with mistletoe extract demonstrated no significant effect. However, a Swiss study showed that half of the 12 patients treated had continuous and complete remission. In vitro and animal studies did show some positive immune-stimulating and antitumor effects with mistletoe. Regarding multiple myeloma, mistletoe extract inhibited cancer cellular proliferation in vitro. Regarding leukemia, an in vitro and in vivo study demonstrated that a mistletoe extract induced apoptosis in acute lymphoblastic leukemia cells and improved survival of test animals. [anticancer]

Other Complementary Approaches

In cases of bone marrow transplant, glutamine supplementation is strongly indicated. One controlled trial involving children receiving stem cell transplant demonstrated that glutamine reduced the duration of fever, decreased the drug-related toxicity, and reduced the incidence of severe mouth sores. Another double-blind, randomized, placebo-controlled study of children receiving stem cell transplant who received a maximum dose of 4 grams of glutamine twice daily during transplant and for one month after experienced a reduction in the need for pain medication and total parenteral (intravenous) nutrition because mouth sores were less severe.

Summary

Blood and lymph freely circulate within their respective channels throughout the entire body. This makes cancers of the blood and lymph complex and sometimes difficult to treat. Currently, research involving nutrients and herbs for these cancers is in its infancy; however, many of these substances may surface as strong complementary treatments for these challenging cancers. An integrated approach that includes diet, lifestyle, nutrients, and conventional treatments may provide enhanced outcomes. Genistein, green tea, and L-carnitine represent some of the most promising natural therapies for these cancers. Nonetheless, cancers of the blood represent a significant challenge to natural therapies, and more research is needed to reveal effective integrated approaches.

twenty-five

Liver Cancer

The body's largest internal organ, the liver, lies in the right side of the abdomen, just under the diaphragm. In addition to filtering toxic waste from the bloodstream, the liver processes and stores nutrients, participates in blood sugar regulation, metabolizes hormones and other compounds, produces clotting factors for the blood, and produces bile, which is secreted into the large intestine to aid in digestion.

A number of different types of tumors can form in the liver and some are not cancerous. Most benign liver tumors do not cause symptoms and do not need to be removed. Although rare, cancer of the liver tissue, or hepatocellular carcinoma, is increasing sharply in incidence. Hepatocellular carcinoma can develop as the result of hepatitis B or hepatitis C infection, and the incidence of these infections has risen sharply over the past several decades. The latency period from the time of infection to the development of liver cancer can be decades, so we are just now seeing the rise in the rate of liver cancer. About 80 to 90 percent of all primary liver cancers worldwide are hepatocellular carcinomas, forming from the main type of liver cell, the hepatocyte. Hepatocellular carcinomas often begin as a single tumor in the liver and spread to other parts of the liver only after an extended period of growth. Approximately 50 to 80 percent of hepatocellular carcinomas are associated with cirrhosis (scarring) of the liver. In addition to resulting from hepatitis B or C infection, hepatocellular carcinoma can also occur as a result of cirrhosis of the liver, and in this situation begins in several locations within the liver simultaneously (this is known as multifocal disease). The other most common form of liver cancer is intrahepatic bile duct carcinoma, or cholangiocarcinoma. Cholangiocarcinoma accounts for approximately 10 to 20 percent of liver cancers. Most cancerous tumors found in the liver are not primary to the liver, but are metastastic tumors from cancers originating elsewhere in the body.

According to the American Cancer Society, more than 22,000 cases of primary liver cancer (which includes bile duct cancer) were diagnosed in 2009, with about twice as many men affected as women. Prognosis is based on the number and size of the tumors and if the cancer has metastasized to other parts of the body. Liver cancer metastasizes to other parts of the liver, the lungs, and bone. Metastasized liver cancer carries a poor prognosis.

Causes, Symptoms, and Diagnosis

Most hepatocellular carcinomas occur in people between 50 and 60 years old, and men are more than twice as likely to be diagnosed. The most common cause of liver cancer is cirrhosis, typically the result of alcohol abuse. Other factors that can lead to the development of liver cancer include exposure to chemical toxins (for example, aflatoxins, which are found in some foods, or vinyl chloride as an occupational exposure) and having viral hepatitis B or C, or other diseases that damage the liver.

Common symptoms of liver cancer include an enlarged abdomen, pain or tenderness in the abdomen (especially in the area of the liver), jaundice (a yellowing of the skin and eyes), and easy bruising or bleeding.

Diagnosis of liver cancer includes physical examination, as the liver may be enlarged and tender. Blood tests are done to look for elevated levels of alpha-fetoprotein (AFP), which is elevated in 50 to 70 percent of patients with hepatocellular carcinoma. An ultrasound-guided biopsy of the liver is the conclusive diagnostic test for liver cancer. An abdominal CT scan, MRI, or radioisotope scan may be done to look for tumor masses and determine the relationship of the mass to major blood vessels in order to decide whether the mass can be surgically removed.

Conventional Treatment

Conventional treatment for liver cancer involves surgery, usually followed by chemotherapy to help prevent a recurrence.

Surgery

Portions of the liver can be removed, and in many cases the liver will regenerate. Surgical removal of a liver cancer tumor is an option with localized, solitary lesions that are not close to major blood vessels and that are within one liver segment. The goal of surgery is to remove all cancerous tissue and obtain a clean surgical margin. As with most cancer surgeries, the margin size depends on the size and location of the tumor. Surgery may include tumor resection (removing just the cancerous tissue), partial hepatectomy (removing part of the liver), or total hepatectomy (removing the entire liver). Cirrhosis of the liver usually rules out resection or partial hepatectomy. If the entire liver is removed, a liver transplant must follow. The transplant may be a partial liver from a healthy donor, usually a relative of the patient, or a whole liver from a cadaver. Transplants may involve long wait times for a donor liver (one year or longer), and must be followed by lifetime use of immune-suppressing antirejection drugs. Surgery is especially beneficial for people with stage I or II tumors.

Surgery is the only form of conventional treatment that offers the potential for a cure from liver cancer. Partial hepatectomy results in a five-year survival rate of 10 to 30 percent. For tumors less than 2 inches in size that cannot be removed, various options exist: cryosugery, in which a probe applies extreme cold to tissue in order to destroy that tissue; percutaneous ethanol injection, in which a specialized needle injects alcohol into the damaged tissue in order to destroy the tissue; and radiofrequency ablation, in which a probe inserted directly into the tumor generates heat by means of high-frequency alternating current that flows between electrodes.

Chemotherapy and Radiation

Because there is high likelihood of relapse after surgery or tumor destruction using other methods, these interventions are typically followed by chemotherapy, either regional or systemic. Disease-free survival in patients treated with chemotherapy is four times that of patients who do not receive chemotherapy, although long-term survival is not significantly changed. Chemotherapy thus delays recurrence or progression of the disease but does not seem to impact overall life span. Doxorubicin has been used to treat liver cancer, but subsequent clinical trials have failed to demonstrate its effectiveness as a single agent. In addition, no clear survival benefit has been documented regarding combination chemotherapy regimens. Fluorouracil combined with interferon has also produced low response rates. However, chemotherapy can produce temporary relief of symptoms, particularly pain, associated with liver tumors and thus provide palliative care. Immunotherapy with lymphocytes (antibody-producing white blood cells) that have been manipulated in the laboratory to be specifically targeted to the cancerous liver cells is administered to the patient along with IL-2, which stimulates the activity of the lymphocytes. This immunotherapy can extend the disease-free time before recurrence. Attempts to use hormone therapy, specifically tamoxifen, have demonstrated a lack of benefit.

Some chemotherapy agents, including doxorubicin, cisplatin, and mitomycin, have demonstrated some effectiveness when given intra-arterially, rather than systemically. However, intra-arterial chemotherapy can only be used when the disease is limited to the liver and the kidneys are functioning properly. For more effective delivery of chemotherapy drugs in multifocal disease, chemoembolization may be used, which injects the drugs directly into the blood vessels feeding the area of the tumor while simultaneously reducing blood supply to the tumor by blocking off the artery with a gelatin sponge. Chemoembolization cannot be used in the presence of hypertension, blood clots, or jaundice. Biodegradable microspheres are also used to deliver the chemotherapy directly to the area of the tumor. Biodegradable microspheres are tiny containers filled with chemotherapy drugs that are injected into the liver or blood vessels supplying the areas of the liver with tumor growth. The containers eventually dissolve in body fluids.

Occasionally, radiation therapy may be used along with chemotherapy in an attempt to shrink tumors so that they can be surgically removed. TheraSpheres and SIR-Spheres are therapeutic devices that deliver radiation directly to tumors in the liver. The tiny spherical beads are embedded with yttrium-90, a radioactive element. Millions of these beads can be injected into the bloodstream and then guided into the hepatic artery, the liver's main blood vessel. When they arrive in the liver, the radiation-laden spheres get stuck within the smaller blood cells that supply tumors. This approach can be effective, as it delivers radiation directly to tumors while sparing healthy tissue. There is also a reduced chance of radiation-associated side effects.

Complementary Approaches

Refer to part II of this book regarding useful complementary approaches for all cancers. The following information is specific to liver cancer.

Lifestyle and Diet

The liver is the major organ of detoxification in the body. As a result, liver cells are repeatedly exposed to toxic and reactive molecules. Liver cells can sustain damage from short-term exposure to large quantities of highly toxic compounds or long-term exposure to other less toxic compounds. Over time, the detoxification and reparative mechanisms in the liver can become overwhelmed, which can result in cirrhosis and can also cause DNA damage and eventually liver cancer. Thus, reducing exposure to chemical toxins is a significant way to reduce the risk of liver cancer. The most common chemical toxins include alcohol, oral estrogens, iron overload, polycyclic aromatic hydrocarbons (formed during charcoal broiling and also found in cigarette smoke), and certain compounds found in petrochemicals, insecticides, and solvents. Nitrosamines are particularly toxic to the liver. There are about 300 different nitrosamine chemicals, and their presence is pervasive; they are found in tobacco smoke, some cosmetics, latex and rubber products, beer, bacon, and cured meats. Also avoid foods with added chemicals, preservatives, and trans fats, as they place increased demands on the liver's detoxification processes; plus, when broken down during detoxification, they may yield more proinflammatory and cell-damaging compounds.

Cruciferous vegetables are especially beneficial for liver function and may reduce symptoms associated with liver cancer. In addition to supporting detoxification, they contain compounds that reduce inflammation and stimulate apoptosis of cancer cells. Cabbage extract was shown in vitro and in vivo to kill liver cancer cells and stimulate immune system activity. Cruciferous vegetables include broccoli, brussels sprouts, cabbage, cauliflower, chard, kale, kohlrabi, mustard greens, parsnips, rutabagas, turnips, and watercress. Because the nutrient value of these foods can be diminished substantially with cooking, it is best to eat them lightly steamed. More research on the actions of these compounds specific to liver cancer is needed; however, given the safety and demonstrated health-promoting benefits of these foods, it is prudent to include them in your diet daily.

Nutrients and Herbs

Both cellular and animal studies have been done on various nutrients and herbs for liver cancer. Here are some of the more notable, recent findings. For information on dosages for the supplements listed below, as well as any potential contraindications, see the appendix.

- *Active hexose correlated compound (AHCC)*: In a prospective cohort placebo-controlled trial, AHCC, a novel compound derived from polysaccharides extracted from mushrooms, enhanced immune function, improved quality of life, and prolonged survival in patients with advanced liver cancer. [anticancer, supportive]

- *Arabinogalactans*: An in vivo study demonstrated that animals who received arabinogalactans had decreased spread of their cancer within the liver. [anticancer]

- *Ginger*: This herb exerted a dose-dependent suppression of liver cancer cell proliferation in vitro and in vivo. [preventive, anticancer]

- *Ginseng*: Earlier studies and a more recent in vitro study indicated that Panax ginseng inhibits the growth of liver cancer by inducing apoptosis of liver cancer cells. [preventive, anticancer]

- *Green tea*: Several studies have demonstrated that green tea is an effective anticancer agent. It was recently demonstrated that the active polyphenol compound in green tea, EGCG, induced apoptosis of liver cancer cells both in vitro and in vivo. [anticancer]

- **Limonene**: Limonene, from citrus fruits, has demonstrated apoptotic effects in liver cancer cells in vitro. [preventive, anticancer]

- **Pine bark extract (pycnogenol)**: In vitro studies showed this herbal antioxidant selectively inhibited growth of human liver cancer cells while slightly promoting the growth of normal, healthy liver cells. [anticancer]

- **Selenium**: This trace mineral provides additional antioxidant activity by regenerating glutathione. It also exerts antiviral effects, which is especially useful when viral hepatitis B or C is implicated in the cancer. [supportive]

- **Silymarin (milk thistle extract)**: This flavonoid complex found in milk thistle has antioxidant activity and helps to stabilize the cell membranes of liver cells. Silymarin also helps to maintain adequate liver levels of glutathione, an amino acid that provides antioxidant protection for healthy liver cells. Silymarin also stimulates apoptosis in liver cancer cells. [supportive, anticancer]

- **Vitamin C**: In vitro and in vivo studies demonstrate that the antioxidant and anti-inflammatory actions of vitamin C exert some protective effects against liver cancer. [preventive]

Other Complementary Approaches

Several homeopathic compounds and formulations have been used for centuries to treat diseases of the liver. Some recent cellular and in vivo research has shown that homeopathic formulas may reduce the symptoms associated with liver cancer and possibly reduce the risk of developing liver cancer. Keep in mind that homeopathy used to treat serious illnesses should be administered by a physician trained in homeopathy. For more information or to find a homeopathic physician in your area, visit the National Center for Homeopathy at www.homeopathic.org.

Summary

The liver is a key organ of detoxification. Avoiding alcohol is essential, as is supporting liver function before, during, and after conventional treatment. All the recommendations in chapter 12 are particularly apt with liver cancer. Antioxidant and anti-inflammatory foods and supplements will help support liver health, support apoptosis of hepatic cancer cells, and assist with the healing process. Utilizing a comprehensive approach will provide the best chance of an enhanced quality of life for those with liver cancer.

twenty-six

Lung Cancer

Enclosed within the protective rib cage, the lungs are a pair of saclike organs responsible for maintaining respiratory functions—the exchange of necessary and waste gases between the inside and outside of the body. The lungs contain a large variety of cell types, and lung cancer can originate in a number of different tissues. The major varieties of lung cancer are known as non-small-cell lung cancer and small-cell lung cancer (also known as oat-cell lung cancer). Accounting for 80 percent of all lung cancers, non-small-cell lung cancers (NSCLC) include squamous-cell lung cancer, adenocarcinoma, and large-cell carcinoma. While they are less common, small-cell lung cancers (SCLC) tend to grow more quickly and be metastasized at diagnosis. Lung cancer is the second most commonly diagnosed cancer in both men and women. According to the American Cancer Society, in 2009, more than 219,000 new cases of lung cancers were diagnosed.

Causes, Symptoms, and Diagnosis

The American Lung Association reports that 87 percent of lung cancer cases are caused by smoking tobacco products. Exposure to secondhand tobacco smoke can also lead to lung cancer, accounting for 3,000 lung cancer deaths each year. The second leading cause of lung cancer is exposure to radon gas. Radon occurs in underground rock and earth and can be found in well water and building materials. Smokers who are exposed to radon are at an even higher risk. Lung cancer can also result from workplace exposure to carcinogenic substances such as asbestos, arsenic, uranium, and some petroleum products. Air pollution may also cause lung cancer.

Symptoms of lung cancer can include a persistent and worsening cough, persistent chest pain, coughing up blood, shortness of breath or wheezing, chronic pneumonia or bronchitis, neck and face swelling, weight loss or loss of appetite, and fatigue.

Diagnosis of lung cancer relies upon a thorough medical history to evaluate the patient's risk, factoring in smoking history, exposure to carcinogenic substances, and family history. A physical exam is performed and X-rays of the lungs may be taken. A computed tomography (CT) scan of the chest is used to confirm the presence of a suspicious mass. A sputum (mucus coughed up from the lungs) sample may be analyzed for the presence of cancer cells. To definitively diagnose lung cancer, a sample of lung tissue must be taken for biopsy. The lung tissue can be removed using a lighted tube inserted through the windpipe (bronchoscopy), by inserting a needle through the chest to remove a sample of the tumor or the fluid surrounding the lungs, or by opening the chest surgically. The location of the tumor and the person's overall health determine how the biopsy is obtained.

Conventional Treatment

Surgery is the primary conventional approach used to treat lung cancer, along with a combination of chemotherapy and radiation for some types of lung cancer.

Surgery

Surgery for lung cancer typically involves removal of the lobe containing the tumor (the right lung has three lobes; because the left lung must coexist with the heart, it has only two). However, removal of a smaller section of the lung may be possible if a clean surgical margin is achievable. Surgery is used in almost all cases of lung cancer, with the goal of removing all cancerous tissue and obtaining a clean surgical margin; margin size depends on the size and location of the tumor. For those with general cardiopulmonary problems who are over 70, surgery becomes more risky. Surgery is curative in many cases for stages I and II of non-small-cell lung carcinoma: tumors less than three centimeters in size with no lymph node involvement or involving only lymph nodes on the same side as the tumor; or a single mass that is larger but without lymph node involvement. During surgery a sampling of lymph nodes will usually be taken. This will help determine how extensively the cancer has spread.

Radiation and Chemotherapy

Radiation is used in most cases of stage III and stage IV NSCLC, in combination with chemotherapy. It is also used in most cases of SCLC, also usually in combination with chemotherapy. It is often used presurgically, to shrink tumors. Because SCLC commonly metastasizes to the brain, prophylactic whole brain radiation is used in many cases. When radiation is used postoperatively, the goal is to reduce tumor-related symptoms and help prevent a recurrence.

Chemotherapy is used in SCLC at all stages and in stage III and stage IV NSCLC. It may be used both preoperatively and postoperatively. Chemotherapy is usually not recommended for stage I NSCLC. Chemotherapy is infrequently recommended for stage II NSCLC when there is concern of micrometastatic spread. Chemotherapy combined with radiation may also be used to treat inoperable lung cancer. New radiation and chemotherapy regimens are presently being studied. Chemotherapy is used to extend survival and to produce improvement in disease-related symptoms. Chemotherapy agents used for NSCLC include paclitaxel, carboplatin, cisplatin, docetaxel, topotecan, irinotecan, vinorelbine, gemcitabine, and pemetrexed. Chemotherapy agents used for SCLC include etoposide, cisplatin, carboplatin, irinotecan, paclitaxel, cyclophosphamide, doxorubicin, vincristine, and topotecan. Either single-agent or combination therapy may be used. Tyrosine kinase inhibitors such as Tarceva (erlotinib) and Iressa (gefitinib) can also improve survival rates in previously treated patients with NSCLC and improve tumor-related symptoms and important aspects of quality of life. For information about how to counteract typical side effects of these medications, consult the chart "Chemotherapy Drugs and Their Nutrient and Herb Interactions" that starts on page 141.

Complementary Approaches

Refer to part II of this book regarding useful complementary approaches for all cancers. The following information is specific to lung cancer.

Lifestyle and Diet

A person who smokes one pack of cigarettes a day is 20 times more likely to develop lung cancer compared to a nonsmoker. Once a person quits smoking, their risk declines but it remains higher than nonsmokers for many years after they've quit. According to *Cancer Management: A Multidisciplinary Approach*, "Several cancer centers have recently reported that more than half of their patients with newly diagnosed lung cancer are former smokers, having quit more than a year before diagnosis." If you smoke, use a proactive approach combining conventional nicotine addiction aids (nicotine gum and nicotine patch) with complementary acupuncture, behavioral modification techniques, and supplements such as vitamin C, thioglycerols, and *Lobelia inflata* (Indian tobacco plant), which can help you quit. The only smokers who quit successfully are those who want to quit. Once you do quit, a supervised detoxification program will help remove residual nicotine and other cigarette by-products and will help rebuild your health. Exposure to secondhand smoke can also cause cancer, so it should be minimized or, hopefully, avoided altogether.

A study featured in the *Journal of the American Medical Association* specifically looking at women and lung cancer found that estrogen plays a role in lung cancer development. Studies have demonstrated that estrogen causes non-small-cell lung cancer to grow, while antiestrogens block that effect. So a woman's chance of developing lung cancer not only increases with cigarette smoke, but also with estrogen replacement therapy. This is especially true for women with a predisposition to developing lung cancer. The report published in the *Journal of the American Medical Association* concludes, "Women who have never smoked are more likely to develop lung cancer than men who have never smoked. Mounting evidence suggests that this could be due, in part, to estrogen signaling." Female smokers who have also been on hormone replacement therapy may want to consider a detoxification diet and gentle cleanse, as outlined in chapter 12. This will help the body eliminate any toxins or excess estrogens.

An earlier small study featuring patients with non-small-cell lung cancer in various stages demonstrated that a diet containing selected vegetables helped improve weight maintenance and survival, even in cases of stage III and stage IV patients. The benefit from a diet high in colorful and green leafy vegetables is likely due to its higher antioxidant content, as previous studies have shown that an increase in dietary antioxidants correlated with a decreased risk of lung cancer. A controlled clinical trial featuring patients with advanced NSCLC demonstrated that daily consumption of a high-quality vegetable soup (Sun Farm brand) over the course of two years significantly increased median survival by four times compared to non–soup drinkers.

People with lung cancer or at risk of it will want to make sure to feed their body foods that are rich in antioxidant nutrients. This means increased consumption of fresh fruits and vegetables, preferably raw or lightly steamed. It is important to stress that the benefit from antioxidant intake is via the diet. The prevention or treatment benefit from supplementation with selected antioxidants is unclear. Several large studies have even found that beta-carotene supplementation increases the risk of lung cancer, most notably in smokers (or past smokers).

Adequate protein is also of critical importance for those with lung cancer. Lung cancer carries a high risk of cachexia (muscle wasting and weight loss), and protein consumption is one of the most powerful ways to delay and reduce cachexia. The best dietary sources of protein from an anticancer point of view are cold-water fish, legumes, lean meats such as chicken and pork, and nuts and seeds. Protein requirements for people with lung cancer can exceed 80 grams daily.

Nutrients and Herbs

A number of nutrients and herbs are showing benefits in the complementary treatment of lung cancer, specifically NSCLC. For information on dosages for the supplements listed below, as well as any potential contraindications, see the appendix.

- *Antioxidants*: Yale University School of Medicine found a strong correlation between *dietary* antioxidant intake and reduced lung cancer in male smokers; antioxidants assessed included carotenoids, flavonoids, vitamin E, selenium, and vitamin C. Of note, *supplemental* beta-carotene appears to increase the risk of lung cancer in smokers. The benefit of supplemented antioxidants in terms of lung cancer is not yet well understood. It does appear that flavonoids and selenium may be of some benefit. [preventive]

- *Ashwagandha*: Animal studies of this herb have demonstrated that it has immune-stimulating properties, and that when used with the chemotherapy drug paclitaxel, it helped suppress proliferation of lung cancer cells. [anticancer, supportive]

- *Astragalus*: Evaluation of 34 randomized trials using astragalus in combination with platinum-based chemotherapy agents such as cisplatin and carboplatin demonstrated that the herb enhanced survival compared to chemotherapy alone even three years after treatment. In addition, quality of life was enhanced in the patients taking the astragalus with chemotherapy versus those taking chemotherapy alone. [anticancer, supportive]

- *Curcumin*: This anti-inflammatory herb has been shown to induce apoptosis in human non-small-cell lung cancer in vitro. [preventive, anticancer]

- *Fermented wheat germ extract (Avemar)*: Avemar reduced the number of liver metastases in animals with lung cancer. In a human trial Avemar improved quality of life in patients with NSCLC receiving chemotherapy. [anticancer, supportive]

- **Green tea**: Green tea and its active compound EGCG have consistently shown benefit for many cancers, including lung cancer. Both in vitro and in vivo studies have shown green tea can induce apoptosis of lung cancer cells. A phase I clinical trial involving 17 patients with advanced lung cancer demonstrated that green tea was well tolerated. [anticancer]

- **Melatonin**: This hormone exerts anticancer effects in vitro. Melatonin also has been shown to improve the quality of life in patients with NSCLC and low performance status (which is determined based on the extent of a person's ability to independently manage various body functions and tasks such as walking, talking, eating, and breathing). Melatonin also improves quality of life and survival in NSCLC patients receiving etoposide and cisplatin chemotherapy. One study showed that both the overall tumor regression rate and the five-year survival rate were significantly higher in patients who were treated with melatonin along with chemotherapy. [anticancer, supportive]

- **Omega-3 fatty acids**: Levels of the omega-3 fatty acids EPA and DHA tend to be reduced in lung cancer. Cold-water fish or fish oil supplements are the best source of these fatty acids. EPA inhibits growth of lung cancer cells in vitro. Preliminary studies of a supplement program that contained fish oil as an anti-inflammatory agent show promise in reversing weight loss, with apparent gains in lean tissue and performance. [preventive, anticancer, supportive]

- **Shark cartilage (Neovastat liquid extract)**: A phase I/II trial involving patients with NSCLC who received high-dose liquid shark cartilage extract demonstrated a significant survival advantage for these patients compared to the low-dose group. There were no observed toxicities. [anticancer]

- **Silymarin**: An antioxidant flavonoid found in the herb milk thistle, silymarin has been shown to inhibit tumor growth and progression of lung cancer cells in animal studies. [anticancer]

- **Vitamin and mineral supplements**: A study from the Mayo Clinic used questionnaires to determine vitamin and mineral use among small-cell lung cancer patients; they found that there was a strong association between vitamin and mineral supplementation and improved survival. [anticancer]

- **Vitamin D**: Among early-stage NSCLC patients, those with higher blood levels of vitamin D had increased overall survival compared to the patients with the lowest blood levels of vitamin D. Additionally, this same clinical trial increased recurrence-free survival. [preventive, anticancer]

Summary

Present smoking, past smoking, and secondhand smoke can all cause lung cancer. In addition, excessive exposure to specific environmental toxins, as well as increased estrogen exposure, can increase the chance of developing lung cancer. Aggressive steps should be taken to reduce exposure to known lung carcinogens. Eating more fruits and vegetables and adding antioxidant nutrients to the diet will also be helpful, as will drinking green tea and perhaps taking additional supplemental EGCG. Supplementation with melatonin, fish oil, and certain other nutrients and herbs may improve quality of life and survival.

twenty-seven

Ovarian Cancer

The ovaries are key organs of the female reproductive system. The two small, almond-shaped organs produce eggs for reproduction and are located at the ends of the fallopian tubes, inside the pelvis on either side of the uterus. Ovaries secrete estrogen and progesterone, hormones critical to reproduction and other body functions.

Several types of tumors can form in the ovaries, fallopian tubes, and peritoneum (the membrane lining the pelvis and abdomen), and not all of them are cancerous. Epithelial ovarian tumors, which develop in the cells that surround the outside of the ovary, are the most common cancerous tumors of the ovary. Stromal tumors, which develop in the connective tissue cells that hold the ovary together, are far less common. Germ cell tumors, which develop in the egg maturation cells of the ovary, account for only about 3 percent of all ovarian cancers. Approximately 5 to 10 percent of ovarian cancers are familial. These cancers are usually associated with inherited mutations of BRCA1 and/or BRCA2 genes. BRCA1 and BRCA 2 gene mutations are inherited defects in genes that are necessary for cell repair. People with these gene mutations are at much higher risk for the development of cancers, particularly cancers of the breast and ovary. According to the American Cancer Society, only about 20 percent of all ovarian cancers are diagnosed in the early stage when it is most treatable.

Ovarian cancer usually spreads by local shedding of malignant cells into the peritoneal cavity (the space between the abdominal wall and the abdominal organs). These shed cells then implant on the organs and tissues within the peritoneal cavity and can locally invade the bladder and bowel.

Up to 25 percent of women with stage I disease have positive lymph nodes (the presence of cancer cells in the lymph nodes indicates metastasis to the lymphatic system). About 50 percent of women with stage II disease have positive lymph nodes, and 75 percent of women with stage III and stage IV have positive lymph nodes. Ovarian metastases can block abdominal lymph vessels, resulting in impairment of lymphatic flow and a condition known as ascites (fluid accumulation in the abdomen).

In 2009, more than 21,000 women were diagnosed with ovarian cancer. According to American Cancer Society statistics, the number of cases of ovarian cancer has been fairly stable over the past several years. Prognosis is most favorable in women diagnosed at a younger age and with smaller amount of disease, women with good performance status at diagnosis (a measure based on the extent of a person's ability to independently manage various body functions and tasks such as walking, talking, eating, and breathing), and is also dependent upon certain cellular characteristics of the tumor. Tumor marker CA-125 may be elevated at diagnosis, but this initial elevation is not as significant in terms of prognosis. However, for women with stage III or stage IV disease, levels of CA-125 after several cycles of chemotherapy and at least one month into active treatment are highly correlated with likelihood of treatment response and survival. If CA-125 normalizes after treatment has begun, subsequent elevations are highly predictive of recurrent, active disease. (For more information on tumor markers, see the sidebar "Tumor Markers in the Blood" on page 36.)

Causes, Symptoms, and Diagnosis

Factors that may heighten a woman's risk of getting ovarian cancer include a family history of ovarian cancer, age (most ovarian cancer occurs after menopause), never having given birth, infertility, use of talcum powder in the genital area, a personal history of breast cancer, and testing positive for the BRCA1 and BRCA2 gene mutation. BRCA2 is less of a risk factor than the BRCA1 mutation, and BRCA2 mutation carriers have an improved survival over BRCA1 mutation carriers.

In its earlier stages, ovarian cancer presents few symptoms. This is why ovarian cancer is usually not diagnosed until its later stages. As the cancer progresses, symptoms can include abdominal pain or cramps; pain in the lower back or pelvis; abnormal vaginal bleeding or discharge; pain or bleeding during intercourse; nausea, loss of appetite, or weight loss; bloating or intestinal gas; enlargement of the belly (ascites); fatigue; constipation or diarrhea; and a change in urinary frequency or urgency.

If it is suspected that a patient may have ovarian cancer, a gynecological oncologist will use imaging scans such as CT scans, MRIs, or ultrasound to look for tumors and to help determine whether the cancer may have spread. CT scans can also be used to help guide a needle to take a biopsy sample. Barium enema X-rays and colonoscopy may also be used to determine whether the cancer has spread to the intestines or rectum, and chest X-rays may be taken to see whether it has metastasized to the lungs. Only a biopsy of a tissue sample from the suspected tumor can definitively diagnose ovarian cancer.

Conventional Treatment

Conventional treatment for ovarian cancer relies heavily on surgery, with radiation and chemotherapy used in recurrent and metastasized cases, respectively.

Surgery

Surgery is used in almost all cases, and usually includes a full hysterectomy, bilateral salpingo-oophorectomy (removal of the ovaries and fallopian tubes), and omentectomy (removal of parts of the tissue that supports the inner organs). There are significant survival advantages to having surgery done by a surgeon who specializes in gynecological oncology. These surgeons have the expertise to properly inspect the abdominal cavity and tissue outside of the ovaries for tumor sites and are also adept at determining what tissue to remove for biopsy. Surgery is typically not considered to be curative in most cases of ovarian cancer, and additional treatment is usually recommended.

Radiation and Chemotherapy

Radiation is used only in recurrent cases. Whole-abdominal radiation may be used between rounds of chemotherapy. Pelvic radiation therapy is also an option in more limited disease. In cases with small residual tumors in the peritoneum, intraperitoneal P-32 radiation is sometimes used; this technique involves infusion of radioactive phosphate-32 solution into the peritoneal cavity for localized radiation treatment.

Women with stage IA and IB ovarian cancer, which is when the cancer is contained within the ovary(ies), do not benefit significantly from chemotherapy, and surgery is considered sufficient treatment. Chemotherapy is used to treat stage IC cancer, which is when the cancer is within one or both of the ovaries and is also present on the outer surface of the ovaries, the ovary(ies) has ruptured, or there are malignant cells found in the fluid or washings from the abdomen. Chemotherapy also plays an important role in the treatment of metastasized ovarian cancer—stage II through stage IV— where it is used postsurgically to reduce risk of recurrence and metastasis. Chemotherapy combinations are often used and sometimes, with cancers that are confined to the peritoneal cavity, intraperitoneal chemotherapy will be given. Typical chemotherapy agents used are cisplatin, paclitaxel, carboplatin, docetaxel, and cyclophosphamide. Recurrent disease is often treated with ifosfamide, etoposide, liposomal doxorubicin, gemcitabine, topotecan, oxaliplatin, 5-FU, or altretamine. For information about how to counteract typical side effects of these medications, consult the chart "Chemotherapy Drugs and Their Nutrient and Herb Interactions" that begins on page 141.

In recurrent advanced cases, chemotherapy may be given in high doses (which destroys bone marrow), followed by stem cell support therapy. In stem cell support, stem cells may be harvested from a healthy donor or from the patient's own blood or bone marrow before chemotherapy treatments. After chemotherapy ends, the healthy stem cells are injected into the patient with the hope that these healthy immune cells will actively recognize and attack cancerous tissue. Receiving stem cells from a donor may require lifetime use of immune-suppressing antirejection drugs. Additionally, hormonal therapy, such as tamoxifen, may play a role in reducing ovarian cancer recurrence, as well as relieving symptoms.

Complementary Approaches

Refer to part II of this book regarding useful complementary approaches for all cancers. The following information is specific to ovarian cancer.

Lifestyle and Diet

Many studies have demonstrated that exercise can help prevent ovarian cancer. Researchers have concluded that exercise prevents ovarian cancer because it stimulates the immune system, positively influences hormonal balance, helps control glucose metabolism, and controls obesity.

Diet can play a big role in the development of ovarian cancer. The American Cancer Society reports, "A number of studies have shown a reduced rate of ovarian cancer in women who ate a diet high in vegetables." Epidemiological studies have also shown that countries that consume higher amounts of fat have higher rates of ovarian cancer. Results from studies regarding dairy products as a cause of ovarian cancer are conflicting. However, many studies point specifically to cow's milk as a potential cause. Researchers have hypothesized that milk from pregnant cows contains estrogens that can be harmful to women. Following a thorough analysis of incidence rates in 40 countries, Japanese researchers concluded in a 2005 issue of *Medical Hypotheses*, "We are most concerned with milk and dairy products, because the milk we drink today is produced from pregnant cows, in which estrogen and progesterone levels are markedly elevated." Hormone-free milk and other dairy products are available, obtained from cows that haven't been given supplemental hormones. If you choose to eat dairy products, consume hormone-free products whenever possible. Organic dairy products, which are also hormone free, are an even better choice.

A recent study in the *Archives of Internal Medicine* demonstrated that drinking green and black tea lowered the risk of developing ovarian cancer. The researchers reported that drinking just one cup of tea per day reduced the risk by 24 percent, and two cups by 46 percent; as you add more cups, you can decrease the risk by another 18 percent per cup per day.

Nutrients and Herbs

There are several nutrients and herbs that can have a significant benefit as a complementary treatment for ovarian cancer. Their effectiveness depends on many variables, including how advanced the disease is. For information on dosages for the supplements listed below, as well as any potential contraindications, see the appendix.

- *Antioxidants*: Vitamins C and E, beta-carotene, and CoQ10 (along with a multivitamin-multimineral complex) were shown to improve the efficacy of chemotherapy and resulted in a normalization of CA-125 levels in two patients. While preliminary, these case studies support previous in vitro data on antioxidants. [supportive]

- *Curcumin*: A recent in vitro study demonstrated that curcumin inhibited the growth of human ovarian cancer cells, which confirms past cellular studies. [preventive, anticancer]

- *Ginkgo biloba*: Researchers at Brigham and Women's Hospital in Boston found that this herb was associated with a 60 percent lower risk of developing ovarian cancer. Ginkgo should not be taken for two weeks prior to surgery, because it can act as a blood thinner and may encourage bleeding. [preventive]

- *Green tea*: A recent cellular study found that EGCG from green tea inhibited ovarian cancer cells and also sensitized them to cisplatin chemotherapy. Another study that combined green tea with lysine, proline, arginine, and vitamin C found that this regimen inhibited the development and growth of ovarian cancer cells. [anticancer, supportive]

- *Melatonin*: This hormone may increase sensitivity of ovarian cancer cells to cisplatin. [supportive]

- *Mushroom polysaccharides*: A human study of 100 patients with cervical, ovarian, or endometrial cancer undergoing chemotherapy treatment demonstrated that a mushroom extract, *Agaricus blazei* Murill

Kyowa (ABMK), improved chemotherapy-associated side effects, including loss of appetite, hair loss, emotional instability, and general weakness. However, in this study, this particular mushroom extract did not appear to stimulate increased immune activity, as mushroom extracts usually do. [supportive]

- **Quercetin**: This phytochemical exerts a dose-dependent inhibition of ovarian cancer cell growth in vitro; quercetin interrupts chemical pathways within the cell that ultimately trigger ovarian cancer cell division, or cell growth. Quercetin also prevents cellular DNA from unwinding, therefore impairing the ability of cancer cells to divide. And finally, quercetin inhibits the tumor cell's ability to consume adequate nutrition. [preventive, anticancer]

- **Soy**: A published case study of a woman with ovarian cancer who appeared to be resistant to platinum-based chemotherapy described how she stabilized and then improved following treatment with a concentrated fermented soy extract. While there is not enough data to warrant routine use of fermented soy extract, this case study does raise the possibility of benefit. Results from in vitro and in vivo studies about soy and ovarian cancer are conflicting; however, a cellular study demonstrated that genistein and daidzein from soy reduce ovarian cancer cell proliferation. [anticancer]

- **Vitamin A**: This antioxidant vitamin inhibits the growth of several ovarian tumor cell lines. Vitamin A appears to block cell cycle progression of human ovarian carcinoma cells. When vitamin A binds to retinoic acid receptors on ovarian cancer cells, apoptosis or cell differentiation is induced, depending on the type and concentration of retinoid. [anticancer]

- **Vitamin D**: Application of activated vitamin D to ovarian cancer cells results in significant growth inhibition. Ovarian cells contain receptors for vitamin D. When these receptors are occupied, along with certain androgen receptors, growth-signaling pathways in ovarian cancer cells are inhibited. [preventive, anticancer]

- **Vitamins C and E**: A study published in the journal *Nutrition and Cancer* demonstrated that women who take vitamins C and E have a lower risk of developing ovarian cancer and that these vitamins may provide some benefit as a complementary treatment. An animal study that utilized intravenous vitamin C at dosages achieved in humans showed decreased growth rates of ovarian tumors. [preventive, anticancer]

Summary

When caught early, ovarian cancer is highly treatable. In advanced cases, a more aggressive integrative approach will help enhance outcomes and quality of life. In any case, making appropriate dietary changes and exercising consistently will help prevent recurrence and will enhance response to treatment. Drinking green tea and even supplementing with EGCG is recommended. Vitamins D and A, quercetin, curcumin, and ginkgo offer additional anticancer potential and may enhance overall treatment.

twenty-eight

Pancreatic Cancer

Located in the abdomen to the rear of the stomach, and surrounded by the liver, intestines, and other organs, the pancreas is a flat, pear-shaped gland that produces insulin and other hormones. The pancreas also releases enzymes that help with the digestion of food. Most cancers of the pancreas begin in the gland's ducts, and most cysts and tumors that develop in the pancreas are found to be cancerous. The American Cancer Society estimated that there were more than 42,000 cases of newly diagnosed pancreatic cancer in 2009. In 2008, more than 35,000 people died of pancreatic cancer, making it the fourth leading cause of cancer death in the United States. The five-year survival rate for all stages is less than 5 percent, and the one-year survival rate for all stages combined is 20 percent. For disease confined to the pancreas, the five-year survival rate is 16 percent, and with stage III and IV disease, the five-year survival rate is 7 percent. If the cancer has already metastasized at the time of diagnosis, the five-year survival rate is 2 percent.

Causes, Symptoms, and Diagnosis

The greatest risk factors for pancreatic cancer are environmental and lifestyle factors, such as smoking, a high-fat diet, obesity, diabetes, and exposure to carcinogenic chemicals. A small number of pancreatic cancers can also be attributed to hereditary factors, such as a family history of polyps or colon cancer, certain types of breast cancer, or hereditary pancreatitis.

In its early stages, pancreatic cancer does not cause symptoms. In its later stages, symptoms may include weight loss, pain in the upper abdomen or upper back, loss of appetite, nausea or vomiting, and jaundice, which results in yellowing of the eyes and skin and a darkening of the urine.

If pancreatic cancer is suspected, a doctor will perform a physical exam to check for signs of jaundice and for abnormal structures, fluid, or pain in the abdomen. Blood, urine, and stool samples may be taken. Elevated blood levels of bilirubin (a breakdown product of hemoglobin) can be caused by a tumor blocking the bile duct and can be a warning sign (though elevated bilirubin levels can also be present with noncancerous conditions). Imaging tests such as CT scans, ultrasound, and endoscopy are required to identify tumors. Either a biopsy (done by inserting a needle into the pancreatic tumor under X-ray or ultrasound guidance) or surgical removal of the tumor will provide tissue for laboratory analysis and definitive diagnosis.

Staging of pancreatic cancer is very important because it determines the most appropriate course of treatment. The staging process considers the size and location of the tumor and if it has spread to nearby tissues or lymphatic vessels. Location is a major factor in whether surgical removal of the tumor is a possibility. Tumors that encase major arteries and veins or are adjacent to them cannot be removed surgically. Additional scans are also done to determine if distant spread has occurred. The most common sites of metastasis are the lymphatic system, liver, and lungs.

Conventional Treatment

Conventional treatment for pancreatic cancer almost always involves radiation and chemotherapy, with surgery in some cases.

Surgery

Surgery is used when possible (10 to 15 percent of the time), with the goal of removing all cancerous tissue and obtaining a clean surgical margin. The close proximity of key arteries and veins makes most tumors too difficult to remove. Surgery is only done if the tumor has not encased critical arteries and veins and has not metastasized outside of the pancreas. Surgery involving the pancreas is very complex and has a high risk of complications. The most common surgical procedure is referred to as a Whipple and involves removal of part of the stomach, part of the pancreas, the gallbladder, and the first portion of the small intestine (the duodenum). This procedure attaches the remainder of the stomach to the next portion of the small intestine. When tumors can be removed, long-term survival rates are 15 to 20 percent, with median survival time of 15 to 24 months. Recurrence is common—85 percent. This is because of the frequent occurrence of sub-clinical hepatic metastases, in which the cancer has spread to the liver but the metastasis isn't detectable.

Radiation and Chemotherapy

Radiation is used in almost all cases, and it is almost always combined with chemotherapy. Fluorouracil is often combined with radiation in an attempt to shrink the tumor mass so that it can be removed surgically. This combination treatment approach also extends expected life span for an additional 6 months on average (from 13 to 19 months).

Chemotherapy may be used alone in the case of inoperable tumors and metastases. Gemcitabine is the most commonly used chemotherapy drug; it is also being studied, along with other chemotherapy agents, for treating pancreatic cancers found at an earlier stage. Gemcitabine is primarily used to improve quality of life, not to extend life. The drug erlotinib has shown minimal benefit to patients with advanced pancreatic cancer. According to the American Cancer Society, studies demonstrated that erlotinib prolonged life by only 12 days, with most of the study participants receiving no benefit. Cetuximab is another drug that is being added to chemotherapy for additional benefits, although these benefits are modest at this point in time. For information about how to counteract typical side effects of these medications, consult the chart "Chemotherapy Drugs and Their Nutrient and Herb Interactions" starting on page 141.

Additional experimental chemotherapy options include intra-arterial chemotherapy, usually with mitomycin and cisplatin sent directly to the liver, as well as systemic chemotherapy with fluorouracil, which may prevent, delay, or treat liver metastases. Another common regimen for pancreatic cancer includes gemcitabine, oxaliplatin, and docetaxel. People with metastatic pancreatic cancer should consider participating in clinical trials with gene therapy and bioimmune therapies. Ask your oncologist if you would be a good candidate for trials that are presently being conducted.

Complementary Approaches

Refer to part II of this book regarding useful complementary approaches for all cancers. The following information is specific to pancreatic cancer.

Lifestyle and Diet

Smoking is an established risk factor for pancreatic cancer. Recent research has also shown that being overweight, eating a high-fat diet, and having diabetes (or insulin resistance), along with a sedentary lifestyle, can contribute to pancreatic cancer. Recent research identified waist-to-hip ratio as a contributor, with individuals who have a larger waist circumference than hip circumference at increased risk. Of note, waist-to-hip ratio is highly predictive of insulin resistance. (Refer to chapter 11 for more information on insulin resistance.)

Diet plays a significant role in the development of pancreatic cancer. A review of 109 pancreatic cancer patients demonstrated that a diet high in fat and cholesterol significantly increased the risk of pancreatic cancer. A recent study featured in the *International Journal of Cancer* confirmed that red meat intake is associated with an increased risk of pancreatic cancer. Conversely, another recent study showed that a diet high in cruciferous vegetables, specifically cabbage, was associated with a reduced risk of pancreatic cancer. Another recent report, which followed nearly 82,000 Swedish men and women, found that dietary intake of folic acid (also known as folate) was associated with a reduced risk of pancreatic cancer. Folic acid is found in beans, asparagus, spinach, and other vegetables. Many nuts are also a good source of folic acid.

Those with pancreatic cancer will need higher amounts of protein in their diet to maintain body weight and muscle mass. Protein requirements may range from 60 to 80 grams daily. People with pancreatic cancer may also need to take supplemental pancreatic enzymes (often in high doses, which many insurance plans cover) to properly digest food and absorb nutrients.

Nutrients and Herbs

The same study that found a link between a high-cholesterol diet and increased risk of pancreatic cancer also discovered that vitamin C intake decreased the risk. Other nutrients and herbs have also been studied regarding pancreatic cancer, including the following.

- *Alpha-lipoic acid*: This compound plays a valuable antioxidant role in the liver. It also induces apoptosis and reduces inflammation, thereby reducing a stimulus for growth of cancer. In a case study of a patient with metastatic pancreatic cancer, intravenous alpha-lipoic acid caused disease stabilization. The researchers state that they are using this treatment as part of a pancreatic cancer protocol for other patients; however, it is too soon to broadly prescribe it, as its effects in a broader range of patients remains unknown. [anticancer]

- *Curcumin*: Both in vitro and in vivo studies demonstrate that curcumin can suppress growth and induce apoptosis of human pancreatic cancer cells. In vitro studies have also shown that curcumin can inhibit NF-kB, a proinflammatory protein; this helps control insulin resistance, which has been linked to cancer development and growth. Recent human trials from the M. D. Anderson Cancer Center demonstrated that patients with advanced pancreatic cancer who received 8 grams of curcumin orally daily had a decrease in several serum markers associated with inflammation and cancer proliferation. Despite these serum changes, only 2 of the 20 patients studied showed actual improvement in their tumor burden. No toxicities were observed. [preventive, anticancer]

- *Genistein*: A cellular study showed that genistein, a soy isoflavone, increased the antitumor activity of the chemotherapy drug gemcitabine while reducing the activity of the proinflammatory protein NF-kB. Inhibiting NF-kB helps control insulin resistance, which has been linked to cancer development and growth. [preventive, supportive]

- *Green tea*: Green tea and one of its active compounds, EGCG, have been studied for both preventing and treating a wide variety of cancers. In regard to pancreatic cancer, cellular studies have demonstrated that EGCG may reduce proliferation and invasion of cancer cells. A cellular study utilizing a combination of green tea, lysine, proline, arginine, and vitamin C also demonstrated antitumor activity against pancreatic cancer. [anticancer]

- *Limonene*: This phytochemical found in the inner rinds of citrus fruits inhibits cell proliferation in vitro by inactivating the mutated K-ras gene; K-ras is commonly mutated in pancreatic cancer cells, and this mutation causes unchecked cell proliferation. [anticancer]

- *Melatonin*: A recent animal study found that melatonin reduced oxidative damage and prevented pancreatic cancer development in response to a cancer-causing agent. [preventive]

- *Mistletoe*: While studies involving mistletoe extract have shown conflicting results, a cellular study on human pancreatic cancer cells that compared mistletoe to gemcitabine revealed mistletoe to have more effective antitumor activity. This result has not, however, been demonstrated in animals or in humans. [anticancer]

- *Omega-3 fatty acids*: EPA, an omega-3 fatty acid, inhibited human pancreatic cancer cell growth in vitro. Human studies have shown that EPA can help improve cachexia (muscle wasting) in those with pancreatic cancer. Other fatty acids have been shown to inhibit pancreatic cancer cell growth, including docosahexaenoic acid (DHA), which induced pancreatic cell apoptosis. [preventive, anticancer, supportive]

Al Alschuler: Pancreatic Cancer Diagnosed at Age 65

The summer before they found the tumor, I had cranked a hand-powered tricycle 624 miles up the hot, humid, hilly East Coast to a family reunion to celebrate my sixty-fifth birthday. I was also gathering material for a book that explored what it means to be an exuberant new senior and prepare to "greet sister death" with a smile and a song. The following February, less than 24 hours after completing the book, my partner, Suzanne, said, "You look terrible. I'm taking you to the emergency room." By midnight, the ER doc told me I had a compromised gallbladder and a suspicious growth on my pancreas.

"Suspicious?"

"Probably cancer."

"And if it is?"

"It's the worst kind. There's no protective sheath around the pancreas. It spreads fast. There is no cure. It's invariably fatal."

"How much time?"

"A few months. Maybe a bit more."

It seemed too coincidental to be accidental. My book was a seminar. Now I had a practicum in dying well. It also was a total shock to a professor who knew he'd die someday, but like most of us, acted as if he'd live forever.

My four children gathered immediately from Spain, Costa Rica, Illinois, and Massachusetts. We all were in tears. Suddenly there was so little time left to enjoy each other. They helped me find a superb doctor who performed a miraculous 12½-hour operation to remove a 3-inch tumor and nearby cancerous nodes. I felt both pessimistic and liberated. Those things that had been important for my security—my work as a professor, my income and home—were now irrelevant. Thoreau said, "The price of anything is the amount of life you exchange for it." Only being with loved ones was important.

At the suggestion of my doctor daughter, Lise (coauthor of this book), one of the world's foremost authorities on naturopathic treatments for cancer, I received a special form of chemotherapy at her hospital that included direct showering of the liver—the first and most likely place the cancer might spread. Although the two treatments nearly killed me—I'd lost nearly 70 pounds by that time—I was optimistic.

Lise gave me a regimen of 15 herbal and natural supplements and 3 liquids to boost my immune system, promote T cell activity, reduce inflammation, and attack the cancer. I increased my workouts, eventually swimming a mile a day. It felt good to be proactive.

A cocktail of chemotherapy drugs failed. The cancer spread. Officially I became stage IV—completely metastasized. The doctor looked me in the eye and said, "Think weeks or a few months. Not years." I was shocked again.

An immunization clinical trial failed. A radically new gene modification clinical trial failed. Yet, miraculously I looked and felt quite well, particularly compared to the medical "fact" that I should have died already. I started to hear my doctors and their residents say things like "You're one in a million, a miracle man, a poster boy for natural approaches to pancreatic cancer."

Thinking about death 24/7 really sucks, but I made friends with this dark companion. I listened to countless stories about what others with cancer had chosen to be and do. Most people continue to do and be what they had done and been: An accountant made a list, prioritized it, committed to a plan, and persisted until his death from brain cancer. A psychologist got therapy and joined several support groups. One man watched his favorite

- **Probiotics**: A randomized controlled trial demonstrated that the use of probiotics before and after removal of the pancreas (Whipple) achieved a significant reduction in infection. [supportive]

- **Selenium**: Deficiency of this trace mineral is associated with increased incidence of pancreatic cancer, especially in men. [preventive]

TV shows and golf tournaments. As a teacher and learner, I listened, talked, and studied the mystical literature on what happens after we drop our body sack.

As my youngest daughter pointed out, "This is not just a problem for you, Dad. It's a problem for all of us." She was right, of course. I've spent time with each of them and asked if there was anything troublesome they were holding that we could discuss and clean up. I didn't want them to carry unnecessary burdens that would be more difficult to resolve after I died. There were some painful moments and honest confessions. We cried together. I asked for forgiveness and was forgiven. All of them said that my "eyes-wide-open" approach to death was helpful. I wanted to give to them what my father had given to me—a model of how dying could be sane, graceful, and loving—to help them get ready to let me go, just as I was preparing to do that myself.

I also consulted with Victor, a spokesperson for a distinguished group of teachers who happen not to have bodies—spiritual beings on "the other side." At first, his disembodied nature bothered me—a lot. However, after 30 years of inner consultation, perspectives that deepened my understanding of problems, inspiration when I was discouraged, and authorization to do what I could to make this world more like that one, Victor's lack of physical existence was a trivial matter. Victor pointed out that the inevitable uncertainty about death means that our belief about it is a choice and a matter of faith. We must exercise our cherished free will. We can fear it or welcome it. It's another opportunity to choose our path Home to The Friend. I'd dropped my mother's body at birth. At "death" I will drop the body that served me well for a lifetime. Victor convinced me that dying is perfectly safe—a second birthday.

Yesterday, when I held my newly born fourth grandchild, a perfect little girl, there were tears at the natural, inevitable passage of generations. I was happy beyond words for her new life, and sad that I might not know much of it.

My continued existence 15 months after my diagnosis has left conventional doctors without explanations. I remain in relative good health, with some modest pain in my liver. I am usually energetic, living with two of my children and their families, involved with an international effort to find ways to treat 450 million untreated people worldwide with diagnosable psychoses, participating in an infusion treatment with a natural substance; and I am quietly, ecstatically participating in the lives of my children and grandchildren, enjoying contacts with many friends, colleagues, and former students. I'm a collection of feelings: at peace with an early death (most of the time); occasionally sad at the loss of time; deeply grateful for the marvelous choices my children have made to become such superb adults; looking forward to seeing my youngest child graduate from college in a month after brilliant endeavors there; thankful for the love that reverberates among my four children and me; completely satisfied with my 40-year career as a professor; enjoying the little things every day that are 99 percent of life. As one of my students said when she was approaching her early death from cervical cancer, "It's all here! It's all right here all the time."

I helped bring Lise into this world. She has returned the gift most abundantly by helping to keep me here a while longer.

Summary

Pancreatic cancer does not typically produce symptoms until the disease has progressed. Treating advanced pancreatic cancer is especially challenging, given the aggressive and fast-growing nature of this cancer. While natural medicine has not revealed any clearly effective anticancer treatments at this time, a variety of natural substances have potential and certainly help to improve quality of life. Until more effective treatment options become available, prevention and early diagnosis will be of paramount importance. Using an integrated treatment approach combining complementary and conventional options may best benefit those with pancreatic cancer.

twenty-nine

Prostate Cancer

The prostate is a gland surrounding the male urethra (the tube that carries urine out of the body from the bladder). It is roughly the size and shape of a walnut. Some cells of the prostate produce various components of seminal fluid. The prostate can often become enlarged in older men, causing difficulty with urination; this is known as benign prostatic hyperplasia. Prostatitis refers to an inflamed prostate.

Most prostate cancer starts in the glandular cells of the prostate and is known as adenocarcinoma. Prostate cancer cells usually grow very slowly, but on occasion they can grow and metastasize quickly. Prostate cancer is the most commonly diagnosed cancer in men. According to the American Cancer Society, the number of prostate cancers diagnosed each year has gone up from 189,000 in 2002 to more than 192,000 in 2008. However, the number of deaths caused by prostate cancer did not increase during that same three-year period. When prostate cancer is diagnosed early (while it is confined to the prostate), long-term disease-free survival is expected. Locally advanced prostate cancer also has a good prognosis for long-term survival. If diagnosed after it has already spread to distant organs, the prognosis is not as good, with an expected survival of one to three years.

Causes, Symptoms, and Diagnosis

Age is a major risk factor for prostate cancer. Two-thirds of all prostate cancers diagnosed occur in men over 65. Race is another factor, with prostate cancer occurring 60 percent more often in African-Americans than in Caucasians and Hispanic-Americans, and less frequently in people of Asian descent than in Caucasians and Hispanics. Hereditary factors affect risk as well; having a brother or father with prostate cancer doubles a man's risk. A diet high in red meat and dairy products and low in fruits and vegetables also puts a man at greater risk, as does leading a sedentary lifestyle. Having a vasectomy may increase the risk slightly.

Prostate cancer may not present any symptoms in its early stages; however, the following symptoms may be cause for concern: increased frequency of urination; urinary incontinence or inability to urinate; weak urinary flow; pain during urination; erection difficulty or painful ejaculation; and recurrent pain in the hips, thighs, or lower back.

Digital rectal examination done as part of routine screening or for suspicious symptoms may identify abnormal swelling or an oversized prostate. Additionally, a blood test to detect prostate-specific antigen (PSA) is used to help screen for prostate cancer. This test is most effective when used with other screening methods (refer to the section "Prostate-Specific Antigen (PSA) Test" on page 33).

The most definitive method of prostate cancer diagnosis is a core needle biopsy, in which a doctor inserts a needle into the prostate gland through the wall of the rectum to remove a tissue sample. Several samples are taken in rapid succession. The needle is inserted with use of a special "biopsy gun" and is usually less uncomfortable than it sounds. If necessary, the doctor may give a local anesthetic to reduce discomfort. The biopsied tissue will be assessed for several characteristics and given a Gleason score (a measure of how well differentiated the cells are). The combination of PSA value, Gleason score, serum acid phosphatase, and extent of disease together predict the likelihood of whether it is confined to the prostate gland at diagnosis and the overall prognosis. An MRI may be ordered to determine if the disease has spread beyond the capsule, which affects treatment options. PSA levels are followed throughout treatment to determine response to treatment and monitored after treatment to assess for recurrence. Some oncologists are now monitoring testosterone levels, which should decrease with treatment, as well as testing for neuron-specific enolase (NSE) and chromogranin A, which help to determine if the cancer is likely to respond to androgen ablation therapy, a type of hormonal drug therapy.

Prostate cancer sometimes progresses very slowly and causes few symptoms. Men who are over 70 years old at diagnosis or those who have PSA levels under 2.5 and who have certain types of low-risk cancers are often advised not to treat the cancer unless its characteristics change significantly for the worse. This is known as watchful waiting or active surveillance. A recent study featured in *Urology* found that men in this category who chose active surveillance including diet, exercise, and stress management intervention had a better perceived quality of life than those who received treatment. For those engaged in watchful waiting, it is important to routinely monitor PSA levels.

Conventional Treatment

Conventional treatment for prostate cancer often involves surgery or radiation therapy.

Surgery

Radical prostatectomy (removal of the entire prostate) is the most common treatment for men who have only localized prostate cancer, who otherwise would have a life expectancy of 10 or more years, and who have no medical conditions that preclude surgery. Surgery may include removal of the neurovascular structures leading to the penis, which can cause temporary or permanent incontinence and erectile dysfunction.

Radiation and Chemotherapy

Radiation therapy is used in many cases, especially those in which prostatectomy is not a good or desired option. It may include external beam radiation therapy and/or brachytherapy, in which radioactive material sealed into pellets, rods, catheters, or wires is placed inside the prostate. New research from the University of Chicago Hospitals reported that external beam radiation enhanced the effects of low-dose brachytherapy in cancer patients.

Radiation of the prostate and surrounding area is associated with gastrointestinal toxicity, so supporting gastrointestinal health during and after radiation is critical to help ease this side effect. According to a 2006 report in the journal *Cancer*, "Lower gastrointestinal toxicity after radiation therapy for prostate cancer continues for at least five years and may be more common than previously reported." Fortunately, there are a number of natural therapies to offset gastrointestinal toxicity. Probiotics, fish oil, and L-glutamine are among the therapies utilized. For more information on supporting and enhancing gastrointestinal health, refer to chapter 12.

Chemotherapy is not generally used for prostate cancer. Even in cases of metastatic prostate cancer, chemotherapy drugs have produced disappointing results and are typically only used if the patient does not respond to hormone drugs. When utilized, chemotherapy consists of flutamide, leuprolide, goserelin, estramustine, etoposide, vinblastine, paclitaxel, docetaxel, liposomal doxorubicin, and thalidomide. For information about how to counteract

Natural Management of Menopause-like Side Effects

When men are given androgen-suppressing drugs, they can experience side effects similar to the symptoms of menopause. Here are some ways to manage these side effects naturally.

■ Follow the dietary recommendations in chapter 8, with a special emphasis on eating lots of fruits, vegetables, and whole grains.

■ For hot flashes and night sweats, try supplementing with a combination of vitamin E and the bioflavonoid hesperidin, which is extracted from the inner rind of citrus fruits. For some men, black cohosh can be quite effective, as can increased intake of soy or soy isoflavones.

■ Gamma oryzanol, an extract of rice bran oil, can help with anxiety-associated hot flashes and anxiety-induced insomnia.

■ Homeopathic remedies such as Sepia, Pulsatilla, and Apis can help reduce hot flashes. Other homeopathic remedies, such as gelsemium, arsenicum, and combination bach flower remedies, can assist with anxiety and insomnia.

■ Stress-reducing herbs, such as chamomile, valerian, and St. John's wort, can reduce insomnia and anxiety. Caution is advised with St. John's wort if the person is taking prescription medications, including some of the drugs commonly prescribed for prostate conditions, such as bicalutamide, dutastaride, or finasteride. St. John's wort should only be taken under the guidance of a qualified health-care provider who can assess any possible adverse interactions.

It is also critical to identify and avoid symptom triggers. Common things that can aggravate symptoms include caffeine, alcohol, spicy foods, lack of sleep, and excessive or ongoing stress.

typical side effects of these medications, consult the chart "Chemotherapy Drugs and Their Nutrient and Herb Interactions" beginning on page 141.

Other Conventional Treatments

There are a few alternatives to surgery and radiation, including the following:

● *Proton therapy*: similar to radiation therapy but uses proton beams

● *Cryotherapy*: freezes the prostate under anesthesia

● *CyberKnife*: a new type of radiation therapy that delivers radiation that more precisely conforms to the area of the prostate

● *HIFU*: high-intensity focused ultrasound, currently undergoing clinical trials in the United States; uses high-intensity focused ultrasound waves to destroy the cancerous tissues of the prostate

Hormone suppression drugs are another conventional treatment option with some forms of prostate cancer. Androgen suppressors (drugs that suppress the production of male hormones, primarily testosterone) are often used, in combination with external beam radiation therapy, in advanced cases or after a prostatectomy in recurrent cases. Common androgen suppression drugs include leuprolide (Lupron), bicalutamide (Casodex), gosereline (Zoladex), and others. Hormone therapy has many side effects including causing menopause-like symptoms such as hot flashes, mood swings, and sleep disturbances. To naturally manage these side effects, refer to the sidebar opposite. Osteoporosis is another potential side effect. Australian researchers who studied prostate cancer patients recommended exercise, smoking cessation, and taking vitamin D and calcium supplements to help prevent osteoporosis induced by androgen suppression therapy.

Treatment for prostate cancer is confusing, as there are often a variety of options to choose from. It is important to get a second or even third opinion, as some medical professionals may frequently recommend one therapy over another, depending upon their specialty. A medical oncologist can frequently discuss all of the options and help educate patients about the pros and cons of surgery versus radiation therapy and whether hormonal therapy might play a role. Prostate cancer is often a cancer that grows slowly enough to allow men to take the time they need to educate themselves and make the most informed choices about their treatment.

Complementary Approaches

Refer to part II of this book regarding useful complementary approaches for all cancers. The following information is specific to prostate cancer.

Lifestyle and Diet

Obesity is not only a risk factor for prostate cancer, it can also increase the risk of recurrence, according to researchers from the M. D. Anderson Cancer Center in Texas. Exercise and physical activity are beneficial for those with prostate cancer by supporting weight loss, enhancing pelvic circulation, improving immunity, and reducing fatigue.

The most effective prostate cancer diet is low in red meat and dairy and high in fruits and vegetables. Broccoli in particular has been shown in clinical trials to specifically help prevent prostate cancer. A vegetarian diet has been shown to be effective in some cases. There is conflicting information on soy and soy isoflavones. Dietary soy is associated with a lower risk of prostate cancer. The effects of concentrated soy extracts and other phytoestrogens are less clear. This may be due to the fact that men eating a Western diet (full of meat and low in vegetables) have a different population of bacteria inhabiting their gut. These bacteria may not effectively break down soy into its active metabolite, genistein. Men eating a traditional Japanese diet tend to experience greater benefit from soy in terms of preventing prostate cancer because they have been eating soy foods as a part of their daily diets for years, and therefore are more likely to have a population of gut bacteria that effectively metabolize soy isoflavones into genistein; men who incorporate soy foods in the diet abruptly may not receive the same benefit. A 2008 study involving men with prostate cancer demonstrated that decreased consumption of saturated fat and increased consumption of vegetable proteins slowed the growth of prostate cancer and increased quality of life.

Studies demonstrate that physical activity is important in preventing prostate cancer. In one large prospective study, men over 65 who exercised the most had the lowest risk of prostate cancer. Exercise will also help maintain normal body weight as obesity is a risk factor. In one study involving men who previously had prostate cancer, those with the highest BMI had the highest risk of developing a recurrence.

Nutrients and Herbs

Many natural substances have been studied both for the prevention and treatment of prostate cancer. Here are some of the highlights:

- *Antioxidants*: A study involving more than 5,000 men evaluated intake of vitamins C and E, beta-carotene, selenium, and zinc and found that these antioxidant nutrients were protective against prostate cancer. [preventive]

- *Artemisinin*: An animal study showed that this herb exerted potent growth inhibition of prostate cancer cells. [anticancer]

- *CoQ10*: In vitro, CoQ10 significantly lowered human prostate cancer cell growth. [anticancer]

- *Curcumin*: A recent in vivo study showed that curcumin can help prevent prostate cancer. [preventive]

- *Essiac tea*: A combination of four herbs (*Rheum palmatum*, *Trifolium pretense*, *Arctium lappa*, and *Rumex acetosella*) was found in vitro to inhibit prostate cancer cell growth. [anticancer]

- *Flavonoids*: A smaller study involving men with a history of prostate cancer showed that soy (isoflavones), lycopene, and silymarin delayed cancer progression as evidenced by a slower rise in PSA levels after conventional treatment. Delphinidin from berries caused apoptosis of prostate cancer cells along with significant inhibition of tumor growth in an animal study. [anticancer]

- **Green tea**: Several studies have confirmed green tea as a potent agent against many cancers, including prostate cancer. A recent small double-blind human trial demonstrated that green tea was effective at treating premalignant prostate lesions and also showed that green tea reduced urinary tract symptoms associated with benign prostatic hyperplasia. Researchers at Louisiana State University conducted a study involving 26 prostate cancer patients. Prior to their scheduled surgery the patients were given a green tea extract containing 800 mg of EGCG (equivalent to 12 cups of tea daily) for an average of 34.5 days. The patients had significant reductions in blood levels of PSA, VEGF, and HGF, all of which are correlated with prostate cancer growth. [anticancer]

- **Melatonin**: In vitro and in vivo studies have demonstrated that melatonin can inhibit growth of prostate cancer cells and may help prevent the resistance to hormonal therapy that can sometimes occur in prostate cancer. [anticancer, supportive]

- **Modified citrus pectin**: This derivative of citrus has been shown in pilot trials to increase PSA doubling time, an indicator of disease progression; the longer the PSA doubling time, the more slowly the cancer is progressing. [anticancer]

- **Omega-3 fatty acids**: Eicosapentaenoic acid (EPA), abundant in fish oil, promotes apoptosis and decreases proliferation in prostate cancer cells, causing decreased PSA doubling time in a mouse model. [anticancer]

- **Pomegranate juice**: A recent human clinical trial featuring men with rising PSA levels demonstrated that drinking just 8 ounces of pomegranate juice daily was effective at stabilizing PSA levels up to four times longer than normal, potentially delaying the growth of prostate cancer cells. Previous in vitro studies have shown that pomegranate juice can inhibit prostate cancer cell proliferation. Pomegranate juice has also been shown to have antioxidant and anti-inflammatory properties. [anticancer]

- **Quercetin**: A preliminary cellular study in the journal *Carcinogenesis* demonstrated that the flavonoid quercetin has potential as both a preventive agent and a complementary treatment for prostate cancer. [preventive, anticancer]

- **Silymarin**: Typically therapeutic to the liver, this phytochemical found in the herb milk thistle was shown in vitro and in vivo to inhibit prostate cancer cell growth. Silymarin actually refers to several different flavonoidal compounds with similar structures; silibinin, the most prevalent form, has been entered into phase I and phase II clinical trials with prostate cancer patients. [preventive, anticancer]

● **Vitamin D**: Several studies have demonstrated that vitamin D can inhibit prostate cancer growth. Presently an international placebo-controlled randomized trial is looking into whether vitamin D has benefits for those with prostate cancer. In a pilot study, 15 patients were given 2,000 IU (50 mcg) of cholecalciferol (a form of vitamin D) daily and monitored prospectively every two to three months. In 9 patients, PSA levels decreased or remained unchanged after they started taking cholecalciferol. This was sustained for as long as 21 months. Also, there was a statistically significant decrease in the rate of PSA rise after administration of vitamin D. The doubling time for PSA was increased by approximately 50 percent in the men taking vitamin D. [preventive, anticancer]

For information on dosages for these supplements, as well as any potential contraindications, see the appendix.

Summary

If prostate cancer is caught early, the prognosis is excellent. In elderly men with a low PSA, adopting a watchful waiting approach is often preferable to surgery. For less aggressive prostate cancers, active surveillance that incorporates diet and lifestyle changes along with some of the supplements mentioned in this chapter may provide the best treatment plan. Many nutrients and herbs show significant promise in helping to treat prostate cancer, slow progression, and reduce recurrence. In more aggressive or advanced cancers, diet and supplements complement conventional treatment to improve response and quality of life.

thirty

Sarcoma (Soft Tissue)

Soft tissue sarcomas are considered fairly rare with about 11,000 cases diagnosed in 2009, which includes both adults and children. Osteosarcomas develop in bone tissue and soft tissue sarcomas develop in fat, nerves, blood vessels, muscle, tendons, and deep in the skin. For more information about osteosarcomas, refer to the section on bone cancer. Sarcomas are malignant tumors that develop in tissues that connect, support, or surround other structures and organs of the body. While soft tissue sarcomas can be found in any part of the body, about 60 percent occur in the arms, legs, hands, and feet. About 20 percent appear in the chest and abdomen. According to the American Cancer Institute, there are about 50 different types of soft tissue sarcomas. Sarcomas should not be confused with lipomas, which are benign tumors of fat tissue. Leiomyosarcomas are the most common abdominal sarcoma and liposarcomas are the most common type of sarcoma found in the legs. When discovered early, soft tissue sarcomas are very treatable, with more than 85 percent of patients surviving more than 5 years after complete surgical removal.

Causes, Symptoms, and Diagnosis

In the early stages, soft tissue sarcomas do not show any signs or symptoms. A lump or swelling may be the first physical sign of a sarcoma. A sarcoma can cause pain if it presses on nerves or muscles. Blockage or bleeding can occur if the tumor is located in the abdomen. Risk factors for soft tissue sarcomas include exposure to certain chemicals in the workplace, including vinyl chloride, arsenic, herbicides, and wood preservatives.

Patients are often the first to discover a sarcoma as a lump or mass that does not go away. Proper diagnosis of sarcomas involves a variety of imaging tests, including X-rays, computed tomography (CT) scans, chest CT, or magnetic resonance imaging (MRI). Examination of a biopsied portion of the suspected tumor provides a conclusive diagnosis.

Conventional Treatment

The goal in treating soft tissue sarcomas is not only to cure the cancer but also to preserve as much function of the affected area as possible. Many factors determine the exact course of treatment, including the patient's age and overall health status; the type, grade, size, and location of the tumor; and if the sarcoma has spread to other parts of the body.

Surgery

Surgery is used to take a tissue sample for biopsy and also to remove cancerous tumors. More than 85 percent of people with successful surgical removal of an early-stage, low-grade sarcoma will survive more than five years. Surgery is not indicated in later stages of the disease.

Radiation and Chemotherapy

In some cases, both chemotherapy and radiation may be used to improve the likelihood that all of the cancer is gone. Radiation may be used prior to surgery to shrink the tumor. Chemotherapy drugs used to treat sarcomas may include mesna, ifosfamide, adriamycin, and dacarbazine. Some sarcomas, such as gastrointestinal stromal tumor (GIST), may be treated with targeted therapies such as imatinib (Gleevac).

Complementary Approaches

Refer to part II of this book regarding useful complementary approaches for all cancers. The following information is specific to sarcoma cancer.

Lifestyle and Diet

There are no studies linking a specific dietary approach or lifestyle practice to the treatment of sarcomas.

Nutrients and Herbs

Research regarding specific nutrients or herbs for the treatment of sarcomas is extremely limited. There are just a few natural substances studied specifically involving sarcomas, including the following:

- *Arabinogalactans*: Pretreatment of arabinogalactans in animal studies demonstrated an antimetastatic effect involving sarcoma spread to the liver. [anticancer]

- *L-glutamine*: Studies of animals with sarcoma have shown that supplementation with glutamine increased glutamine levels in skeletal muscle and blood, which, in turn, helped to preserve body weight and to decrease muscle wasting. [supportive]

- *Melatonin*: This natural hormone has been shown to induce rapid regression of implanted human leiomyosarcoma (cancer of the smooth muscles within organs) in animal studies. [anticancer]

- *N-acetylcysteine (NAC)*: NAC inhibits invasion and metastasis of malignant cells, such as Kaposi's sarcoma cells (a form of skin cancer). Additionally, NAC reduces angiogenesis in vitro and in vivo. [anticancer]

- *Quercetin*: In vitro, this bioflavonoid causes intense damage selectively on malignant liposarcoma cells (cancer arising from fat cells). [anticancer]

- *Tea*: Black and green tea have been shown in animal studies to inhibit rhabdomyosarcoma (a muscle cancer more common in children than adults) formation and progression. [prevention, anticancer]

- *Vitamin A*: Vitamin A in the form of retinoic acid has been shown to arrest the growth and to encourage the differentiation of human rhabdomyosarcoma cells (cancer of skeletal muscles). [prevention, anticancer]

Summary

Sarcomas represent a diverse group of relatively rare cancers. More research involving these cancers and their treatment is warranted and several clinical trials are ongoing. While natural substances are as likely to be of benefit in sarcoma as in other malignancies, more research is needed.

thirty-one

Skin Cancer and Melanoma

Skin Cancer (Excluding Melanoma)

The skin, which may be considered the largest organ of the body, serves as a protective shield against light, heat, infection, and injury. The skin also regulates body temperature; stores water, fat, and vitamin D; and senses pain and pleasure. The three layers of the skin are the epidermis (outer), dermis (middle), and subcutaneous (inner).

Collectively, skin cancers are the most common forms of cancer. More than 1 million cases of nonmelanoma skin cancers are diagnosed each year: between 800,000 and 900,000 are basal-cell carcinoma, a tumor of the epidermis, usually with a molelike appearance, that is seldom metastatic; the remainder are squamous-cell skin cancer, tumors originating from the most superficial layer of the epithelium. Melanoma, a far more serious type of skin cancer, is less common; it is discussed separately, later in this chapter.

Causes, Symptoms, and Diagnosis

The single greatest risk factor for all forms of skin cancer is exposure to ultraviolet radiation from the sun. Other risk factors include having a fair complexion; workplace exposure to carcinogenic substances such as coal tar, pitch, creosote, arsenic, or radium; a family history of skin cancer; atypical moles; and repeated severe sunburns during childhood.

Symptoms of skin cancer include scaliness, discharge, changes in pigmentation, pain, tenderness, itchiness, and new or changing skin growths or changes in moles or other areas of the skin. Nonmelanoma skin cancer lesions usually do not cause symptoms until later stages, when they may bleed or cause pain. Skin biopsy is the definitive method of diagnosing skin cancer.

Conventional Treatment

Suspected and isolated lesions are surgically removed. Occasionally, depending upon the size of the lesion, regional lymph nodes will also be removed and tested for the presence of metastatic cells. A topical treatment of imiquimod, a drug that stimulates the body's production of interferon, and fluorouracil can be used to treat certain superficial skin cancers. In addition, the growth may be scraped off or surgically removed. Laser surgery can also be done, as well as cryosurgery, where liquid nitrogen is applied to the growth to freeze it off. Radiation can be used in cases where surgery is not appropriate.

Complementary Approaches

Refer to part II of this book regarding useful complementary approaches for all cancers. The following information is specific to skin cancer.

Diet, Lifestyle, Nutrients, and Herbs

Protecting the skin with sunblock, clothing, a hat, and shade is the best way to prevent skin cancer and help ensure it doesn't recur. A diet high in antioxidant nutrients, such as vitamins A, C, and E and beta-carotene, may have a protective effect. One study, published in the *Journal of the National Cancer Institute*, found that chronic stress also increased susceptibility to skin cancer. Stress reduction techniques may be helpful, and they are also beneficial in enhancing immunity.

A diet high in arachidonic acid was shown to increase risk of squamous-cell skin cancer. This unsaturated fatty acid found in animal fats is a precursor to inflammation, which can promote carcinogenic events.

Drinking tea is associated with a reduced risk of developing squamous-cell skin cancer. One study evaluated citrus peel and strong hot black tea and found both to be protective against squamous-cell skin carcinoma.

In vitro and in vivo studies involving curcumin demonstrated that it inhibited skin cancer growth, but more research is needed to confirm these results.

According to a Continuing Medical Education report featured in the *Journal of the American Academy of Dermatology*, several nutrients available orally or topically have been identified as effective agents against skin cancer. These include EGCG (from green tea), grape seed extract, silymarin (from milk thistle), genistein (from soy), curcumin (from turmeric), lycopene, vitamin E, beta-carotene, and selenium.

While there are no human population studies on herbs for skin cancer, two botanical agents are especially promising based on preliminary experimental data. Silymarin inhibited skin tumor promotion of human skin cancer cells in vivo, and resveratrol was shown to decrease tumor activity in skin cancers induced by chemical carcinogens in vivo.

Melanoma

Melanoma is a malignant tumor originating in the melanocytes—the skin cells that produce the pigment melanin, which is responsible for skin, hair, and eye color. Because they are formed from pigment-producing cells, melanomas are usually (though not always) black or dark brown. Though melanoma is the most dangerous type of skin cancer, if it is diagnosed and treated in its early stages, before it metastasizes, it is almost always curable. After metastasis, however, it is more difficult to treat and is potentially fatal. According to the American Cancer Society, more than 68,000 new cases of melanoma were reported in 2009. Melanoma accounts for less than five percent of all skin cancers; however, it is responsible for the largest number of skin cancer deaths.

Causes, Symptoms, and Diagnosis

The most common risk factor for melanoma is exposure to ultraviolet radiation from the sun, particularly during peak hours and at high altitudes. Frequenting tanning salons also increases risk. Other risk factors include a family history of melanoma, the presence of atypical moles, or an impaired immune system.

Melanoma usually presents itself as a change in an existing mole, though it can also appear in the form of a new one. Changes in shape, size, or color may be indications of melanoma. If you have a suspicious mole, you should have it examined by a doctor.

Biopsy is the only method by which melanoma can be diagnosed definitively. When removing tissue suspected of being a melanoma, the doctor will try to remove all of the suspicious tissue with a margin of healthy tissue in all dimensions. If, due to the growth's size, this isn't possible, a sample will be removed for study. Biopsy for melanoma can usually be done on an outpatient basis under local anesthetic.

Staging the cancer is important and helps determine the course of treatment. Melanoma can metastasize to any other part of the body, but the lungs and liver are the most common sites. After successful treatment, the risk of metastasis decreases over time, but it never completely disappears.

Conventional Treatment

Conventional treatment for melanoma usually involves surgery, with radiation sometimes used as a palliative therapy.

Surgery

Surgery is used in most cases, with the goal of removing all cancerous tissue and obtaining a clean surgical margin. The margin size depends on the size and location of the melanoma, but averages 1 to 4 centimeters. Metastasis occurs in advanced cases, oftentimes in the lymph nodes, so lymph nodes may be biopsied or removed. Tumors sometimes occur in the tissue between the initial lesion and nearby lymph nodes, in which case lumpectomy (removal of the cancerous tissue plus a clean margin) is used. With many early-stage melanomas, surgery and careful follow-up are all that is needed.

Radiation and Chemotherapy

Radiation is not indicated as treatment for melanoma, as melanomas are largely resistant to radiation therapy. However, radiation therapy is sometimes used as palliative therapy for stage III and IV melanoma patients to shrink metastatic lesions, particularly in the central nervous system, to relieve symptoms and improve the quality of life. If the tumor is 2 to 4 millimeters thick and has spread to one or more lymph nodes, high-dose interferon is used. Chemotherapy is typically only used in advanced metastatic cases (stage IV). Chemotherapy has not been shown to cure late-stage melanoma; however, it may be used to help control metastasis. Chemotherapy agents used with stage IV disease include dacarbazine and temozolomide.

Biological immunotherapy agents are also important treatments. IL-2 is a commonly used treatment for stage IV melanoma. Canvaxin is a vaccine that has been studied as a therapy for stage IV patients. Clinical trial results have been mixed; earlier trials show significant promise in terms of increasing survival, but more recent clinical trials have failed to show significant clinical benefit. The jury is still out on Canvaxin. In the meantime, several other trials investigating the therapeutic potential for other immunotherapy and vaccine agents are under way.

Complementary Approaches

Refer to part II of this book regarding useful complementary approaches for all cancers. The following information is specific to melanoma.

Diet and Lifestyle

A strong immune system is especially important for those with melanoma; therefore, all of the diet and lifestyle recommendations in chapter 8 will be helpful. Reducing sun exposure is critical. A diet high in fruits and vegetables and whole grains is recommended.

A study featured in *Cancer Epidemiology, Biomarkers, and Prevention* found that a diet consisting of foods rich in vitamin D and carotenoids, coupled with low alcohol consumption, was associated with a reduced risk of melanoma. Dark green leafy vegetables and cold-water fish are good sources of vitamin D.

Nutrients and Herbs

While human clinical studies regarding nutrients and herbs for melanoma are lacking, preliminary test tube and animal studies have identified specific natural substances that show promise as complementary therapies. For information on dosages for the supplements listed below, as well as any potential contraindications, see the appendix.

- **Carnosol**: A phytochemical derived from rosemary, carnosol has been shown to restrict the invasive activity of melanoma cells in vivo. This action is attributed to the down-regulation of NF-kB by carnosol. NF-kB is a mediator of inflammation, and its reduction decreases the invasiveness of melanoma cells. [anticancer]

- **CoQ10**: A prospective study of 117 melanoma patients demonstrated that serum levels of CoQ10 were lower in people with melanoma and in people who experienced metastasis. The researchers concluded that plasma CoQ10 is a powerful and independent prognostic factor that can be used to estimate risk for melanoma progression. Extrapolating from this study, it may be beneficial to supplement with CoQ10 to raise serum levels (and tissue levels) of CoQ10 in order to reduce risk of disease and disease progression. [preventive, anticancer]

- **Curcumin**: This phytochemical from the spice turmeric was shown to inhibit lung metastasis induced by melanoma skin cancer cells in vivo. [anticancer]

- **Fermented wheat extract (Avemar)**: In a clinical trial, melanoma patients receiving chemotherapy were randomized to receive Avemar and were followed for seven years. In the Avemar group there were no recurrences in an average of 56 months versus 30 months in the other group, and the overall survival of the Avemar group was 66 months versus 45 months in the other group. [anticancer]

- *Green tea*: In animal experiments, green tea extract alone reduced lung metastases in mice with induced melanomas. [anticancer]

- *Melatonin*: Both in vitro and in vivo studies have found that melatonin exerts a direct inhibitory effect on melanoma cells and that it may be synergistic with IL-2. Caution is advised in using melatonin with high-dose IL-2, though, as the side effects from IL-2 may be increased. A qualified health-care practitioner can provide the best guidance on whether or not melatonin may be appropriate. [anticancer, supportive]

- *Mistletoe*: Several in vivo research studies demonstrate that mistletoe suppressed melanoma cell growth. [anticancer]

- *Modified citrus pectin*: The Michigan Cancer Foundation found that modified citrus pectin inhibited melanoma in vivo. [anticancer]

- *Panax ginseng*: Animal studies have shown that this herb inhibits the growth of melanoma cells as well as stimulates NK-cell-mediated melanoma tumor destruction. [preventive, anticancer]

- *Quercetin*: The flavonoid quercetin was shown in vivo studies to inhibit the invasiveness of melanoma cells. [anticancer]

- *Vitamin D*: An in vitro study from Saarland University Hospital, in Germany, found that vitamin D suppresses melanoma cell proliferation by up to 50 percent; this result has been confirmed in other studies. [anticancer]

Summary

Basal- and squamous-cell skin carcinomas are common and generally quite treatable. High-risk individuals need to be especially diligent about reducing sun exposure, particularly when the sun is most direct, at midday. Nutrients and herbs can also help protect and treat these common skin cancers. In particular, prevention and treatment benefits may be derived from antioxidants such as vitamin C and E, along with plant extracts with concentrated flavonoids such as milk thistle, soy, and green tea.

Melanoma is a very serious form of skin cancer, much more so than the more common skin cancers. When caught early, melanoma can be treated, but it poses a more challenging threat if it has spread. Utilizing specific natural substances that reduce the growth of melanoma can be a valuable component in the successful treatment of melanoma. CoQ10, melatonin, quercetin, and vitamin D are among some of the promising natural agents in the fight against melanoma.

thirty-two

Testicular Cancer

The testicles are egg-shaped male sex glands located inside the scrotum, which is the loose skin sac located directly below the penis. The testicles produce both the hormone testosterone and sperm—the male reproductive cells. Although the testicles are made up of many types of cells, the vast majority of testicular tumors begin in the germ cells—the cells that form sperm. In 2009, just over 8,000 cases of testicular cancer were diagnosed.

Causes, Symptoms, and Diagnosis

The largest risk factor for testicular cancer is having an undescended testicle (cryptorchidism), an unusual condition in which one or both of the testicles fail to descend from the abdomen into the scrotum during the prebirth period inside the womb. Other factors that slightly increase risk of testicular cancer include a family history of testicular cancer or a personal history of cancer in the other testicle; HIV infection; age, with the majority of cases occurring in males between the ages of 15 and 40; and race, with Caucasians having double the risk of Asian-Americans and 5 to 10 times the risk of African-Americans. The risk for Hispanic men is greater than that for Asian-American men, but less than for Caucasians.

Warning signs of possible testicular cancer include enlargement of or lumps in one testicle, which may be painless; a heavy feeling in the scrotum; pain, aches, or discomfort in the scrotum, groin, or abdomen; general fatigue; enlargement or tenderness of the breasts; and loss of sex drive due to abnormal production of hormones by the germ cell tumor (this side effect is rare).

Diagnosis includes a complete medical history and physical examination of the testicle to observe any pain, swelling, or growths. The abdominal lymph nodes are also examined to look for possible metastasis. If a growth appears to be present, the doctor may examine the area with ultrasound to better determine whether the growth may be cancerous. Blood tests may be done to look for tumor-induced changes in levels of certain hormones—alpha-fetoprotein (AFP) and human chorionic gonadotropin (HCG). If cancer is determined to be present, the entire testicle will likely be removed to prevent spreading of the tumor to other parts of the body. A biopsy of the removed tumor will be done to confirm the presence and nature of the cancer.

Imaging tests to look for metastases may include chest X-rays, CT scans, MRI, lymphangiogram (the insertion of a lighted tube into the lymph nodes), or PET scans. If testicular cancer metastasizes, it typically spreads to the lymph system, liver, bone, or brain. Fortunately, prognosis for testicular cancer is excellent, with a cure rate of 90 to 100 percent depending on the type of testicular cancer.

Early diagnosis is important, so a self-exam during or right after a warm shower or bath, when the skin is relaxed, is recommended. Teenage boys should also be performing regular self-exams. It is important for men to ask their doctor how to properly perform a testicular self-exam.

Conventional Treatment

Conventional treatment for testicular cancer usually involves surgery and radiation, with chemotherapy used less frequently.

Surgery

Orchiectomy (removal of the entire affected testicle) is used in almost all cases. Lymphadenectomy (removal of nearby lymph nodes) is also common. Surgery is often curative if the cancer is isolated to the testicle.

Radiation and Chemotherapy

Radiation of adjacent lymph nodes is standard. According to the American Cancer Society, some research is showing that those with stage I disease may not require radiation, especially if they are followed closely with blood tests after surgery. This approach is just as effective as radiation treatment for tumors less than 2.5 inches in size and where there is no evidence that the cancer has spread.

Chemotherapy is used only after surgery and radiation have failed and in cases of metastasis, but it offers an 80 percent success rate in those cases. Carboplatin is the chemotherapy drug often used for stage I tumors that have invaded the blood vessels. Stage II tumors are typically treated with three cycles of chemotherapy drugs, namely, cisplatin, etoposide, and bleomycin. Additional chemotherapy agents such as vinblastine and ifosfamide are used with recurrent testicular cancer. For information about how to counteract typical side effects of these medications, consult the chart "Chemotherapy Drugs and Their Nutrient and Herb Interactions" beginning on page 141.

Treatment for testicular cancer can cause infertility. Those who wish to have children can work with a sperm bank prior to treatment.

Complementary Approaches

Refer to part II of this book regarding useful complementary approaches for all cancers. The following information is specific to testicular cancer.

Lifestyle and Diet

According to the American Cancer Society, testicular cancer survivors have a higher chance of getting other cancers. For this reason, an overall health-promoting lifestyle is important. Exercise on a regular basis, drink alcohol only in moderation (if at all), don't smoke, and eat a healthy whole foods diet (see chapter 4 for specific dietary advice).

Environmental toxins can affect testicular health even while a baby boy is still in his mother's womb. Research on how toxins affect wildlife, as well as other animal studies, have demonstrated that certain chemical toxins can damage the testes. According to a report in the *British Medical Journal*, "A recent study that reported higher levels of organochlorine chemicals in mothers of men with testicular cancer, and new discoveries about phthalates, have reawakened interest in the possible aetiological involvement of environmental chemicals and testicular dysgenesis syndrome." Testicular dysgenesis syndrome results from disruption of embryonal programming and gonadal development during fetal life and results in a variety of problems including undescended testicles (cryptorchidism), low sperm counts, and testicular cancer. For information on cancer-related toxins, refer to the chart "Evaluating Your Exposure to Environmental Toxins," beginning on page 24.

Other Risk Factors

Preliminary research from Vanderbilt University speculates that use of performance-enhancing supplements may increase a man's risk of developing testicular cancer. While the link is inconclusive, Vanderbilt researchers found that 20 percent of the 129 testicular cancer patients questioned used some form of exercise enhancement supplements. More research in this area is needed.

Synthetic steroid hormone use has been shown to cause the testes to atrophy (shrink); however, there are no studies linking synthetic steroid use directly to testicular cancer. Synthetic steroids can cause many serious side effects and should be avoided unless prescribed by your doctor.

There has been debate regarding whether dietary phytoestrogens impact risk of testicular cancer. While studies are conflicting, researchers from the M. D. Anderson Cancer Center in Houston, Texas, evaluated 159 cases of testicular cancer and found there was no effect—that phytoestrogens neither increase nor decrease risk.

Other Complementary Approaches

Researchers at Johns Hopkins reviewed more than 30 years of testicular cancer research to evaluate the effects of heat on these cancers. They concluded that the heat sensitivity of testicular cancer cells makes them more vulnerable and applying heat can enhance the effects of conventional radiation and chemotherapy treatments. Because heat can weaken testicular cancer cells, there may be an application for complementary hyperthermia therapy.

Summary

Testicular cancer is highly treatable and typically comes with a positive prognosis. While more than 8,000 cases of testicular cancer were diagnosed in 2009, less than 400 men died of the disease in that same year. Early diagnosis and surgery remain the cornerstones of successful treatment. A healthy lifestyle, including following the dietary recommendations in chapter 4, will also help prevent testicular cancer or its recurrence. Evidence for complementary therapies for the treatment of testicular cancer is generally lacking, thus a reliance on conventional treatment is appropriate.

thirty-three

Thyroid Cancer

The thyroid gland is a small butterfly-shaped gland located in the lower front of the neck alongside the trachea. It produces hormones to regulate metabolism. The thyroid gland absorbs iodine from food sources and combines it with the amino acid tyrosine to make thyroxine (T4) and triiodothyronine (T3). T3 and T4 are released into the blood and travel to cells throughout the body where they stimulate metabolism, the conversion of oxygen and calories to energy. Thyroid hormones are essential for all metabolic activity in the body.

Nodules, which may be solid or filled with fluid, can form in the thyroid. Nodules are usually noncancerous and do not cause symptoms, but malignant tumors are possible. Although thyroid cancer is the most common cancer of the endocrine system, it only represents about 1 percent of all malignancies. In 2009, more than 37,000 new cases of thyroid cancer were diagnosed, with more than twice as many women as men being affected. The four different types of thyroid cancer are anaplastic, follicular, medullary, and papillary. Papillary and follicular tumors are highly treatable and usually curable. Medullary and anaplastic tumors are much less common but are more aggressive, metastasizing early, and have a poorer prognosis. Younger people diagnosed with thyroid cancer have a better prognosis, in general, than people diagnosed over the age of 45. Overall, papillary or follicular tumors that are small (less than ½ inch) and contained within the thyroid have a 20-year survival rate of 98 percent among women younger than 50 or men younger than 40.

Causes, Symptoms, and Diagnosis

People who have been exposed to high doses of radiation, including X-rays, are at a greater risk of developing thyroid cancer. Those exposed to nuclear fallout are at the greatest risk. People with a family history of thyroid disease have an increased risk of developing thyroid cancer, and certain inherited genetic mutations can elevate the risk of developing some forms of thyroid cancer. New research also indicates that people with celiac disease may have an increased risk of developing thyroid cancer, and this increased risk is evident even when these people avoid eating wheat. People who ingest insufficient quantities of iodine may also be at greater risk.

Possible signs of thyroid cancer can include pain in the throat or neck, hoarseness, painful swallowing, and a lump in the area of the thyroid gland. If a new lump in the lower front region of the neck moves up and down with swallowing, it could be a thyroid nodule, which should be evaluated for malignancy.

In addition to palpation of the neck region for lumps and swelling, tests to detect thyroid cancer include scans of the blood for abnormal levels of the hormones calcitonin and thyroid-stimulating hormone. A thyroid scan may be conducted; this involves injecting a small amount of radioactive isotopes into the thyroid, which is then viewed through a special imaging device. Ultrasound imaging may also be used. Definitive diagnosis of thyroid cancer requires a biopsy. Tissue is obtained from the nodule with a fine needle or after surgical removal of the nodule. Approximately 10 percent of biopsied nodules are cancerous.

Conventional Treatment

Conventional treatment for thyroid cancer involves surgery in nearly every case, with radiation and chemotherapy used in more advanced cases.

Surgery

Because most thyroid nodules are not malignant, it is very important to confirm a cancer diagnosis. While there has been some debate as to the extent of surgery for malignant thyroid tumors, surgery is performed in nearly all cases and is usually the only required treatment. Surgical options include lobectomy, near-total thyroidectomy, and total thyroidectomy. Lobectomy involves removal of only the side of the thyroid gland where the cancer is located. Near-total thyroidectomy entails removal of all but a small part of the thyroid; leaving a small portion is beneficial, as any thyroid tissue left intact has the ability to continue to produce T3 and T4 to help support the metabolic needs of the body. As the name indicates, total thyroidectomy involves removal of the entire thyroid gland, with or without lymph node dissection, which is removal of the lymph nodes in the neck if they have been determined to contain malignant cells, or for biopsy to determine this. Those who have a near-total thyroidectomy or total thyroidectomy will require thyroid hormone replacement for the rest of their life in order to maintain metabolism.

Radiation and Chemotherapy

If the original thyroid tumor was large or extended into regional lymph nodes, or if there is a high risk of recurrence, additional treatment is required beyond surgery. The most common treatment is the use of radioactive iodine. The person minimizes intake of dietary and supplemental iodine, and thyroid hormone replacement is withheld until the doctor determines that any residual thyroid cancer cells are deficient enough in iodine to be ready to take up any iodine that is administered. At this point, a whole body iodine scan is done by administering a small dose of radioactive iodine (iodine-131) to determine if there are remaining thyroid cells that need to be destroyed. If enough cancer cells show up on the whole body iodine scan, a large dose of radioactive iodine is given. The thyroid cancer cells take up this iodine and are destroyed by its radioactivity. Afterward, thyroid hormone replacement medication is resumed. This treatment is generally well tolerated.

External beam radiation is infrequently used to shrink cancerous thyroid tumors. Most medullary and anaplastic tumors do not benefit from radiation therapy. External beam radiation is only used if radioactive iodine treatment is unsuccessful.

Chemotherapy is typically only used in cases of advanced anaplastic and medullary thyroid cancer or recurrent papillary or follicular cancers. Chemotherapy for thyroid cancer is considered somewhat experimental, and varying responses have been reported in the medical literature. Chemotherapy agents used include doxorubicin and cisplatin.

Complementary Approaches

Refer to part II of this book regarding useful complementary approaches for all cancers. The following information is specific to thyroid cancer.

Lifestyle and Diet

There are no studies linking a specific dietary approach to the treatment of thyroid cancer. However, a diet deficient in iodine and other key nutrients can contribute to illnesses associated with the thyroid, including cancer. Foods that can inhibit the utilization of iodine include turnips, cabbage, soybeans, peanuts, and pine nuts. Foods high in zinc and vitamins A and E will assist with proper manufacture of thyroid hormones. Pumpkin seeds, whole wheat, rye, and certain nuts are great sources of zinc. Animal studies have demonstrated that a diet high in soy, when combined with iodine deficiency, can increase the risk of thyroid cancer. Therefore, a diet high in soy products may be contraindicated for those diagnosed with thyroid cancer or at high risk of thyroid cancer.

Exercise has been shown to support proper thyroid function. According to Dr. Michael Murray's book *Encyclopedia of Nutritional Supplements*, "Many health benefits of exercise may be a result of improved thyroid function."

Nutrients and Herbs

Several nutrients and herbs show promise in the prevention and treatment of thyroid cancer, particularly melatonin, quercetin, resveratrol, CoQ10, and vitamins A and E. Following is a review of the scientific studies associated with these nutrients and herbs.

- *Melatonin*: Oxidative stress is one factor involved in the development of thyroid cancer. There is preliminary evidence that melatonin can reduce oxidative damage associated with many thyroid diseases, including cancer. [preventive, supportive]

- *Quercetin*: The flavonoid quercetin has been shown to inhibit thyroid peroxidase, a stimulator of thyroid cells, including malignant thyroid cells. Thus, quercetin may inhibit the growth of thyroid cancer. [preventive, anticancer]

- *Resveratrol*: A cellular study featured in the *Journal of Clinical Endocrinology and Metabolism* demonstrated that resveratrol induced apoptosis and reduced tumor growth signaling in human thyroid cancer cell lines, specifically in papillary and follicular cancers. [preventive, anticancer]

- *Vitamin A*: In preliminary studies, retinoic acid, a form of vitamin A, has demonstrated an ability to inhibit the growth of thyroid cancers. It encourages malignant cells to differentiate into cells that behave normally. Retinoic acid may be especially beneficial in follicular thyroid cancers. [anticancer]

- *Vitamin E and CoQ10*: Japanese researchers discovered that patients with follicular and papillary thyroid tumors had higher levels of vitamin E and a lower concentration of CoQ10 in the thyroid tissue. These levels were correlated with their free radical scavenging activities. This research suggests that these two antioxidant nutrients may play a role in prevention and treatment of thyroid cancers by reducing the oxidative damage to the thyroid cells. [preventive, anticancer]

Summary

The thyroid is an important hormone-producing gland. Because most thyroid nodules are noncancerous, proper diagnosis is critical. If cancer develops in the thyroid, the outlook is generally optimistic since these tumors can often be removed. Surgery and radioactive iodine treatment are generally well tolerated and allow the person to resume a high quality of life after treatment. There are several nutrients that appear to have potential for thyroid cancer prevention and treatment, but more research in this area is needed.

thirty-four

Uterine Cancer

The uterus is a small, hollow organ located in a woman's pelvis, between the rectum and bladder. It is where a fetus develops in the event of a pregnancy. In addition to pregnancy, the uterus lining responds to estrogen and progesterone hormones. As these hormone levels increase on a monthly basis, the uterine lining thickens in preparation for implantation of a fertilized egg. If no implantation occurs, the hormone levels drop off rapidly and the uterine lining sheds, a process known as menstruation.

Most uterine cancers start in the tissue of the endometrium, which lines the inside of the uterus; this is known as endometrial cancer. Cancer can also start in the muscle tissue of the uterus, in which case it is called uterine sarcoma. There are several different microscopically classified types of uterine cancer: between 75 and 80 percent of all endometrial cancers are endometrioid carcinomas; about 10 percent are papillary serous adenocarcinomas; 2 to 5 percent are sarcomas; and 4 to 5 percent are clear cell adenocarcinomas. While papillary and clear cell cancers are more rare, they also tend to be more aggressive. In 2009, the American Cancer Society reported that more than 42,000 new cases of uterine cancer were diagnosed.

Causes, Symptoms, and Diagnosis

Risk factors for endometrial cancer include age (with most cases occurring between the ages of 60 and 70), obesity, high blood pressure, polycystic ovarian disease, and endometrial polyps or growths. Early onset or late cessation of menstruation, infertility, and never having been pregnant are also associated with increased risk, as is the use of estrogen replacement therapy to reduce symptoms of menopause. For women under the age of 50, body mass index (BMI), parity, type of menstrual cycles, history of polycystic ovarian (PCO) syndrome, and diabetes are related to endometrial cancer; of these, increased BMI was the strongest relationship. In menopausal women with a history of breast cancer, use of the drug tamoxifen is also a risk factor.

Symptoms of uterine cancer can include unusual vaginal bleeding or discharge, problems with urination, pain during intercourse, and pain in the pelvis. Presently, there are no good screening methods available. When postmenopausal women experience vaginal bleeding, which is abnormal for this age group, a physician should be consulted, as this could be a sign of uterine cancer.

In order to diagnose endometrial cancer, a sample of endometrial tissue must be taken for biopsy, which can be done in the doctor's office. A dilation and curettage (D&C) procedure may be done in a hospital setting if more tissue is needed to get an accurate diagnosis. Transvaginal ultrasound can also be used to help diagnose endometrial cancer.

Conventional Treatment

Conventional treatment for endometrial cancer usually involves surgery and sometimes radiation. Other treatments, such as hormonal therapy, are indicated in some cases.

Surgery

Surgery is used in most cases, with the goal of removing all cancerous tissue and obtaining a clean surgical margin. Surgery is also often necessary for proper staging of the cancer, which determines what other treatments are required, if any. The extent of the surgery depends on the size and location of the tumor. Surgery may include hysterectomy, bilateral salpingo-oophorectomy (removal of both ovaries and both fallopian tubes), lymph node removal, and diagnostic techniques, such as lymph node sampling and pelvic washing (bathing the abdominal cavity in a fluid and then testing the fluid). Surgery alone can be curative if the cancer is contained within the uterus. If the cancer has spread beyond the uterus, additional chemotherapy and/or radiation will be required. The best outcomes occur when the surgery is performed by a gynecological oncologist.

Radiation and Chemotherapy

Radiation is used in cases that are higher risk, inoperable, or recurrent, and for women who choose not to have surgery. External beam radiation or brachytherapy may be used (brachytherapy involves sealing radioactive material into pellets, rods, catheters, or wires that can be inserted into the cancerous area and left in place). Both low-dose-rate and high-dose-rate brachytherapy can be used for endometrial cancer. IMRT (intensity-modulated radiotherapy) is also an equally effective option when indicated.

Chemotherapy is not a significant treatment option for most cases of endometrial cancer. It is only used after surgery and/or radiation and in cases of advanced or recurrent illness. Chemotherapy agents used in these cases include cisplatin, carboplatin, doxorubicin, liposomal doxorubicin, and paclitaxel. For information about how to counteract typical side effects of these medications, consult the chart "Chemotherapy Drugs and Their Nutrient and Herb Interactions" that starts on page 141.

Other Conventional Treatments

In very advanced cases of endometrial cancer with progesterone-positive (PR+) tumors, hormonal therapy may be indicated. These medications are also used for patients who are not healthy enough to undergo surgery or radiation. According to the National Cancer Institute, up to 30 percent of women who receive progesterone therapy for PR+ endometrial cancer experience a significant slowing of cancer growth.

Complementary Approaches

Refer to part II of this book regarding useful complementary approaches for all cancers. The following information is specific to uterine cancer.

Lifestyle and Diet

Obesity is associated with an increased risk of endometrial cancer. Diabetes and increased body mass index are independent risk factors for uterine cancer. A diet high in animal fats has been linked to the development of endometrial cancer, too. Conversely, a diet high in fruits and vegetables is believed to provide some protection against endometrial cancers. Several reports have indicated that exercise and physical activity are associated with a reduced risk of many cancers, including endometrial cancer.

Nutrients and Herbs

There is limited research on nutrients and herbs to treat uterine cancer. However, it is important to note that herbs with estrogenic activity, such as red clover, dong quai, and possibly licorice, may be contraindicated in estrogen-related endometrial cancers. For information on dosages for the supplements listed below, as well as any potential contraindications, see the appendix.

- *Melatonin*: In vitro studies demonstrated that melatonin has antiproliferative effects on estrogen-related endometrial cancer. [anticancer]

- *Mushroom polysaccharides*: A human study of 100 patients with cervical, ovarian, or endometrial cancer undergoing chemotherapy treatment demonstrated that a mushroom extract, *Agaricus blazei* Murill Kyowa (ABMK), improved chemotherapy-associated symptoms, including loss of appetite, hair loss, emotional instability, and general weakness. However, in this study, this particular mushroom extract did not appear to stimulate increased immune activity, as mushroom extracts usually do. [supportive]

- *Resveratrol*: This phytonutrient from red grapes was found in vitro to stop human endometrial cancer cells from rapidly reproducing. Another in vitro study that combined resveratrol with green tea (specifically, EGCG) inhibited angiogenesis of human endometrial tumor cells. [anticancer]

- *Soy isoflavones*: While data on soy isoflavones is conflicting, an animal study using genistein and daidzein from soy demonstrated a protective effect against estrogen-related endometrial cancers. [preventive]

Summary

Those with uterine cancer can benefit from losing weight, improving blood sugar control, and reducing animal fat in the diet, while increasing physical activity and consumption of fruits and vegetables. If the cancer is caught early, surgery can be curative. Estrogenic herbs should be avoided. Melatonin, resveratrol, and medicinal mushroom extracts are among the most promising natural agents for uterine cancer.

Conclusion: The Future of Cancer Care

Cancer is more than a physical disease. Cancer is a mental-emotional-physical phenomenon. During the many months we researched and wrote this book, we dealt with our own emotions and personal experiences surrounding cancer. Eclipsing our fears and sadness was the awe that comes from interacting with people diagnosed with cancer and their loved ones. We continue to be inspired by the countless individuals who choose not to be identified solely by their diagnosis—individuals who step beyond their cancer to capture all that life has to offer. With tenacity and grace, these people do not allow cancer to define them, their existence, and even their future. While they are diverse in terms of how they handle their health, treatment, and emotions, they share a common characteristic—the need to *thrive*, not just survive.

We appreciate the numerous cancer "thrivers" we have met who continue to live beyond their diagnosis and prognosis. We have also come to respect those who have died at the hands of this illness. And we honor the strength and joy of loved ones—the people who bear witness to the lives of their beloved family members and friends with cancer.

It is tempting to rant about what is wrong with medicine today because there surely is a long list of things that must change. But let us first recognize the value of the many health-care professionals—the researchers, lab technicians, nurses, doctors, and many others—who devote their lives to the field of cancer care. These professionals, who are at the core of cancer care, have chosen to help people when they are most helpless and afraid.

What Is the Purpose of Medicine?

By Jeremy Geffen, MD

In oncology, where life-and-death issues and costly diagnosis and treatment options loom, emotions often run high. In response, many physicians choose to deal only with technical issues that can be clearly defined, measured, and treated. This can leave everyone feeling frustrated and dissatisfied.

What is the solution? It is time to enlarge our vision of medicine—not just for cancer patients but for all patients. In this new vision, medicine has two distinct purposes. The relative purpose of medicine is to relieve symptoms and to cure disease to the fullest extent possible. But there is an ultimate purpose of medicine, which extends beyond the physical realm to include the mind, heart, and spirit of every patient, and their loved ones as well.

With this view, it is understood that cancer patients are asking two things from their physicians. On the relative level, patients most definitely want their illness cured. But this is not the whole story. On a deeper level, people want to be cured in order to feel whole and fully alive, to feel connected with their deepest self and purpose, and to experience love and joy in the deepest parts of their being. Quite often patients are convinced that their capacity to feel and experience these essential, life-affirming states and emotions has been violently stripped away by their diagnosis. Many cancer patients believe that they simply cannot experience the deepest levels of wholeness, love, and joy again until the doctor has gotten rid of the cancer. Fundamentally, they feel separated from the love, joy, meaning, inspiration, and fulfillment that make life worth living, and they feel that

Presently, there is a shocking trend in oncology. According to the American Society of Clinical Oncology, 40 percent of cancer specialists in the United States are 55 years of age or older. Many will retire in the next decade. The rate of new oncologists presently will not keep pace with the rate of retirement, causing a shortage of nearly 4,000 oncologists by the year 2030. And yet, the number of people diagnosed with cancer in the United States is estimated to increase by 45 percent by 2030. Obviously, this is a dangerous trend. As we brace ourselves for a major change in health care, we must consider this serious issue that will soon plague oncology. Patients can become more proactive in choosing their doctors and be receptive to embracing an integrative approach that may include a team of health-care professionals working together to ease the burden of the oncologist.

Importance of Integrative Cancer Care

What causes a survivor to become a thriver? Some might say hope, and specifically the hope for a cure. Yes, hope is important. But from our perspective, it is not the hope for a cure that encourages us as much as hope for a change—a change in the way cancer, cancer treatment, and healing are viewed. Our hope is that collaboration becomes the cornerstone of cancer care in the future. Not just collaboration between patient and doctor, but collaboration that mirrors our very own internal systems—a web

bridging the separation depends on the clinical work of the doctor.

In light of this, I believe the ultimate purpose of medicine must be to foster the emotional and spiritual fulfillment that is a shared aspiration of all human beings. Moreover, medicine must empower patients to find that fulfillment *within themselves*—regardless of their diagnosis, current condition, or clinical outcome.

I describe the ultimate purpose of medicine as follows: to assist all beings to experience unbounded love, joy, and inner peace, and to know this is the essence of who we truly are. This purpose deserves attention fully equal to the relative purpose of treating symptoms and curing disease.

The two purposes of medicine correspond to the two domains of existence in which we abide simultaneously. The domain of *doing* encompasses all our worldly activities, efforts, identities, and endeavors. It includes everything we do to try to heal when we are sick, including chemotherapy, radiation, herbs, vitamins, massage, or acupuncture. But the domain of *being* is equally important. This domain encompasses who we really are beyond our thoughts, individual identities, successes, failures, sickness, or health. The domain of being is where the ultimate purpose of medicine leads.

Regardless of where you are on the journey through cancer, understanding and embracing the ultimate—as well as the relative—purpose of medicine can bring comfort, peace, and deep healing, and can transform all aspects of the experience. I am confident the time is coming when all patients and all medicine will settle for nothing less.

This has been adapted with permission from Dr. Geffen's book The Journey through Cancer: Healing and Transforming the Whole Person, *second edition (*Three Rivers Press, 2006*).*

of interconnectedness, a rhythmic flow that comes naturally. This is not simply teamwork involving treatment. It is an alliance that encompasses body, mind, and spirit. It is a consistent, overarching effort that combines the best of conventional and complementary medicine with the proactive efforts of the patient, which must include a healthy diet, positive lifestyle choices, and appropriate dietary supplements. This is integrated medicine, and it is the future of cancer care.

Conventional medicine has delivered many advances over the past decade. Areas that hold promise for the future of cancer treatment include utilizing nanotechnology for more pinpointed treatments and the study of the biological actions of proteins, known as proteomics. Just as genomics has helped medical science in many ways, proteomics is quickly becoming an important focus in cancer diagnosis and treatment.

In the future, diet, lifestyle, and dietary supplements will go beyond merely supporting and sustaining. These controllable factors will be viewed as significant complementary treatment techniques to reverse cancer. More funding is needed for researching integrative approaches. Our present system primarily rewards those who can substantiate the performance of isolated synthetic drugs that can be patented. Research into combined approaches or utilizing a healthy diet, positive lifestyle choices, and supplements, all of which cannot be patented, is presently not being supported as much as it could be, or should be.

Over the years, we have talked to many leaders in the field of integrative medicine and we hear a consistent, positive message that things are shifting. Conventional medicine, medical schools, and research facilities are beginning to pay attention to the broader aspects that make up an integrated approach to cancer treatment and healing. But we cannot wait until everyone is truly on the same page. Until that time, people must be proactive about using an integrative approach for both prevention and healing.

Throughout history, long-lasting change has come from the masses—groups of people who take the initiative. Our health-care system is in dire need of such an initiative. True and lasting change will come from patients and their loved ones. Our doctors are so pressured by managed care, insurance directives, and other constraints that they are limited as to the degree of change they can invoke. Patients and loved ones need to work in partnership with the system that is in place while also searching for information on complementary approaches to healing and staying healthy. Each of us must take the lead in our own health care. The system will then be forced to change to keep up with the demands of its customers, the patients.

The New View

It is our goal that health-care professionals, patients, loved ones, politicians, and all people of influence begin to look at cancer differently. It is time to set aside the desperate search for a magic bullet that will cure all cancers. Back in the 1960s, President Richard Nixon declared a "war on cancer." The strategy was to find a cure, some type of amazing chemical or machine that could zap cancer out of existence. Cancer has proven to be a formidable opponent.

It is time to pause, take a deep breath, and reevaluate our war on cancer. It is time to methodically and logically approach cancer treatment and healing from a multifaceted standpoint. To win the war on cancer, we must utilize a systems approach that addresses cancer on many biological levels and includes healing of the body, mind, and spirit.

If we are to transform cancer care, we must begin by transforming ourselves. Let's broaden our view with the hope that we can find true collaboration, and thereby create true healing.

Appendix

Glossary

adjuvant therapy. Treatment used in addition to and following the primary treatment to cure, reduce, control, or palliate cancer.

anemia. A condition where the bone marrow produces a deficit of red blood cells. Anemia can also be the result of cancer treatment.

angiogenesis. The development of blood vessels.

antiangiogenesis. Prevention or impairment of the development of blood vessels, used therapeutically to inhibit blood supply to tumors.

antibodies. Proteins produced by the body's immune system to bind to foreign substances (antigens) and destroy them or "tag" them for recognition and destruction by other parts of the immune system.

antioxidants. Substances that help inhibit or prevent oxidative damage caused by free radicals.

apoptosis. Disintegration of cells into small particles that can be digested and removed by other cells without causing inflammation.

autologous bone marrow transplant. Removal, storage, treatment, and restoration of the bone marrow of a cancer patient. It can be done as a treatment or as a method to enhance treatment. For example, in leukemia, the marrow is removed from the patient, purged of cancer cells, and then returned to the patient.

benign tumor. An abnormal, noncancerous growth of tissue that does not spread to other parts of the body, as a cancerous tumor can do.

biological drugs. Substances that are made from living organisms used to prevent, diagnose, or treat cancer. These can include vaccines, interleukins, or antibodies.

biopsy. The microscopic examination of tissue or cells removed from the body to determine if cancer cells are present.

bone marrow. The spongy substance in the center of the bone that produces all of the body's red blood cells and platelets and most of the white blood cells.

bone scan. An image taken after the injection of a radioactive tracer substance into the blood, which carries it to the bones. Cancerous areas in the bone where cells are dividing rapidly will pick up more of the radioactive substance, resulting in "hot spots" on the developed film image.

brachytherapy. A type of radiation therapy where radioactive pellets or cathodes are placed in or near a tumor to provide a high dose of radiation to the tumor while minimizing exposure of the surrounding healthy tissues.

cachexia. A condition including malnourishment and muscle wasting that can accompany cancer.

chemotherapy. The treatment or control of cancer using anticancer drugs that destroy cancer cells by interfering with their growth or reproduction.

clinical trial. Systematic evaluation of a possible new treatment conducted with patients after the treatment has shown some benefits in animal testing or laboratory testing.

COX-1 and COX-2. Enzymes produced during inflammation; some anti-inflammatory drugs block these enzymes but in doing so they impede production of prostaglandins, which play an important role in many body functions.

CT scan (computed tomography scan). Also called computerized axial tomography (CAT) scan. A diagnostic procedure using a computer linked to an X-ray machine to produce highly detailed cross-sectional pictures of the body.

cytokines. Proteins produced by lymphocytes and monocytes (white blood cells) to help control the intensity and duration of the inflammatory response; cytokines include interleukin-1 (IL-1), interleukin-6 (IL-6), and tumor necrosis factor (TNF).

cytotoxic. Something that is destructive to cells.

DNA (deoxyribonucleic acid). One of the two nucleic acids found in all cells. DNA is the part of a cell that contains and controls all of the cell's genetic information. The genes in DNA are responsible for passing on traits from generation to generation.

enteral nutrition. Nutrition delivered as a liquid, by drinking or by tube feeding, which may be via nasogastric (NG tube), gastrostomy (G tube), or jejunostomy (J tube).

free radical. An unstable, highly reactive molecule that has one or more unpaired electrons that can damage healthy cells. Free radical molecules are found or formed as a result of UV radiation, smoking, aging, stress, disease, and many other circumstances and substances.

hormone. A substance produced in the body that travels through the blood to another area of the body in order to increase or decrease some activity of other tissues or organs; hormones include estrogen, testosterone, and cortisol.

hormone receptor. A structure on the surface of or inside a cell that combines with a hormone to alter the function of that cell; for example, an estrogen receptor.

hormone therapy. The use or manipulation of hormones to treat disease or imbalance.

hyperthermia therapy. A procedure still undergoing investigation that uses heat to kill cancer cells or make them more sensitive to chemotherapy and/or radiation.

immunoglobulins. Another name for antibodies. Each lymphocyte produces a specific antibody, or immunoglobulin. There are five main types of immunoglobulins, grouped according to their concentration in the blood: IgG, IgA, IgM, IgD, and IgE.

in situ cancer. Noninvasive cancer; the earliest stage of cancer, confined to the original site.

integrative oncology. A comprehensive, evidence-based, multidisciplinary approach to cancer care that attempts to fully support all participants by combing scientifically valid treatments from both conventional and complementary and alternative medicine.

interferon. A class of protein produced in miniscule amounts by white blood cells, which boosts the immune system response to malignant cell infection.

interleukins. A type of cytokine that enables communication among leukocytes and other cells active in an inflammatory or immune response.

invasive cancer. A stage of cancer in which cells have spread to healthy tissue adjacent to the original tumor.

leukocytes. White blood cells activated in response to malignant cellular changes and infection and inflammation. These cells destroy malignant or infected cells and also play a role in post-inflammation cleanup and repair.

lumpectomy. Removal of a cancerous breast lump and the surrounding tissue.

lymph fluid. Fluid that flows throughout the body in the lymphatic vessels, helping to maintain the fluid level of cells. It delivers nutrients to cells and carries waste products to the bloodstream for elimination. The human body has one to two quarts of lymph fluid, accounting for 1.5 to 3 percent of body weight.

lymph node. One of many small, bean-shaped organs of the immune system linked by lymphatic vessels throughout the body. They make and store many different immune cells that fight infections.

lymphedema. An accumulation of fluid that may collect in the arms or legs when lymph vessels or lymph nodes are blocked or removed, which can result from cancer or treatment for cancer.

lymphocytes. White blood cells that travel through the lymph system as part of the immune and inflammatory response; they include T cells, B cells, and antibiodies.

macrophages. The mature form of the white blood cells known as monocytes. They are produced in the bone marrow, then circulate in the bloodstream for a few days before entering tissues, where they develop into macrophages. Macrophages "swallow" germs and foreign proteins, then release an enzyme that chemically damages, kills, or neutralizes whatever is ingested. The name means "big" (*macro*) "swallower" or "eater" (*phage*). Macrophages are the filter feeders of the immune system, ingesting everything that is not normal, healthy tissue—even old body cells or cancer cells.

malignant tumor. A cancerous tumor that's likely to penetrate the tissues or organ in which it originated and can spread to other sites.

mammogram. An X-ray procedure used in the screening and diagnosis of breast cancer that can reveal a tumor in the breast long before it can be felt.

mastectomy. Surgical removal of the breast.

metastasis. The spread of cancer from one part of the body to another.

MRI (magnetic resonance imaging). An imaging technique used in the diagnosis and evaluation of disease and to monitor for the recurrence of cancer. MRI produces internal pictures of the body using radio waves and a powerful electromagnet linked to a computer.

natural killer cells. Also known as NK cells, a type of nonspecific, free-ranging immune cell produced in the bone marrow and matured in the thymus gland. NK cells can recognize and quickly destroy virus and cancer cells on first contact. Armed with an estimated 100 different biochemical poisons for killing foreign proteins, they can kill target cells without having encountered them previously. As with antibodies, their role is surveillance, to rid the body of foreign or aberrant cells. NK cells can destroy cancerous cells before they multiply and cause disease. Decreased numbers of NK cells have been linked to the development and progression of cancer, as well as chronic and acute viral infections and other deficiencies of the immune system.

naturopathy (also ***naturopathic medicine).*** A comprehensive system of health care emphasizing the use of natural therapies for the promotion of health and prevention of disease.

neutrophils. The most common type of white blood cell, which is responsible for much of the body's protection against infection.

NF-kB (nuclear factor kappa B). A gene found in all cell types involved in cellular responses to stimuli such as stress, cytokines, free radicals, ultraviolet irradiation, and bacterial or viral antigens. NF-kB plays a key role in regulating the immune response to infection and activates enzymes and cytokines during the inflammatory process.

oxidation. A chemical reaction resulting from exposure to oxygen or other electron-seizing atoms. On the cellular level, oxidative reactions are a source of energy, but oxidative reactions generate free radicals and other oxidizing agents that can damage cellular components, such as membranes, and interfere with cells' regulatory systems.

palliative treatment. The use of medical remedies to relieve pain and symptoms, and/or prevent further complications rather than to cure.

peripheral neuropathy. Damage to nerves that results in muscle weakness, numbness, or tingling, particularly in the hands and feet; this can occur as a result of chemotherapy toxicity or from other medications, as well as other health conditions, including some types of cancer.

phagocytes. White blood cells that ingest and destroy microorganisms, cell debris, and other particulates.

platelets. Blood cells that help the blood clot.

probiotics. Dietary supplements containing potentially beneficial bacteria and yeasts that favor the growth of "good" bacteria in the body while inhibiting harmful microbes. Lactobacillus is one of the most commonly studied and used probiotics.

prostaglandins. Biologically active chemicals derived from essential fatty acids with many functions; for example, they are involved in vasodilation, bronchodilation, inflammatory reactions, regulation of cell proliferation, regulation of fluid balance, platelet aggregation, gastrointestinal activity, neurotransmission, and glucose metabolism.

prostate-specific antigen (PSA). A protein in the blood produced by prostate tissue that serves as a tumor marker.

protocol. The outline or plan for a treatment program.

radiation therapy. The use of high-energy penetrating rays or subatomic particles to treat or control disease.

radical prostatectomy. Surgical removal of the prostate and the surrounding tissue.

recurrence (relapse). The reappearance of an illness and its symptoms after a period of improvement.

red blood cells. The blood cells that carry oxygen from the lungs throughout the body.

remission. The decrease or disappearance of disease.

staging or stage of disease. Description of a period in the course of a disease; in cancer, the stage of solid tumors is determined based on the size and location of the initial tumor, presence or absence of cancer in the lymph nodes, and whether the cancer has traveled to distant parts of the body.

systemic. Pertaining to the whole body rather than just one part.

T cells. Cells whose specialized immune function takes three forms: helper T cells, suppressor T cells, or natural killer cells. Helper T cells facilitate the production of antibodies by the B cells. Suppressor T cells suppress B cell activity. Natural killer cells recognize and destroy virus and cancer cells on contact.

tumor marker. Any substance found in increased amounts in the body fluids of people with cancer. The presence of a tumor marker for a specific cancer can be an indication that cancer is present in the body. Tumor markers can be used as part of the diagnostic process but generally cannot provide a definitive diagnosis. Tumor markers are also used to monitor the progress of treatment as well as possible recurrence of cancer after treatment.

white blood cells. A general term for a variety of cells in the blood that play a major role in the body's immune system. A low level of white blood cells can make a person susceptible to infections.

Source: Portions of this glossary are used with the permission of Cancer Treatment Centers of America (www.cancercenter.com).

Dosage Ranges

This section lists daily dosage ranges, as well as additional information about each substance recommended in this book. For more information about interaction with chemotherapy drugs, refer to the "Chemotherapy Drugs and Their Nutrient and Herb Interactions" chart, which begins on page 141. Remember, all of your doctors should be informed about the supplements you're taking. To develop the best and most effective supplement program, consult with a licensed naturopathic doctor, dietician, or health-care practitioner knowledgeable in the use of supplements for cancer prevention and treatment and for supporting conventional therapies. Always purchase supplements made by reputable manufacturers.

Please note: Self-diagnosis and self-treatment are not recommended for any illness, especially cancer. The information in this chart is intended for educational purposes only. Please see a qualified health-care professional if you have questions about your health or the supplements you should take or are taking. Also, it is critical that you disclose supplement use to your doctor.

Nutrient/Herb	Daily Dosage Range	Comments
5-hydroxy tryptophan	100 mg to 300 mg	Obtain health-care provider supervision and monitoring when also taking antidepressant medications.
Acetyl-L-carnitine	1,000 mg to 2,000 mg	
Activated charcoal	2,000 mg to 3,000 mg	Bowel movements will darken while taking charcoal. Contraindicated with oral chemotherapy drugs.
Active hexose correlated compound (AHCC)	3 g to 6 g	
Aloe vera	Aloe extract: 50 mg to 200 mg	Aloe latex should not be ingested orally as it can cause kidney failure.
Alpha-lipoic acid	300 mg to 600 mg	Contraindicated with some chemotherapy drugs. Caution with drugs that lower blood sugar. Supplement thiamin if taking high doses.
Anthocyanidins	Tincture (1:5) of bilberry extract: 6 ml to 15 ml Standardized extract with 25% anthocynanidins: 200 mg to 500 mg	
Arabinogalactans	2 g to 6 g	
Artemisinin (from *Artemisia annua*)	400 mg to 800 mg daily with food but at least 3 hours away from iron-containing food or supplements	Exact dosage for artemisinin has not been determined and concentration of artemisinin varies between products. Artemisinin should be avoided during and for an additional 30 days after radiation therapy. Artemisinin is not safe the first trimester of pregnancy due to possible toxicity to the fetus.
Ashwagandha (*Withania somnifera*)	3 g to 6 g Tincture(1:5): 12 ml to 25 ml Standardized extract with 1.5% withanolides: 500 mg to 1,500 mg	May have additive effects with other sedative drugs. May interfere with some chemotherapy drugs.
Astragalus (*Astragalus membranaceus*)	Dried root: 1 to 2 g Tincture (1:5): 15 ml Standardized extract with 0.5% 4-hydroxy-3-methoxy isoflavone: 500 mg to 2 g	

Nutrient/Herb	Daily Dosage Range	Comments
Beta-carotene	15 mg to 30 mg 10,000 IU to 100,000 IU	May be associated with increased risk of lung cancer, especially in smokers. High doses can cause yellowing of skin (not permanent).
Beta-glucans	40 mg to 60 mg	
Black cohosh (*Actea racemosa*)	Standardized extract with 1 mg 27-deoxyactein triterpene: 40 mg to 80 mg	
Bromelain	Standardized to ≥ 2,000 MCU (milk-clotting units): 500 mg to 2,000 mg	Caution with anticoagulant medications. Caution with gastrointestinal ulceration.
Calcium	500 mg to 1,500 mg	Use calcium citrate for enhanced absorption.
Calcium D-glucarate	200 mg to 1,200 mg	
Calendula	Dried flower: 1 g to 2 g Tincture (1:5): 3 ml to 15 ml Liquid extract (1:1): 2 ml to 4 ml Topical ointment: 2 g to 5 g (herb)/100 g (ointment)	
Carnosol	Dried leaf (rosemary): 4 g to 6 g Tincture (1:5): 6 ml to 15 ml	Concentrated volatile oil should not be taken internally; long-term use may prevent iron absorption and aggravate anemia.
Cayenne (*Capsicum annuum*)	Standardized extract with ≥ 0.25% capsaicin: 400 mg to 1,200 mg	Contraindicated with gastrointestinal ulceration.
Chasteberry (*Vitex agnus-castus*)	Tincture(1:5): 3 ml Standardized extract with 0.5% agnuside and 0.6% aucubin: 400 mg	Caution with levodopa, hormone replacement therapy, and oral contraceptives.
Chromium	100 mcg to 500 mcg	Normal dose can cause cognitive and motor dysfunction in some cases.
Coenzyme Q10	100 mg to 300 mg	May interfere with some chemotherapy drugs.
Colostrum	500 mg to 3,000 mg	
Conjugated linoleic acid	1 g to 3 g	

Nutrient/Herb	Daily Dosage Range	Comments
Curcumin	Standardized extract with 95% curcuminoids: 500 mg to 6,000 mg	May interfere with some chemotherapy drugs. Caution with anticoagulation medication and in people with bleeding disorders.
Daidzein	10 mg to 20 mg	Caution with ER+ cancers
Deglcyrrhizinated licorice (DGL)	Chewable tablets: 2,280 mg to 4,560 mg	Best taken before meals. Obtain medical supervision and monitoring when taking oral chemotherapy.
DHEA	25 mg to 50 mg	Use under care of a licensed health-care practitioner.
Diindolylmethane (DIM)	60 mg to 180 mg	
dl-Phenylalanine	500 mg to 1,000 mg daily	Obtain health-care provider supervision and monitoring when also taking antidepressant or antianxiety medications.
Dong quai (*Angelica sinensis*)	Tincture(1:5): 3 ml to 10 ml Standardized extract with 0.8% to 1.1% ligustilide: 200 mg to 600 mg	Phytoestrogenic: caution with ER+ cancers. Caution with anticoagulant medications.
Echinacea spp.	Tincture (1:5): 5 ml to 20 ml Standardized extract with 4% echinacosides or 4% sesquiterpene esters: 1,000 mg to 1,500 mg	May interfere with some chemotherapy drugs.
Ellagic acid	40 mg to 500 mg (therapeutic range)	
Essiac tea	4 oz to 8 oz	Contraindicated with breast cancer.
Fermented soy products	1 oz to 4 oz	
Fermented wheat germ	9 g	
Flaxseed lignans	2 to 3 tablespoons of ground flaxseeds; high-lignan flax oil providing 600 mg to 1,800 mg lignans	
Folic acid (folate)	400 mcg to 5,000 mg	Supplementation may mask B_{12} deficiency. High doses may be contraindicated with certain chemotherapy drugs.
Gamma oryzanol	300 mg	

Nutrient/Herb	Daily Dosage Range	Comments
Garlic	Fresh garlic: 1 g to 3 g Standardized extract with an allicin yield of 12,000 mcg to 1,000 mg: 300 to 1,000 mg	Obtain medical supervision and monitoring when also taking anticoagulant medications.
Genistein	20 mg to 80 mg	
Ginger	Standardized extract with 4% volatile oils: 250 mg to 1,000 mg	Caution with bleeding disorders.
Ginkgo biloba	Standardized extract with 24% ginkgo flavone glycosides and 6% triterpenes: 40 mg to 160 mg	Caution with anticoagulant medications. Caution with ER+ cancers. May interfere with some chemotherapy drugs.
Ginseng, Panax (*Panax* spp.)	Dried root: 500 mg to 3,000 mg Tincture (1:5): 2 ml to 10 ml Standardized extract with 4% to 7% ginsenosides: 100 to 400 mg	Caution with ER+ cancers.
Ginseng, Siberian (*Eleutherococcus senticosus*)	Tincture (1:5): 5 ml to 10 ml Standardized extract with 0.8% to 1% eleutherosides B and E: 200 mg to 600 mg	
Ginsenosides	See ginseng, panax	
Green tea (*Camellia sinensis*)	Standardized extract with 50% to 97% polyphenols and $\geq$ 50% epigallocatechin gallate (EGCG): 1,000 mg to 2,000 mg	
Gymnema (*Gymnema sylvestre*)	Dried herb: 1 g to 3 g Tincture (1:2): 5 ml to 10 ml Standardized extract with 25% gymnemic acids: 500 mg to 1,500 mg	
Hesperidin	500 mg to 1,500 mg	
Honey	1 tablespoon two to four times daily	Use pasteurized honey to avoid potential microbiological contamination from raw honey.
Indole-3-carbinol	300 mg to 800 mg	
Iodine	Dosage is based upon iodine status; RDA = 150 mcg; up to 20 x RDA (3 mg) has no known side effects	Obtain health-care provider supervision and monitoring to establish deficiency and for appropriate dosing.

Nutrient/Herb	Daily Dosage Range	Comments
Kava	Standardized extract with 70% kava lactones: 100 mg to 300 mg	May cause digestive upset; may cause severe liver damage in rare cases.
L-carnitine	1 g to 2 g	
L-glutamine	3 g to 30 g	
L-glutathione	500 mg to 3,000 mg	
Licorice	Dried root: 1 g to 3 g Tincture (1:5): 3 ml to 10 ml Standardized extract with 20% glycyrrhizinic acid: 500 mg to 1,000 mg Deglycyrrhizinated licorice (DGL) with $\leq$ 2% glycyrrhizinic acid: 1 g to 4 g	Avoid in individuals with liver or kidney impairment. May cause sodium and water retention and may deplete potassium. Avoid with diuretics, digoxin, and certain antihypertensives. May interfere with some chemotherapy drugs. Caution with ER+ cancers.
Limonene	Optimal dosage range yet to be established; up to 12 g safely used in one phase I study. Suggested minimum dose: 800 mg.	
Lutein	5 mg to 30 mg	
Lycopene	15 mg to 45 mg	
Magnesium	250 mg to 1,000 mg	
Melatonin	3 mg to 20 mg	May cause sedation and drowsiness. Avoid in bipolar disorder.
Mistletoe	Standardized extract with lectin-I in a subcutaneous injection: 1 ng/kg (nanograms per kilogram of body weight) Iscador: 5 mg three times weekly	Use must be supervised by a licensed health-care practitioner. (Iscador is a trade name.)
Modified citrus pectin	8 g to 15 g	
Mushroom polysaccharides	1,3- and 1,6-beta-glucans: 0.5 to 1 mg per kg body weight	
N-acetylcysteine	600 mg to 1,500 mg	Contraindicated with some chemotherapy drugs.
Omega-3 fatty acids (from fish oil)	Standardized to eicosapentaenoic acid (EPA) and docosahexaenoic acid (DHA): 1,000 mg to 5,000 mg	Obtain medical supervision and monitoring when also taking anticoagulant medications.

Nutrient/Herb	Daily Dosage Range	Comments
Omega-3 fatty acids (from flaxseed oil)	Cold-pressed seed oil: 58% to 60% omega-3 fatty acids: 15 ml (1 tablespoon)	
Phosphatidylcholine	500 mg to 3,000 mg	
Phosphatidylserine	200 mg to 300 mg	
Pine bark extract (Pycnogenol)	200 mg to 300 mg	Pine bark is marketed under the trade name Pycnogenol.
Pomegranate	8 oz glass of pomegranate juice	
Potassium	Less than 3,500 mg (including dietary sources)	Supplement under medical supervision only.
Probiotics	*Lactobacillus acidophilus* or *Lactobacillus rhamnosus* GG: 3 to 10 billion CFU (colony forming units)	Extreme caution in immunosuppressed individuals: use under guidance of a licensed health-care provider.
Quercetin	500 mg to 4,000 mg	May interfere with some chemotherapy drugs.
Resveratrol	15 mg to 200 mg	
Rhodiola (*Rhodiola rosea*)	Standardized extract with 3% rosavins: 100 mg to 300 mg	Caution with radiation therapy.
Selenium	50 mcg to 200 mcg	Caution in individuals with liver and kidney insufficiency.
Shark cartilage (Neovastat liquid extract)	240 ml	
Silymarin (from milk thistle)	Standardized extract with ≥ 70% silymarin: 250 mg to 500 mg	May interfere with some chemotherapy drugs.
Slippery elm (*Ulmus fulva*)	1 tablespoon mixed into ¼ oz applesauce, yogurt, or warm water twice daily	
Sodium bicarbonate	2 grams diluted in 250 ml of water; sip every 2 hours	
Soy isoflavones (for example, genistein)	50 mg to 150 mg	May interfere with tamoxifen. Caution with ER+ cancers.
Spleen polypeptides	300 mg to 1,000 mg	

Nutrient/Herb	Daily Dosage Range	Comments
St. John's wort (*Hypericum perforatum*)	Tincture (1:5): 3 ml to 12 ml Standardized extract with 0.3% to 0.5% hypericin and 3% to 5% hyperforin: 300 mg to 900 mg	Interferes with many medications, including chemotherapy drugs Use under the supervision of a licensed health-care practitioner only.
Sterols and sterolins	Plant sterols (100 sterol: 1 sterolin): 800 mg to 1000 mg	
Sulfurophane	200 to 400 µg of sulfurophane	Contraindicated with chemotherapy drugs and targeted therapies.
Vitamin A	5,000 IU to 25,000 IU	Caution with liver disease. Caution with radiation therapy. Use under the guidance of a licensed health-care professional.
Vitamin B$_1$	2 mg to 30 mg	
Vitamin B$_2$	5 mg to 400 mg	High doses may cause diarrhea.
Vitamin B$_3$	1,200 mg to 3,000 mg	May cause vasodilation and flushing.
Vitamin B$_6$	25 mg to 300 mg	
Vitamin B$_{12}$	1,000 mcg to 2,000 mcg	
Vitamin C	500 mg to 2,000 mg	Caution in individuals with a history of kidney stones.
Vitamin D	400 IU to 4,000 IU	Use under medical supervision if parathyroid disease present. Use for more than two months should be under the guidance of a licensed health-care professional.
Vitamin E	400 IU to 800 IU	Caution with anticoagulant medications.
Vitamin K	50 mcg to 65 mcg	Caution with anticoagulant medications; use under medical supervision.
Willow bark	Standardized extract: 120 mg to 240 mg	
Yarrow (*Achillea millifolium*)	Infuse 1 tablespoon dried yarrow flowers in 8 oz hot water covered x 20 min. Sip 1 teaspoon as needed up to every 20 minutes.	Contraindicated with some chemotherapy drugs.
Zinc	15 mg to 45 mg	Prolonged supplementation requires additional copper supplementation (ratio of 2 mg copper to 15 mg zinc).

Endnotes

Introduction

American Cancer Society. 2006. Special section: Environmental pollutants and cancer. In *Cancer Facts and Figures 2006*, 22–31. Atlanta, GA: American Cancer Society. www.cancer.org /downloads/STT/CAFF2006PWSecured.pdf (accessed November 14, 2006).

American Cancer Society. www.cancer.org/docroot/MIT/content/MIT_3_2X_Costs_of _Cancer.asp (accessed June 19, 2009).

Engel, J., et al. 2003. Communication, quality of life and age: Results of a five-year prospective study in breast cancer patients. *Annals of Oncology* 14(3):421–27.

Mumber, Matthew P., ed. 2006. *Integrative Oncology: Principles and Practice.* Abingdon, Oxon, UK: Taylor & Francis.

Smith, B. D., et al. 2009. Future of cancer in the United States: Burdens upon an aging, changing nation. *Journal of Clinical Oncology* 27(17):2758–65.

Chapter One The Cancer Experience

American Cancer Society. 2009. www.cancer.org/docroot/STT/STT_0.asp (accessed June 2009).

Awale, S., et al. 2006. Identification of arctigenin as an antitumor agent having the ability to eliminate the tolerance of cancer cells to nutrient starvation. *Cancer Research* 66(3):1751–57.

Gazella, K., and S. Snyder. 2006. Rachel Naomi Remen, MD: Recovering the soul of medicine. *Alternative Therapies in Health and Medicine* 12(3):87–93.

McCulloch, M., et al. 2006. Diagnostic accuracy of canine scent detection in early- and late-stage lung and breast cancers. *Integrative Cancer Therapies* 5(1):30–39.

Murphy, G. P., W. Lawrence, and R. Lenhard, eds. 1995. *American Cancer Society Textbook of Clinical Oncology.* 2nd edition. Atlanta, GA: The American Cancer Society.

Murphy, G. P., L. P. Morris, and D. Lange. 1997. *Informed Decisions: The Complete Book of Cancer Diagnosis, Treatment, and Recovery.* New York: Viking.

National Center for Injury Prevention and Control. 10 leading causes of death, United States, 2003, all races, both sexes. Access via http://webappa.cdc.gov/sasweb/ncipc/leadcaus10. html (accessed June 2009).

Remen, Rachel Naomi. Personal interview February 2006.

Rountree, Robert, and Carol Colman. 2000. *Immunotics: A Revolutionary Way to Fight Infection, Beat Chronic Illness, and Stay Well.* New York: Putnam Adult.

Yance, D. R., and S. M. Sager. 2006. Targeting angiogenesis with integrative cancer therapies. *Integrative Cancer Therapies* 5(1):9–29.

Chapter Two Causes and Diagnosis of Cancer

41st Annual Meeting of the American Society of Clinical Oncology, Orlando, Fla., May 13–17, 2005. Wendy Chen, MD, PhD, instructor in medicine, Harvard Medical School, Dana-Farber Cancer Institute, Boston. Len Lichtenfeld, MD, deputy chief medical officer, American Cancer Society, Atlanta.

American Cancer Society. 2009. Special section: Environmental pollutants and cancer. In *Cancer Facts and Figures 2009*, 22–31. Atlanta, GA: American Cancer Society. www.cancer.org /downloads/STT/CAFF2009PWSecured.pdf.

American Nuclear Society. Radiation dose chart. www.ans.org/pi/resources/dosechart/ (accessed November 2006).

Bergstrom, Anna, et al. 2001. Overweight as an avoidable cause of cancer in Europe. *International Journal of Cancer* 91(3):421–30.

Boffetta, P. 1997. Infection with *Helicobacter pylori* and parasites, social class and cancer. *IARC Scientific Publications* 138:325–29.

Boffetta, P., and M. Hashibe. 2006. Alcohol and cancer. *Lancet Oncology* 7(2):149–56.

Calle, E. E., et al. 2003. Overweight, obesity, and mortality from cancer in a prospectively studied cohort of U.S. adults. *New England Journal of Medicine* 348(17):1625–38.

Centers for Disease Control and Prevention. 2005. Annual smoking-attributable mortality, years of potential life lost, and productivity losses—United States, 1997–2001. *Morbidity and Mortality Weekly Report* 154(25):625–28.

Charlton, B. G. 1996. Senescence, cancer and "endogenous parasites": A salutogenic hypothesis. *Journal of the Royal College of Physicians of London* 30(1):10–12.

Christie, Wanda, and Carol Moore. 2005. The impact of humor on patients with cancer. *Clinical Journal of Oncology Nursing* 9(2):211–18.

Donn, Jeff, et al. AP probe finds drugs in drinking water. *Associated Press*. March 10, 2008.

Dork, T., J. H. Karstens, and C. Sohn. 2002. Genetic predisposition towards breast cancer and cellular radiosensitivity. A review. [In German.] *Geburtshilfe und Frauenheilkunde* 62(12):1162–69.

Environmental Working Group Staff. 2003. Bodyburden: The pollution in people. January. www.ewg.org (accessed June 2009).

Evans, Nancy, ed. 2006. *State of the Evidence 2006: What Is the Connection between the Environment and Breast Cancer.* 4th edition. San Francisco: Breast Cancer Fund, Breast Cancer Action.

Gaynor, Mitchell. 2006. Dangerous toxins may be lurking in your home. *Bottom Line Health Newsletter*, February.

Health Media Ltd. 2003. Anxious people may be more prone to cancer. May 30. (Available at www.cancercompass.com/cancer-news/1,4620,00.htm; accessed June 2009.)

Iwamatsu, Yumi, et al. 2003. Differences in emotional distress between breast tumor patients with emotional inhibition and those with emotional expression. *Psychiatry and Clinical Neurosciences* 57(3):289–94.

Kroenke, C. H., et al. 2006. Depressive symptoms and prospective incidence of colorectal cancer in women. *American Journal of Epidemiology* 162(9):839–48.

Lichtenstein, Paul, et al. 2000. Environmental and heritable factors in the causation of cancer—Analyses of cohorts of twins from Sweden, Denmark, and Finland. *New England Journal of Medicine* 343(2):78–85.

Lowe, Rachel Myers. 2003. Emphasis on healthy weight urged to reduce cancer risk. *CancerPage.com*, March 5. www.cancerpage.com/news/article.asp?id=5614 (accessed June 2009).

Menegaux, F., et al. 2006. Household exposure to pesticides and risk of childhood acute leukaemia. *Occupational and Environmental Medicine* 63(2):131–34.

Modugno, F., et al. 2006. Obesity, hormone therapy, estrogen metabolism and risk of postmenopausal breast cancer. *International Journal of Cancer* 118(5):1292–301.

Mokdad, Ali H., et al. 2004. Actual causes of death in the United States, 2000. *Journal of the American Medical Association* 291(10):1238–45.

Murphy, G. P., L. P. Morris, and D. Lange. 1997. *Informed Decisions: The Complete Book of Cancer Diagnosis, Treatment, and Recovery.* New York: Viking.

Murray, Michael, et al. 2002. *How to Prevent and Treat Cancer with Natural Medicine.* New York: Riverhead Books.

Nelson, Nancy. 2004. The majority of cancers are linked to the environment. *BenchMarks* 4(3). www.cancer.gov/newscenter/benchmarks-vol4-issue3/page1 (accessed June 2009).

NewsRx. 2003. Information may help identify early environmental exposures that increase risk. June 26. (Available at www.cancercompass.com/cancer-news/1,4806,00.htm; accessed June 2009.)

Nickerson, Krista. 2006. Environmental contaminants in breast milk. *Journal of Midwifery and Women's Health* 51(1):26–34.

Organic Consumers Association. 2006. Organic Consumers Association home page. www .organicconsumers.org (accessed November 15, 2006).

Pedersen, A., C. Johansen, and M. Gronbaek. 2003. Relations between amount and type of alcohol and colon and rectal cancer in a Danish population based cohort study. *Gut* 52(6):861–67.

Putnam, Judy, Jane Allshouse, and Linda Scott Kantor. 2002. U.S. per capita food supply trends: More calories, refined carbohydrates, and fats. *FoodReview* 25(3):2–15.

Rauscher, Megan. 2005. High number of cancers due to obesity: Study. *Reuters Health*, November 1. (Available at www.cancerpage.com/news/article.asp?id=9009; accessed June 2009).

Rayner, M., and P. Scarborough. 2005. The burden of food related ill health in the U.K. *Journal of Epidemiology and Community Health* 59(12):1054–57.

Reuters Health. 2005. Depression raises colorectal cancer risk. *Reuters Health*, November 3. (Available at www.cancerpage.com/news/article.asp?id=9026; accessed November 15, 2006).

Schlosser, Eric. 2005. *Fast Food Nation: The Dark Side of the All-American Meal.* New York: Harper Perennial.

Soffritti, Morando, et al. 2006. First experimental demonstration of the multipotential carcinogenic effects of aspartame administered in the feed to Prague-Dawley rats. *Environmental Health Perspectives* 114(3):379–85.

Szutorisz, H., et al. 2003. A chromosome 3-encoded repressor of the human telomerase reverse transcriptase (hTERT) gene controls the state of hTERT chromatin. *Cancer Research* 63(3):689–95.

The Organic Center. www.organic-center.org/science.nutri.php?action=view&report_id=145 (accessed September 2009).

Tufts E-News. Are environmental toxins causing breast cancer? *Tufts E-News.* www.tufts.edu /communications/stories/102802AreEnvironmentalToxinsCausingBreastCancer.htm (accessed June 2009).

U.S. Preventive Services Task Force. 2006. Genetic risk assessment and BRCA mutation testing for breast and ovarian cancer susceptibility: Recommendation statement. *American Family Physician* 73(5):869–74.

Wigle, Donald T., and Bruce P. Lanphear. 2002. Human health risks from low-level environmental exposures: No apparent safety thresholds. *PLoS Medicine* 2(12):e350.

Diagnosis and Screening

Abeloff, M. D., et al., eds. 2004. *Clinical Oncology.* 3rd edition. Philadelphia: Elsevier/Churchill Livingstone.

American Cancer Society. 2006. HPV vaccine approved; prevents cervical cancer. June 8. www .cancer.org/docroot/NWS/content/NWS_1_1x_HPV_Vaccine_Approved_Prevents_Cervical_Cancer.asp (accessed November 15, 2006).

American Cancer Society. 2006. Screening guideline for the early detection of cancer in asymptomatic people. In *Cancer Facts and Figures* 2006:52. Atlanta, GA: American Cancer Society. www.cancer.org/downloads/STT/CAFF2006PWSecured.pdf (accessed November 15, 2006).

Church, Timothy R. 2006. Screening for colorectal cancer by colonoscopy: Adding to the evidence. *Journal of the American Medical Association* 295(20):2411–12.

Corsetti, V., et al. 2006. Role of ultrasonography in detecting mammograpically occult breast carcinoma in women with dense breasts. *La Radiologia Medica* 111(3):440–48.

Di Matteo, L., and R. Di Matteo. 2005. Does testing for prostate-specific antigen contribute to declining prostate cancer mortality? Estimating the broader economic influences on aggregate prostate cancer mortality rates. *European Journal of Health Economics* 6(1):270–300.

Dillon, M. F., et al. 2006. Predictors of invasive disease in breast cancer when core biopsy demonstrates DCIS only. *Journal of Surgical Oncology* 93(7):559–63.

Hay, J. L., K. D. McCaul, and R. E. Magnan. 2006. Does worry about breast cancer predict screening behaviors? A meta-analysis of the prospective evidence. *Preventative Medicine* 42(6):401–8.

Hoffman, R. M. 2006. Viewpoint: Limiting prostate cancer screening. *Annals of Internal Medicine* 144(6):438–40.

Kristal, A. R., et al. 2006. Associations of demographic and lifestyle characteristics with prostate-specific antigen (PSA) concentration and rate of PSA increase. *Cancer* 106(2):320–28.

Le-Petross, H. T. 2006. Breast MRI as a screening tool: The appropriate role. *Journal of the National Comprehensive Cancer Network* 4(5):523–26.

Lin, O. S., et al. 2006. Screening colonoscopy in very elderly patients: Prevalence of neoplasia and estimated impact on life expectancy. *Journal of the American Medical Association* 295(20):2411–12.

Michaelson, J. S., et al. 2003. The effect of tumor size and lymph node status on breast carcinoma lethality. *Cancer* 98(10):2133–43.

Murphy, G. P., L. P. Morris, and D. Lange. 1997. *Informed Decisions: The Complete Book of Cancer Diagnosis, Treatment, and Recovery.* New York: Viking.

National Cancer Institute. 2006. Cancer screening overview. National Cancer Institute, www.cancer.gov/cancertopics/pdq/screening/overview/healthprofessional (accessed June 2009).

Pacific Chiropractic and Research Center. 2006. Mammography/thermography/ultrasound: What's the difference? www.breastthermography.com/mammography_thermography.htm (accessed May 03, 2006).

Parisky, Y. R., et al. 2003. Efficacy of computerized infrared imaging analysis to evaluate mammographically suspicious lesions. *American Journal of Roentgenology* 180(1):263–69.

Rosenthal, A., and I. Jacobs. 1998. Ovarian cancer screening. *Seminars in Oncology* 25(3):315–25.

Rosenthal, Thomas C., and Stirling M. Puck. 1999. Screening for genetic risk of breast cancer. *American Family Physician* 59(1):99–104.

Rotham, Julie. 2003. Gene study gives new hope in identifying aggressive breast cancer. *Sydney Morning Herald*, March 17. www.smh.com.au/articles/2003/03/17/1047749721304.html (accessed June 2009).

Sanchini, M. A., et al. 2005. Relevance of urine telomerase in the diagnosis of bladder cancer. *Journal of the American Medical Association* 294(16):2052–56.

Seattle Times. 2003. Research stirs hope of earlier diagnosis for ovarian cancer. June 25. (Available at www.cancercompass.com/cancer-news/1,4849,00.htm; accessed June 2009.)

Singh, H., et al. 2006. Risk of developing colorectal cancer following a negative colonoscopy examination: Evidence for a 10-year interval between colonoscopies. *Journal of the American Medical Association* 295(20):2411–12.

Smith, L. H., et al. 2005. Ovarian cancer: Can we make the clinical diagnosis earlier? *Cancer* 104(7):1398–407.

U.S. Nuclear Regulatory Commission. 2004. Fact sheet on biological effects of radiation. www.nrc.gov/reading-rm/doc-collections/fact-sheets/bio-effects-radiation.html (accessed May 15, 2006).

USA Today. 2003. New breast self-exam guidelines stir debate. May 19. (Available at www.cancercompass.com/cancer-news/1,4555,00.htm; accessed November 15, 2006.)

Walter, L. C., C. L. Lewis, and M. B. Barton. 2005. Screening for colorectal, breast, and cervical cancer in the elderly: A review of the evidence. *American Journal of the Medical Sciences* 118(10):1078–86.

Yahara, Toshiro, et al. 2003. Relationship between microvessel density and thermographic hot areas in breast cancer. *Surgery Today* 33(4):243–48.

Chapter Three Prevention Is Paramount

Bennett, M. P., et al. 2003. The effect of mirthful laughter on stress and natural killer cell activity. *Alternative Therapies in Health and Medicine* 9(2):38–45.

Bernstein L., et al. 2005. Lifetime recreational exercise activity and breast cancer risk among black women and white women. *Journal of the National Cancer Institute* 97(22):1671–79.

Biever, Celeste. 2003. Knockout broccoli fights cancer. *New Scientist* (2389).

Byers, Ted, et al. 2002. American Cancer Society guidelines on nutrition and physical activity for cancer prevention: Reducing the risk of cancer with healthy food choices and physical activity. *CA: A Cancer Journal for Physicians* 52(2):92–119.

Carney, Caroline P., et al. 2003. Relationship between depression and pancreatic cancer in the general population. *Psychosomatic Medicine* 65(5):884–88.

Chan, J. M., F. Wang, and E. A. Holly. 2005. Vegetable and fruit intake and pancreatic cancer in a population-based case-control study in the San Francisco Bay Area. *Cancer, Epidemiology, Biomarkers, and Prevention* 14(9):2093–97.

Cho, E., et al. 2003. Premenopausal fat intake and risk of breast cancer. *Journal of the National Cancer Institute* 95(14):1079–85.

Eli, R., and J. A. Fasciano. 2006. An adjunctive preventative treatment for cancer: Ultra-violet light and ginkgo biloba, together with other antioxidants, are a safe and powerful, but largely ignored, treatment option for the prevention of cancer. *Medical Hypotheses* 66(6):1152–56.

Fan, S., et al. 2006. BRCA1 and BRCA2 as molecular targets for phytochemicals indole-3-carbinol and genistein in breast and prostate cancer cells. *British Journal of Cancer* 94(3): 407–26.

Folsom, Aaron R., and Ching Ping Hong. 2006. Magnesium intake and reduced risk of colon cancer in a prospective study of women. *American Journal of Epidemiology* 163(3):232–35.

Fowke, J. H., C. Longcope, and J. R. Hebert. 2000. Brassica vegetable consumption shifts estrogen metabolism in healthy postmenopausal women. *Cancer, Epidemiology, Biomarkers, and Prevention* 9(8):773–79.

Franceshi, Silvia, et al. 1997. Food groups and risk of colorectal cancer in Italy. *International Journal of Cancer* 72(1):56–61.

Fung, T., et al. 2003. Major dietary patterns and the risk of colorectal cancer in women. *Archives of Internal Medicine* 163(3):309–14.

Fung, T., et al. 2006. Diet quality is associated with the risk of estrogen receptor-negative breast cancer in postmenopausal women. *Journal of Nutrition* 136(2):466–72.

Garland, Cedric F., Frank C. Garland, and Edward D. Gorham. 2006. The role of vitamin D in cancer prevention. *American Journal of Public Health* 96(2):252–61.

Gaudet, Tracy. 2006. Interviewed on "The Science of Emotions." *The New Medicine, a PBS Documentary.* March 29. www.thenewmedicine.org.

Gaynor, Mitchell L. 2005. *Nurture Nature, Nurture Health: Your Health and the Environment.* New York: Nurture Nature Press.

Gaynor, Mitchell L., Jerry Hickey, and William Fryer. 2000. *Dr. Gaynor's Cancer Prevention Program.* New York: Kensington Publishing.

Giovannucci, E. 2002. Modifiable risk factors for colon cancer. *Gastroenterology Clinics of North America* 31(4):925–43.

Glaser, Janice, and Ronald Glaser. 2006. Interviewed on "The Science of Emotions." *The New Medicine, a PBS Documentary.* March 29. www.thenewmedicine.org.

Greenwald, Peter, and Sharon S. McDonald. 1997. Cancer prevention: The roles of diet and chemoprevention. *Cancer Control* 4(2):118–27.

Ingels, Darin. 2001. Nutrients reduce risk of some cancers. *Healthnotes Newswire*, November 8 (Available at www.cncahealth.com/nutritional-news.htm?org=cnca&page=newswire /newswire_2001_11_08_3.cfm; accessed June 2009.)

Kabat-Zinn, Jon. 2005. Bringing mindfulness to medicine. Interview by Karolyn A. Gazella. *Alternative Therapies in Health and Medicine* 11(3):56–64.

Kirsh, V. A., et al. 2006. Supplementary and dietary vitamin E, beta-carotene, and vitamin C intakes and prostate cancer risk. *Journal of the National Cancer Institute* 98(4):245–54.

Kleiner, S. M. 1999. Water: An essential but overlooked nutrient. *Journal of the American Dietary Association* 99(2):200–6.

Kleiner, S. M. 2004. The art and science of hydration. *Acta Pediatrica Española* 93(12):1557–58.

Kruk, J., and H. Y. Aboul-Enein. 2006. Physical activity in the prevention of cancer. *Asian Pacific Journal of Cancer Prevention* 7(1):11–21.

Kushi, L., and E. Giovannucci. 2002. Dietary fat and cancer. *American Journal of Medicine* 113(suppl.9B):63S–70S.

Liu, X., et al. 2005. Relationship between body size and prostate cancer in a sibling based case-control study. *Journal of Urology* 174(6):2169–73.

Marchione, Marilynn. 2006. Vitamin D may help prevent breast cancer: Studies. *Globe and Mail*, April 4. www.theglobeandmail.com.

McTiernan A., et al. 2003. Recreational physical activity and the risk of breast cancer in post-menopausal women: The Women's Health Initiative Cohort Study. *Journal of the American Medical Association* 290(10):1331–36.

Menendez, J. A., et al. 2006. A genomic explanation connecting "Mediterranean diet," olive oil and cancer: Oleic acid, the main monounsaturated fatty acid of olive oil, induces formation of inhibitory "PEA3 transcription factor-PEA3 DNA binding site" complexes at the Her-2/neu (erbB-2) oncogene promoter in breast, ovarian and stomach cancer cells. *European Journal of Cancer* 42(15):2425–32.

Morgan, James. 2005. Vitamin D reduces risk of common cancers: Study shows dramatic drops. *RedOrbit Breaking News*, December 28. www.redorbit.com/news/health/341755/vitamin_d_reduces_risk_of_common_cancers_study_shows_dramatic/index.html# (accessed June 2009).

Murray, Michael, Joseph A. Pizzorno, and Lara Pizzorno. 2005. *The Encyclopedia of Healing Foods.* New York: Atria Books.

Nagata, C., et al. 2005. Associations of mammographic density with dietary factors in Japanese women. *Cancer, Epidemiology, Biomarkers, and Prevention* 14(12):2877–80.

National Cancer Institute. 2006. Cancer prevention overview. National Cancer Institute, www.cancer.gov/cancertopics/pdq/prevention/overview/healthprofessional (accessed November 15, 2006).

National Institutes of Health. 2005. Dietary supplement fact sheet: Vitamin D. http://dietary-supplements.info.nih.gov/factsheets/VitaminD_pf.asp (accessed November 15, 2006).

Navarro-Peran, Enma, et al. 2005. The antifolate activity of tea catechins. *Cancer Research* 65(6):2059–64.

Newswise. 2003. More vitamin B-6 may protect against cancer. *Newswise Medical News*, April 30. www.newswise.com/articles/view/?id=VITB6.WSU (accessed June 2009).

Ngoan, L. T., et al. 2002. Dietary factors and stomach cancer mortality. *British Journal of Cancer* 87(1):37–42.

Penedo, F. J., and J. R. Dahn. 2005. Exercise and well-being: A review of mental and physical health benefits associated with physical activity. *Current Opinion in Psychiatry* 18(2):189–93.

Reibel, K., et al. 2001. Mindfulness-based stress reduction and health-related quality of life in a heterogenous patient population. *General Hospital Psychiatry* 23(4):183–92.

Remen, Rachel Naomi. 2000. *My Grandfather's Blessings.* New York: Riverhead Books.

Rosenszweig S., et al. 2003. Mindfulness-based stress reduction lowers psychological distress in medical students. *Teaching and Learning in Medicine* 15(2):88–92.

Ryan, Susan W. 2005. Exercise as medicine. Presentation at Complementary and Natural Health Care Expo West. October 7.

Safe, S., et al. 1999. Symposium on mechanisms of action of naturally occurring anticarcinogens. *Toxicological Sciences* 52(1):1–8.

Sternberg, Ester. 2006. Interviewed on "The Science of Emotions." *The New Medicine, a PBS Documentary.* March 29. www.thenewmedicine.org.

Tanaka, S., et al. 2006. Aged garlic extract has potential suppressive effect on colorectal adenomas in humans. *Journal of Nutrition* 136(suppl.3):821S–26S.

Thune, I., and A. S. Furberg. 2001. Physical activity and cancer risk: Dose-response and cancer, all sites and site specific. *Medicine and Science in Sports and Exercise* 33(suppl.6):S530–50.

Vineas, P., P. Schulte, and A. J. McMichael. 2001. Misconceptions about the use of genetic tests in populations. *Lancet* 357:709–12.

Yeh, C. C., et al. 2005. Vegetable/fruit, smoking, glutathione S-transferase polymorphisms and risk for colorectal cancer in Taiwan. *World Journal of Gastroenterology* 11(10):1473–80.

Zhao, X., et al. 2006. Modification of lymphocyte DNA damage by carotenoid supplementation in postmenopausal women. *American Journal of Clinical Nutrition* 83(1):163–69.

Chapter Four Building a Strong Foundation with Diet, Nutrition, and Stress Reduction

Aggarwal, B. B., and S. Shishodia. 2006. Molecular targets of dietary agents for prevention and therapy of cancer. *Biochemical Pharmacology* 71(10):1397–421.

Alexander, S, et al. 1999. Phase I/II study of stage III and IV non-small cell lung cancer patients taking a specific dietary supplement. *Nutrition and Cancer* 34(1):62–69.

Almadori, G., et al. 2006. Pilot phase IIA study for evaluation of the efficacy of folic acid in the treatment of laryngeal leucoplakia. *Cancer* 107(2):328–36.

American Institute for Cancer Research. 2006. Saturated fats are worse than you think: They affect not only cholesterol, but can also raise risk of cancer, diabetes. *MSNBC.com.* www.msnbc.msn.com/id/12867692 (accessed January 29, 2007).

Bauer, J., et al. 2005. Compliance with nutrition prescription improves outcomes in patients with unresectable pancreatic cancer. *Clinical Nutrition* 24(6):998–1004.

Bravi, F., et al. 2006. Self-reported history of hypercholesterolaemia and gallstones and the risk of prostate cancer. *Annals of Oncology* 17(6):1014–17.

Brignall, M. S. 2001. Prevention and treatment of cancer with indole-3-carbinol. *Alternative Medicine Review* 6(6):580–89.

Colomer, R., and J. A. Menendez. 2006. Mediterranean diet, olive oil and cancer. *Clinical and Translational Oncology* 8(1):15–21.

Daniells, Stephan. 2006. Garlic, onions could protect against stomach cancer. *NutraIngredients-USA. Breaking News on Supplements and Nutrition,* May 16. www.nutraingredients-usa.com/news/ng.asp?id=67704 (accessed June 2009).

Dietary Guidelines for Americans. 2005. www.healthierus.gov/dietaryguidelines (accessed January 29, 2007).

Donaldson, Michael. 2004. Nutrition and cancer: A review of the evidence for an anti-cancer diet. *Nutrition Journal* 3:19.

Environment News Service. 2006. Curried cauliflower effective against prostate cancer. *ENS Newswire,* January 16. www.ens-newswire.com/ens/jan2006/2006-01-16-01.asp (accessed June 2009).

European Society for Medical Oncology. 2006. New research finds direct link between high cholesterol and prostate cancer. *Science Daily Press Releases,* April 12. www.sciencedaily.com/releases/2006/04/060411231430.htm (accessed November 16, 2006).

Fontana, L., et al. 2006. Effect of long-term calorie restriction with adequate protein and micronutrients on thyroid hormones. *Journal of Clinical Endocrinology and Metabolism* 91(8):3232–35.

Food Nutritional Chart. http://whatscookingamerica.net/NutritionalChart.htm (accessed January 29, 2007).

Gaby, Alan R. 2003. Guidelines issued for cancer treatments. *Healthnotes Newswire,* March 6. www.healthnotes.com/online/newswire_2003_03_06_1.htm (accessed November 19, 2006).

Gasper, A. V., et al. 2005. Glutathione S-transferase M1 polymorphism and metabolism of sulforaphane from standard and high-glucosinolate broccoli. *American Journal of Clinical Nutrition* 82(6):724.

Gaynor, M. L. 2003. Isoflavones and the prevention and treatment of prostate disease: Is there a role? *Cleveland Clinic Journal of Medicine* 70(3):203–4, 206, 208–9.

Gaynor, M. L. 2005. *Nurture Nature, Nurture Health: Your Health and the Environment.* New York: Nurture Nature Press.

Gill, C. I., et al. 2005. Potential anti-cancer effects of virgin olive oil phenols on colorectal carcinogenesis models in vitro. *International Journal of Cancer* 117(1):1–7.

Giovannucci, E. 2003. Diet, body weight, and colorectal cancer: A summary of the epidemiologic evidence. *Journal of Women's Health* 12(2):173–82.

Gonzalez, C. A., et al. 2006. Fruit and vegetable intake and the risk of stomach and oesophagus adenocarcinoma in the European prospective investigation into cancer and nutrition (EPIC-EURGAST). *International Journal of Cancer* 118(10):2559–66.

Jones, Charisse, and Nanci Hellmich. 2006. NYC bans trans fats in restaurants. *USAToday.com.* (Available at www.usatoday.com/news/health/2006-12-04 trans-fat-ban_x.htm; accessed December 6, 2006.)

Jones, J. M., et al. 2004. Becoming proactive with the whole-grain message. *Nutrition Today* 39(1):10–17.

Khor, T. O., et al. 2006. Combined inhibitory effects of curcumin and phenethyl isothiocyanate on the growth of human PC-3 prostate xenografts in immunodeficient mice. *Cancer Research* 66(2):613–21.

Kuriyama, I., et al. 2005. Inhibitory effect of glycolipids fraction from spinach on mammalian DNA polymerase activity and human cancer cell proliferation. *Journal of Nutritional Biochemistry* 16(10):594–601.

Kushi, L. H., et al. 2001. The macrobiotic diet in cancer. *Journal of Nutrition* 131(suppl.11):3056S–64S.

Lamson, Davis W., and Matthew S. Brignall. 2000. Antioxidants and cancer III: Quercetin. *Alternative Medicine Review* 5(3):196–208.

Larsson, S. C., et al. 2005. Whole grain consumption and risk of colorectal cancer: A population-based cohort of 60,000 women. *British Journal of Cancer* 92(9):1803–7.

Liebman, Bonnie. 2005. Keeping abreast: The latest on diet and breast cancer. *Nutrition Action Healthletter* 32(7):3–7. (Available at http://findarticles.com/p/articles/mi_m0813/is_7_32/ai_n15342942; accesssed June 2009.)

MacLean, H., et al. 2006. Effects of omega-3 fatty acids on cancer risk: A systematic review. *Journal of the American Medical Association* 295(16):403–15.

Michels, Karin B. 2004. The role of nutrition in cancer development and prevention. *International Journal of Cancer* 114(2):163–65.

Murray, Michael. 1996. *Encyclopedia of Nutritional Supplements: The Essential Guide for Improving Your Health Naturally.* New York: Three Rivers Press.

Murray, Michael, et al. 2002. *How to Prevent and Treat Cancer with Natural Medicine.* New York: Riverhead Books.

Murray, Michael, Joseph Pizzorno, and Lara Pizzorno. 2005. *The Encyclopedia of Healing Foods.* New York: Atria Books.

National Cancer Institute. 2006. Nutrition in cancer care. www.cancer.gov/cancertopics/pdq/supportivecare/nutrition/healthprofessional/allpages (accessed November 15, 2006).

Piller, R., J. Chang-Claude, and J. Linseisen. 2006. Plasma enterolactone and genistein and the risk of premenopausal breast cancer. *European Journal of Cancer Prevention* 15(3):225–32.

Ravasco, Paula, et al. 2005. Dietary counseling improves patient outcomes: A prospective, randomized, controlled trial in colorectal cancer patients undergoing radiotherapy. *Journal of Clinical Oncology* 23(7):1431–38.

Reuters Health. 2005. Dietary fish oil curbs breast cancer progression in animal study. *Reuters Health*, November 24. (Available at www.oncolink.org/resources/article.cfm?c=3&s=8&ss=23&id=12555&month=11&year=2005; accessed November 16, 2006.)

Reuters Health. 2005. Virgin olive oil blocks cancer cells in lab. *Reuters Health*, October 26. (Available at www.upmccancercenters.com/news/reuters/reuters.cfm?article=6224; accessed November 16, 2006.)

Schatzkin, A., et al. 2000. Lack of effect of a low-fat, high-fiber diet on the recurrence of colorectal adenomas. Polyp prevention trial study group. *New England Journal of Medicine* 342(16):1149–55.

Slavin, J. L., et al. 2001. The role of whole grains in disease prevention. *Journal of the American Dietetic Association* 101(7):780–5.

Stein, Rob. 2005. Diet, exercise and reduced stress slow prostate cancer, study finds. *Washington Post*, August 11.

Thompson, Henry J., et al. 1999. Effect of increased vegetable and fruit consumption on markers of oxidative cellular damage. *Carcinogenesis* 20(12):2261–66.

U.S. Department of Agriculture. Anatomy of MyPyramid. www.mypyramid.gov/professionals /pdf_anatomy.html (accessed November 16, 2006).

Williams, M. T., and N. G. Hord. 2005. The role of dietary factors in cancer prevention: Beyond fruits and vegetables. *Nutrition in Clinical Practice* 20(4):451–9.

Wu, M., et al. 2005. Omega-3 polyunsaturated fatty acids attenuate breast cancer growth through activation of a neutral sphingomyelinase-mediated pathway. *International Journal of Cancer* 117(3):340–48.

Lifestyle

Ahmed, R. J., et al. 2006. Randomized controlled trial of weight training and lymphedema in breast cancer survivors. *Journal of Clinical Oncology* 24(18):2765–72.

Aktas, G., and F. Ogce. 2005. Dance as a therapy for cancer prevention. *Asian Pacific Journal of Cancer Prevention* 6(3):408–11.

American Cancer Society. 2006. Make exercise work for you. www.cancer.org/docroot/PED /content/PED_6_1X_Tips_on_Maintaining_Your_Exercise_Program.asp (accessed November 16, 2006).

Andersen, C., et al. 2006. The effect of a multidimensional exercise programme on symptoms and side-effects in cancer patients undergoing chemotherapy: The use of semi-structured diaries. *European Journal of Oncology Nursing* 10(4):247–62.

Barnes, D. E., et al. 2003. A longitudinal study of cardiorespiratory fitness and cognitive function in healthy older adults. *Journal of the American Geriatric Society* 51(4):570–71.

Bennett, Mary P., et al. 2003. The effect of mirthful laughter on stress and natural killer cell activity. *Alternative Therapies in Health and Medicine* 9(2):38–44.

Benson, Herbert. 2005. Are you working too hard? A conversation with mind/body researcher Herbert Benson. *Harvard Business Review* 83(11):53–58, 165.

Berman, Jeff, Gran Fleegler, and John Hanc. 2001. *The FORCE Program: The Proven Way to Fight Cancer through Physical Activity and Exercise.* New York: Ballantine Books.

Bower, Julienne, et al. 2005. Yoga for cancer patients and survivors. *Cancer Control* 12(3):165–71.

Carlson, L. E., and S. N. Garland. 2005. Impact of mindfulness-based stress reduction (MBSR) on sleep, mood, stress and fatigue symptoms in cancer outpatients. *International Journal of Behavioral Medicine* 12(4):278–85.

Carlson, L. E., et al. 2004. Mindfulness-based stress reduction in relation to quality of life, mood, symptoms of stress and level of cortisol, dehydroepiandrosterone sulfate (DHEAS) and melatonin in breast and prostate cancer outpatients. *Psychoneuroendocrinology* 29(4):448–74.

Cohen, L., et al. 2004. Psychological adjustment and sleep quality in a randomized trial of the effects of a Tibetan yoga intervention in patients with lymphoma. *Cancer* 100(10):2253–60.

Cooper, C. L., and E. B. Faragher. 1993. Psychosocial stress and breast cancer: The interrelationship between stress events, coping strategies and personality. *Psychological Medicine* 23(3):653–52.

Corbin, Lisa. 2005. Safety and efficacy of massage therapy for patients with cancer. *Cancer Control* 12(3):158–64.

Culos-Reed, S. N., et al. 2006. A pilot study of yoga for breast cancer survivors: Physical and psychological benefits. *Psycooncology* 15(10):891–97.

Davidson, Richard J., et al. 2003. Alterations in brain and immune function produced by mindfulness meditation. *Psychosomatic Medicine* 66(1):564–70.

Demark-Wahnefried, Wendy, et al. 2005. Riding the crest of the teachable moment: Promoting long-term health after diagnosis of cancer. *Journal of Clinical Oncology* 23(24):5814–30.

Field, T., et al. 2005. Cortisol decreases and serotonin and dopamine increase following massage therapy. *International Journal of Neuroscience* 115(10):1397–413.

Giovannucci, E., et al. 2005. A prospective study of physical activity and incident and fatal prostate cancer. *Archives of Internal Medicine* 165(9):1005–10.

Gordon, James S., and Sharon Curtin. 2000. *Comprehensive Cancer Care*. New York: Perseus Publishing.

Graham, J. E., L. M. Christian, and J. K. Kiecolt-Glaser. 2006. Stress, age, and immune function: Toward a lifespan approach. *Journal of Behavioral Medicine* 29(4):380–400.

Grossman, P., et al. 2004. Mindfulness-based stress reduction and health benefits. A meta-analysis. *Journal of Psychosomatic Research* 57(1):35–43.

Gu, Mingtong. 2006. Personal interview by Karolyn A. Gazella. May 12.

HERA Organization. www.heraorganization.org.

Hernandez-Reif, M., et al. 2005. Natural killer cells and lymphocytes increase in women with breast cancer following massage therapy. *International Journal of Neuroscience* 115(4): 495–510.

Hoffman, Lisa, and Alison Freeland. 2002. *The Healing Power of Movement: How to Benefit from Physical Activity during Your Cancer Treatment*. Cambridge, MA: Perseus Publishing.

Holmes, Michelle D., et al. 2005. Physical activity and survival after breast cancer diagnosis. *Journal of the American Medical Association* 293(20):279–86.

Inoue, M., et al. 2004. Impact of body mass index on the risk of total cancer incidence and mortality among middle-aged Japanese: Data from a large-scale population-based cohort study—The JPHC study. *Cancer Causes and Control* 15(7):671–80.

Jonas, Wayne B., and Cindy C. Crawford. 2003. Science and spiritual healing: A critical review of spiritual healing, "energy" medicine, and intentionality. *Alternative Therapies in Health and Medicine* 9(2):56–61.

Khalsa, Dharma Singh, and Cameron Stauth. 2001. *Meditation as Medicine: Activate the Power of Your Natural Healing Force*. New York: Pocket Books.

Michaud, D. S., et al. 2001. Physical activity, obesity, height, and the risk of pancreatic cancer. *Journal of the American Medical Association* 286(8):967–68.

Nainis, N., et al. 2006. Relieving symptoms in cancer: Innovative use of art therapy. *Journal of Pain and Symptom Management* 31(2):162–69.

Ornish, D., et al. 2005. Intensive lifestyle changes may affect the progression of prostate cancer. *Journal of Urology* 174(3):1065–69, discussion 1069–70.

Ott, M. J., R. L. Norris, and S. M. Bauer-Wu. 2006. Mindfulness meditation for oncology patients: A discussion and critical review. *Integrative Cancer Therapies* 5(2):98–108.

Ouattrin, R., et al. 2006. Use of reflexology foot massage to reduce anxiety in hospitalized cancer patients in chemotherapy treatment: Methodology and outcomes. *Journal of Nursing Management* 14(2):96–105.

Pardini, R. S. 2006. Nutritional intervention with omega-3 fatty acids enhances tumor response to anti-neoplastic agents. *Chem Biol Interact* 162(2):89–105.

Pinto, Bernadine M., and Joseph J. Trunzo. 2004. Body esteem and mood among sedentary and active breast cancer survivors. *Mayo Clinic Proceedings* 79(2):181–86.

Plews-Ogan, M., et al. 2005. A pilot study evaluating mindfulness-based stress reduction and massage for the management of chronic pain. *Journal of General Internal Medicine* 20(12):1136–38.

Remen, Rachel Naomi. 2000. *My Grandfather's Blessings*. New York: Riverhead Books.

Rockhill, B., et al. 2001. Physical activity and mortality: A prospective study among women. *American Journal of Public Health* 91(4):578–83.

Sandel, Susan L., et al. 2005. Dance and movement program improves quality-of-life measures in breast cancer survivors. *Cancer Nursing* 28(4):301–9.

Saper, Robert H., et al. 2004. Prevalence and patterns of adult yoga use in the United States: Results of a national survey. *Alternative Therapies in Health and Medicine* 10(2):44–49.

Savard, J., et al. 1999. Association between subjective sleep quality and depression on immunocompetence in low-income women at risk for cervical cancer. *Psychosomatic Medicine* 61(4):496–507.

Simonsick, E. M. 2003. Fitness and cognition: Encouraging findings and methodological considerations for future work. *Journal of the American Geriatric Society* 51(4):459–65.

Sinha, Arushi. 2002. Art of healing. *Cure* 1(3):46–51.

Smith, J. E., et al. 2005. Mindfulness-based stress reduction as supportive therapy in cancer care: Systematic review. *Journal of Advanced Nursing* 52(3):315–27.

Stein, Rob. 2005. Diet, exercise and reduced stress slow prostate cancer, study finds. *Washington Post*, August 11.

Thompson, L.U., et al. 2005. Dietary flaxseed alters tumor biological markers in postmenopausal breast cancer. *Clinical Cancer Research* 11(10):3828–35.

Torpy, J. M., C. Lynm, and R. M. Glass. 2005. JAMA patient page. Fitness. *Journal of the American Medical Association* 294(23):3048.

Weiger, W. A., et al. 2003. Advising patients who seek complementary and alternative medical therapies for cancer. *Annals of Internal Medicine* 139(2):152.

White, M., and M. Verhoef. 2006. Cancer as part of the journey: The role of spirituality in the decision to decline conventional prostate cancer treatment and to use complementary and alternative medicine. *Integrative Cancer Therapies* 5(2):117–22.

Chapter Five Treatment Approach Overview

American Cancer Society. 2001. *Clinical Oncology.* Edited by Robert T. Osteen, Ted S. Gansler, and Raymond E. Lenhard. Malden, MA: Blackwell Publishers.

Cancer Treatment Centers of America. 2006. 3D conformal radiation. www.cancercenter.com /conventional-cancer-treatment/3d-conformal-radiation.cfm (accessed November 15, 2006).

Cancer Treatment Centers of America. 2006. Chemotherapy. www.cancercenter.com /conventional-cancer-treatment/chemotherapy.cfm (accessed November 15, 2006).

Cancer Treatment Centers of America. 2006. External beam radiation. www.cancercenter.com /conventional-cancer-treatment/external-beam-radiation.cfm (accessed November 15, 2006).

Cancer Treatment Centers of America. 2006. HDR brachytherapy. www.cancercenter.com /conventional-cancer-treatment/hdr-brachytherapy.cfm (accessed November 15, 2006).

Cancer Treatment Centers of America. 2006. Managing side effects. www.cancercenter.com /after-care-services/managing-side-effects.cfm (accessed November 15, 2006).

Denmeade, Samuel R., and John T. Isaacs. 1996. Programmed cell death (apoptosis) and cancer chemotherapy. *Cancer Control* 3(4):303–9.

Gilliland, D. Gary, and Tom Fagan. 2005. Your health in the 21st century: Do stem cells cause cancer? *Newsweek* 145(26A):20.

Grana, G. 2006. Adjuvant aromatase inhibitor therapy for early breast cancer: A review of the most recent data. *Journal of Surgical Oncology* 93(7):585–92.

Greten, Tim F., and Elizabeth M. Jaffee. 1999. Cancer vaccines. *Journal of Clinical Oncology* 17(3):1047–60.

Jani, A. B., et al. 2006. Role of external beam radiotherapy with low-dose-rate brachytherapy in treatment of prostate cancer. *Urology* 67(5):1007–10.

Kalb, Claudia. 2005. Your health in the 21st century: The next revolution. *Newsweek* 145(26A):21.

Kim, Edward S., and Waun Ki Hong. 2005. An apple a day . . . does it really keep the doctor away? The current state of cancer chemoprevention. *Journal of the National Cancer Institute* 97(7):468–70.

Klinger, B., et al. 2000. Suggested curriculum guidelines on complementary and alternative medicine: Recommendations of the Society of Teachers of Family Medicine group on alternative medicine. *Family Medicine* 31(10):30–3.

Lerner, Michael. 2003. Medicine and the environment. Interview by Bonnie Horrigan. *Alternative Therapies* 9(2):81–88.

Murphy, G. P., L. P. Morris, and D. Lange. 1997. *Informed Decisions: The Complete Book of Cancer Diagnosis, Treatment, and Recovery.* New York: Viking.

Murray, Michael, et al. 2002. *How to Prevent and Treat Cancer with Natural Medicine.* New York: Riverhead Books.

National Cancer Institute. 2006. Drug dictionary. www.cancer.gov/drugdictionary (accessed May 7, 2006).

National Cancer Institute. 2006. Trastuzumab (Herceptin). www.cancer.gov/clinicaltrials /digestpage/herceptin (accessed July 4, 2006).

Northwest Biotherapeutics. 2006. Brain cancer patients living longer and doing better after personalized vaccine therapy. Press release, February 22. (Available at www.nwbio.com /press2006.02.22.php.)

Radiological Society of North America (refer to radiation therapy for cancers). 2006. www .radiologyinfo.org (accessed July 4, 2006).

Raymond, Joan, and Barbara Kantrowitz. 2005. Your health in the 21st century: Making chemo easier to take. *Newsweek* 145(26A):16–20.

Integrative Treatment

American Association of Naturopathic Physicians. 2005. www.naturopathic.org (accessed November 15, 2006).

American Cancer Society. 2002. *American Cancer Society's Complementary and Alternative Cancer Methods Handbook.* Atlanta, GA: American Cancer Society.

Barnes, Patricia M., et al. 2004. Complementary and alternative medicine use among adults: United States, 2002. *Advance Data* 343:1–19.

Basch, E. M., J. C. Servoss, and U. B. Tedrow. 2005. Safety assurances for dietary supplements policy issues and new research paradigms. *Journal of Herbal Pharmacotherapy* 5(1):3–15.

Cohen, L. 2006. Randomized trial of yoga in women with breast cancer undergoing radiation treatment. Presentation given at the annual meeting of the American Society of Clinical Oncology, June 5.

Cohen, L., et al. 2004. Psychological adjustment and sleep quality in a randomized trial of the effects of a Tibetan yoga intervention in patients with lymphoma. *Cancer* 100(10):2253–60.

Cohen, M. H., et al. 2005. Policies pertaining to complementary and alternative medical therapies in a random sample of 39 academic health centers. *Alternative Therapies in Health and Medicine* 11(1):36–40.

Deng, G., and B. R. Cassileth. 2005. Integrative oncology: Complementary therapies for pain, anxiety, and mood disturbance. *CA: A Cancer Journal for Clinicians* 55(2):109–16.

Fink, D., et al. 2006. Hyperbaric oxygen therapy for delayed radiation injuries in gynecological cancers. *International Journal of Gynecological Cancer* 16(2):638–42.

Fred Hutchinson Cancer Research Center. 2002. More than 70 percent of adults with cancer use alternative therapies: Nearly all report improved sense of well-being. Fred Hutchinson Cancer Research Center home page, September 4. www.fhcrc.org/about/ne /news/2002/09/04/alternative.html (accessed June 2009).

Geffen, Jeremy. 2006. *The Journey through Cancer: Healing and Transforming the Whole Person.* 2nd edition. New York: Three Rivers Press.

Haller, C. A., and N. L. Benowitz. 2000. Adverse cardiovascular and central nervous system events associated with dietary supplements containing ephedra alkaloids. *New England Journal of Medicine* 343(25):1833–38.

Jemal, A., et al. 2006. Cancer statistics, 2006. *CA: A Cancer Journal for Clinicians* 56(2):106–30.

Lengacher, C. A., et al. 2006. Relief of symptoms, side effects, and psychological distress through use of complementary and alternative medicine in women with breast cancer. *Oncology Nursing Forum* 33(1):97–104.

Levy, R. L., and N. R. Miller. 2006. Hyperbaric oxygen therapy for radiation-induced optic neuropathy. *Annals of the Academy of Medicine, Singapore* 35(30):151–57.

Marwick, Charles. 2002. Adverse reactions to dietary supplements under investigation by FDA. *British Medical Journal* 325(7359):298.

Miles, P. 2003. Living in relation to mystery: Addressing mind, body, and spirit. *Advances in Mind-Body Medicine* 19(2):22–23.

Miles, P. 2006. *Reiki: A Comprehensive Guide.* New York: Tarcher/Penguin.

Miller, S. C., et al. 2006. The role of melatonin in immuno-enhancement: Potential application in cancer. *International Journal of Experimental Pathology* 87(2):81–87.

Molassiotis, A. P., et al. 2005. Use of complementary and alternative medicine in cancer patients: A European survey. *Annals of Oncology* 16(4):655–63.

Mumber, Matthew P., ed. 2006. *Integrative Oncology: Principles and Practice.* Abingdon, Oxon, UK: Taylor and Francis.

Murray, Michael T. 1999. *Natural Alternatives to Over-the-Counter and Prescription Drugs.* New York: HarperCollins.

National Cancer Institute. 2006. Laetrile/amygdalin: Evaluation of CAM approaches. www .cancer.gov/cancertopics/pdq/cam/laetrile (accessed November 15, 2006).

National Center for Complementary and Alternative Medicine. 2006. Get the facts: 10 things to know about evaluating medical resources on the web. http://nccam.nih.gov/health/webresources (accessed November 15, 2006).

National Center for Complementary and Alternative Medicine. 2006. What is complementary and alternative medicine? http://nccam.nih.gov/health/whatiscam/#4 (accessed November 17, 2006).

Orlando, Carolyn Williams. 2001. Re: Study of alternative medicine usage by cancer patients. *HerbClip,* April 22. Available at www.herbalgram.org/iherb/herbclip/review.asp?i=42449 (accessed January 29, 2007).

Ott, M. J., R. L. Norris, and S. M. Bauer. 2006. Mindfulness meditation for oncology patients: A discussion and critical review. *Integrative Cancer Therapies* 5(2):98–108.

Patterson, Ruth E., et al. 2002. Types of alternative medicine used by patients with breast, colon, or prostate cancer: Predictors, motives, and costs. *Journal of Alternative and Complementary Medicine* 8(4):477–85.

Pelletier, Kenneth R. 2002. *The Best Alternative Medicine.* West Albany, NY: Fireside Press.

Richardson, Mary Ann, et al. 2000. Complementary/alternative medicine use in a comprehensive cancer center and the implications for oncology. *Journal of Clinical Oncology* 18(13):2505–14.

Rubin, Daniel. 2005. Naturopathic oncology: An emerging discipline. *Hematology and Oncology News and Issues* 4(8):19–22.

Scherwitz, L. W., P. McHenry, and R. Herrero. 2005. Interactive guided imagery therapy with medical patients: Predictors of health outcomes. *Journal of Alternative and Complementary Medicine* 11(1):69–83.

Shaw, B. R., et al. 2006. An exploratory study of predictors of participation in a computer support group for women with breast cancer. *Computers, Informatics, Nursing* 24(1):18–27.

Shaw, D., et al. 1997. Traditional remedies and food supplements: A 5-year toxicological study (1991–1995). *Drug Safety* 17(5):342–56.

Siwek, J., et al. 2001. How to write an evidence-based clinical review article. *American Family Physician* 65:251–58.

Szabo, Liz. 2006. Kids with cancer bond online. *USA Today,* April 11.

Tindle, H. A., et al. 2005. Trends in use of complementary and alternative medicine by U.S. adults: 1997–2002. *Alternative Therapies in Health and Medicine* 11(1):42–49.

Vapiwala, N., et al. 2006. Patient initiation of complementary and alternative medical therapies (CAM) following cancer diagnosis. *Cancer Journal* 12(6):467–74.

Weiger, Wendy, and David Eisenberg. 2002. Cancer: Easing the treatment. *Newsweek* 140(23):49.

Weiger, Wendy A., et al. 2003. Advising patients who seek complementary and alternative medical therapies for cancer. *Annals of Internal Medicine* 139(2):155.

Wysowski, D. K., and L. Swartz. 2005. Adverse drug event surveillance and drug withdrawals in the United States, 1962–2002: The importance of reporting suspected reactions. *Archives of Internal Medicine* 165(12):1363–69.

Yates, J. S., et al. 2005. Prevalence of complementary and alternative medicine use in cancer patients during treatment. *Support Care Cancer* 13(10):806–11.

Yu, Stella M., Reem M. Ghandour, and Zhihuan J. Huang. 2004. Herbal supplement use among U.S. women, 2000. *Journal of the American Medical Women's Association* 59(1):17–24.

Chapter Six Supporting Your Body during Conventional Treatment

Alschuler, Lise. 2006. Implications of inflammation and cancer development. Lecture presented at the New Hampshire Association of Naturopathic Physicians Pharmaceutical Perspectives Conference. November.

American Cancer Society. 2002. *American Cancer Society's Complementary and Alternative Cancer Methods Handbook.* Atlanta, GA: American Cancer Society. 2002.

American Society of Health-System Pharmacists. 2004. Warfarin. www.nlm.nih.gov /medlineplus/druginfo/medmaster/a682277.html (accessed June 6, 2006).

Argiles, J. M. 2005. Cancer-associated malnutrition. *European Journal of Oncology Nursing* 9 (suppl.2):S39–50.

Argyriou, A. A., et al. 2006. A randomized controlled trial evaluating the efficacy and safety of vitamin E supplementation for protection against cisplatin-induced peripheral neuropathy: Final results. *Supportive Care in Cancer* 14(11):1134–40.

Blask, D. E., R. T. Dauchy, and L. A. Sauer. 2005. Putting cancer to sleep at night: The neuroendocrine/circadian melatonin signal. *Endocrine* 27(2):179–88.

Blumenthal, Rosalyn D., et al. 2000. Anti-oxidant vitamins reduce normal tissue toxicity induced by radio-immunotherapy. *International Journal of Cancer* 86(2):276–80.

Borek, C. 2004. Dietary antioxidants and human cancer. *Integrative Cancer Therapies* 3(4):333–41.

Bozzetti, F., et al. 1997. Glutamine supplementation in cancer patients receiving chemotherapy: A double-blind randomized study. *Nutrition* 13(7–8):748–51.

Bushman, J. L. 1998. Green tea and cancer in humans: A review of the literature. *Nutrition and Cancer* 31(3):151–59.

Capodice, J. L., et al. 2009. Zyflamend in men with high-grade prostatic intra epithelial neoplasia: Results of a phase I clinical trial. *Journal of the Society of Integrated Oncology* 7(2): 43–51.

Cascinu, Stefano, et al. 2002. Neuroprotective effects of reduced glutathione on oxaliplatin-based chemotherapy in advanced colorectal cancer: A randomized, double-blind, placebo-controlled trial. *Journal of Clinical Oncology* 20(16):3478–83.

Chicago Daily Herald. 2003. Alternative approach: Nontraditional therapies may boost chemo. June 17. (Available at www.mycancercompass.com/public.cfm/4761/9457; accessed June 23, 2006.)

Chirnomas, D., et al. 2006. Chemosensitization to cisplatin by inhibitors of the Fanconi anemia/BRCA pathway. *Molecular Cancer Therapeutics* 5(4):952–61.

Daniele, B., et al. 2001. Oral glutamine in the prevention of fluorouracil induced intestinal toxicity: A double-blind, placebo controlled, randomised trial. *Gut* 48(1):28–33.

Ezzo, J. M., et al. 2006. Acupuncture-point stimulation for chemotherapy-induced nausea or vomiting. *Cochrane Database of Systematic Reviews* no. 2: CD002285.

Filshie, J., et al. 2005. Acupuncture and self-acupuncture for long-term treatment of vasomotor symptoms in cancer patients—Audit and treatment algorithm. *Acupuncture in Medicine* 23(4):171–80.

Folkers, K. 1996. Relevance of the biosynthesis of coenzyme Q10 and of the four bases of DNA as a rationale for the molecular causes of cancer and a therapy. *Biochemical and Biophysical Research Communications* 224(2):358–61.

Folkers, K., et al. 1997. Activities of vitamin Q10 in animal models and a serious deficiency in patients with cancer. *Biochemical and Biophysical Research Communications* 234(2):296–99.

Fujisawa, S., and Y. Kadoma. 2006. Anti- and pro-oxidant effects of oxidized quercetin, curcumin or curcumin-related compounds with thiols or ascorbate as measured by the induction period method. *In Vivo* 20(1):39–44.

Giovannucci, E., et al. 2006. Prospective study of predictors of vitamin D status and cancer incidence and mortality in men. *Journal of the National Cancer Institute* 98(7):428–30.

Goldberg, Burton, John W. Anderson, and Larry Trivieri. 2002. *Alternative Medicine: The Definitive Guide.* 2nd edition. Berkeley, CA: Celestial Arts.

Harle, L., et al. 2005. Omega-3 fatty acids for the treatment of cancer cachexia: Issues in designing clinical trials of dietary supplements. *Journal of Alternative and Complementary Medicine* 11(6):1039–46.

HealthNotes. 2000. *Drug-Herb-Supplement Depletions/Interactions.* Volume 1 of *Healthnotes Clinical Essentials: Science-Based Reference of Supplementary and Alternative Medicine.* Portland, OR: HealthNotes.

Hrushesky, William J. M., David Blask, and Paolo Lissoni. 2003. Melatonin, chronobiology, and cancer. Paper presented at the National Cancer Institute Office of Cancer Complementary and Alternative Medicine Invited Speaker Series. February 28.

Johanning, G. L., D. C. Heimburger, and C. J. Piayathilake. 2002. DNA methylation and diet in cancer. *Journal of Nutrition* 132(12):3814S–18S.

Josefson, A., and M. Kreuter. 2003. Acupuncture to reduce nausea during chemotherapy treatment of rheumatic diseases. *Rheumatology (Oxford)* 42(10):1149–54.

Jung, Y. D., and L. M. Ellis. 2001. Inhibition of tumour invasion and angiogenesis by epigallocatechin gallate (EGCG), a major component of green tea. *International Journal of Experimental Pathology* 82(6):309–16.

Kokkinakis, D. M. 2006. Methionine-stress: A pleiotropic approach in enhancing the efficacy of chemotherapy. *Cancer Letters* 233(2):195–207.

Ladas, Elena J., et al. 2004. Antioxidants and cancer therapy: A systematic review. *Journal of Clinical Oncology* 22(3):517–28.

Lamson, Davis W., and Matthew S. Brignall. 2000. Antioxidants and cancer therapy II: Quick reference guide. *Alternative Medicine Review* 5(2):152–59.

Lev-Ari, S., et al. 2006. Down-regulation of prostaglandin e2 by curcumin is correlated with inhibition of cell growth and induction of apoptosis in human colon carcinoma cell lines. *Journal of the Society for Integrated Oncology* 4(1):21–26.

Liebens, F., et al. 2009. Breast cancer seeding associated with core needle biopsies: A systematic review. *Maturitas* 62(2):113–23.

Lindsey, Heather. 2005. Data show benefits for use of acupuncture in alleviating cancer pain, nausea and xerostomia. *Oncology Times*, February 25.

Lissoni, P., et al. 1996. Increased survival time in brain glioblastomas by a radioneuroendocrine strategy with radiotherapy plus melatonin compared to radiotherapy alone. *Oncology* 53(1):43–6.

McCully, K. S. 1994. Chemical pathology of homocysteine. II. Carcinogenesis and homocysteine thiolactone metabolism. *Annals of Clinical and Laboratory Science* 24(1):27–59.

McCully, K. S. 1998. Personal interview by Karolyn Gazella. June/July.

Morrow, Gary R., et al. 2005. Management of cancer-related fatigue. *Cancer Investigation* 23(3):229–39.

Murphy, G. P., L. P. Morris, and D. Lange. 1997. *Informed Decisions: The Complete Book of Cancer Diagnosis, Treatment, and Recovery.* New York: Viking.

Murray, Michael T. 1994. *Natural Alternatives to Over-the-Counter and Prescription Drugs.* New York: William Morrow and Company.

Murray, Michael, et al. 2002. *How to Prevent and Treat Cancer with Natural Medicine.* New York: Riverhead Books.

Na, H. K., and Y. J. Surh. 2006. Intracellular signaling network as a prime chemopreventive target of (-)-epigallocatechin gallate. *Molecular Nutrition and Food Research* 50(2):152–59.

National Cancer Institute. 2006. Coenzyme Q10. www.cancer.gov/cancertopics/pdq/cam /coenzymeQ10/healthprofessional (accessed June 23, 2006).

Navarro-Peran, E., et al. 2005. The antifolate activity of tea catechins. *Cancer Research* 65(18):8573.

The New Medicine, a PBS Documentary. March 29, 2006. www.thenewmedicine.org.

Pace, A., et al. 2003. Neuroprotective effect of vitamin E supplementation in patients treated with cisplatin chemotherapy. *Journal of Clinical Oncology* 21(5):927–31.

Persson, C., et al. 2005. Impact of fish oil and melatonin on cachexia in patients with advanced gastrointestinal cancer: A randomized pilot study. *Nutrition* 21(2):170–78.

Prasad, Kedar N., et al. 1999. High doses of multiple antioxidant vitamins: Essential ingredients in improving the efficacy of standard cancer therapy. *Journal of the American College of Nutrition* 18(1):13–25.

Reaney, Patricia. 2006. Anti-cancer compound in green tea identified. *Reuters Health*, March 16. (Available at www.worldhealth.net/p/243,6690.html; accessed June 6, 2006.)

Rock, Cheryl L. 2006. Dietary counseling is beneficial for the patient with cancer. *Journal of Clinical Oncology* 23(7):1348–49.

Seeley, B. M., et al. 2006. Effect of homeopathic Arnica Montana on bruising in face-lifts: Results of a randomized, double-blind, placebo-controlled clinical trial. *Connecticut Facial Plastic Surgery* 8(1):54–9 Jan-Feb.

Sener, G., et al. 2003. Melatonin ameliorates ionizing radiation-induced oxidative organ damage in rats. *Life Sciences* 74(5):563–72.

Singh, S., and A. Khar. 2006. Biological effects of curcumin and its role in cancer chemoprevention and therapy. *Anti-cancer Agents in Medicinal Chemistry* 6(3). 259–70.

Stanford Comprehensive Cancer Center. 2006. Information about cancer: Chemotherapy drugs and side effects. http://cancer.stanford.edu/information/cancerTreatment/methods /chemotherapy/ (accessed June 9, 2006).

Sterba, J., et al. 2006. Pretreatment plasma folate modulates the pharmacodynamic effect of high-dose methotrexate in children with acute lymphoblastic leukemia and non-Hodgkin lymphoma: "Folate overrescue" concept revisited. *Clinical Chemistry* 52(4):692–700.

Tamayo, C., et al. 2000. The chemistry and biological activity of herbs used in Flor-Essence herbal tonic and Essiac. *Phytotherapy Research* 14(1):1–14.

Van Bokhorst-de van der Schueren, M. A. 2005. Nutritional support strategies for malnourished cancer patients. *European Journal of Oncology Nursing* 9(suppl.2):S74–83.

Yin, L. H., et al. 2005. Role of acupuncture anesthesia in operation of rectal cancer. [In Chinese.] *Zongguo Zhen Jiu* [Chinese Acupuncture and Moxibustion] 25(12):876–88.

Yoo, H. G., et al. 2002. Induction of apoptosis by the green tea flavonol (-)-epigallocatechin-3-gallate in human endothelial cells. *Anticancer Research* 22(6A):3373–78.

Chapter Seven Healing Support after Conventional Treatment

Irwin, M. L., et al. 2008. Influence of pre-and postdiagnosis physical activity on mortality in breast cancer survivors: The health, eating, activity, and lifestyle study. *Journal of Clinical Oncology* 26(24):3958–64.

Jung-won, L., and Zebrack, B. 2004. Caring for family members with chronic physical illness: A critical review of caregiver literature. *Health Quality of Life Outcomes* 2:50.

Chemotherapy

Abd-Allah, A. R., et al. 2005. L-carnitine halts apoptosis and myelosuppression induced by carboplatin in rat bone marrow cell cultures (BMC). *Archives of Toxicology* 79(7):406–13.

Abdel-Latif, M. M., et al. 2005. Vitamin C enhances chemosensitization of esophageal cancer cells in vitro. *Journal of Chemotherapy* 17(5):539–49.

Adeyemo, D., et al. 2001. Antioxidants enhance the susceptibility of colon carcinoma cells to 5-fluorouracil by augmenting the induction of the bax protein. *Cancer Letters* 164(1):77–84.

Aebi, S., et al. 1997. All-trans retinoic acid enhances cisplatin-induced apoptosis in human ovarian adenocarcinoma and in squamous head and neck cancer cells. *Clinical Cancer Research* 3(11):2033–38.

Ahn, W. S., et al. 2004. Natural killer cell activity and quality of life were improved by consumption of a mushroom extract, *Agaricus blazei* Murill Kyowa, in gynecological cancer patients undergoing chemotherapy. *International Journal of Gynecological Cancer* 14(4):589–94.

Alleva, R., et al. 2006. Alpha-tocopheryl succinate alters cell cycle distribution sensitising human osteosarcoma cells to methotrexate-induced apoptosis. *Cancer Letters* 232(2):226–35.

Arrigoni-Martelli, E., and V. Caso. 2001. Carnitine protects mitochondria and removes toxic acyls from xenobiotics. *Drugs under Experimental and Clinical Research* 27(1):27–49.

Asaum, J. 2000. Effects of quercetin on the cell growth and the intracellular accumulation and retention of adriamycin. *Anticancer Research* 20(4):277–83.

Barni, S., et al. 1990. A study of the pineal hormone melatonin as a second line therapy in metastatic colorectal cancer resistant to fluorouracil plus folates. *Tumori* 76(1):58–60.

Bokemeyer, C., et al. 1996. Silibinin protects against cisplatin-induced nephrotoxicity without compromising cisplatin or ifosfamide anti-tumour activity. *British Journal of Cancer* 74(12):2036.

Borek, C. 2004. Antioxidants and radiation therapy. *Journal of Nutrition* 134(11):3207S–3209S.

Borek, C. 2004. Dietary antioxidants and human cancer. *Integrative Cancer Therapy* 3(4):333–41.

Borghardt, J., et al. 2000. Effects of a spleen peptide preparation as supportive therapy in inoperable head and neck cancer patients. *Arzeimittelforschung* 50(2):178–84.

Boros, L.G., Nichelatti, M., and Shoenfeld, Y. 2005. Fermented wheat germ extract (Avemar) in the treatment of cancer and autoimmune diseases. *Annals of the New York Academy of Sciences* 1051:529–42.

Brivio, F., et al. 1995. Preoperative neuroimmunotherapy with subcutaneous low-dose interleukin-2 and melatonin in patients with gastrointestinal tumors: Its efficacy in preventing surgery-induced lymphocytopenia. *Oncology Reports* 2:597–99.

Calviello, G., et al. 2005. Docosahexaenoic acid enhances the susceptibility of human colorectal cancer cells to 5-fluorouracil. *Cancer Chemotherapy and Pharmacology* 55(1):12–20.

Cerea, G., et al. 2003. Biomodulation of cancer chemotherapy for metastatic colorectal cancer: A randomized study of weekly low-dose irinotecan alone versus irinotecan plus the oncostatic pineal hormone melatonin in metastatic colorectal cancer patients progressing on 5-fluorouracil-containing combinations. *Anticancer Research* 23(2C):1951–54.

Cersosimo, R. J. 2005. Oxaliplatin-associated neuropathy: A review. *Annals of Pharmacotherapy* 39(1):128–35.

Chan, M. M., et al. 2003. Inhibition of growth and sensitization to cisplatin-mediated killing of ovarian cancer cells by polyphenolic chemopreventive agents. *Journal of Cellular Physiology* 194(1):63–70.

Chang, B., et al. 2002. L-carnitine inhibits cisplatin-induced injury of the kidney and small intestine. *Archives of Biochemistry and Biophysics* 405(1):55–64.

Cheradame, S., et al. 1997. Relevance of tumoral folylpolyglutamate synthetase and reduced folates for optimal 5-fluorouracil efficacy: Experimental data. *European Journal of Cancer* 33(6):950–59.

Choi, C. H., G. Kang, and Y. D. Min. 2003. Reversal of P-glycoprotein-mediated multidrug resistance by protopanaxatriol ginsenosides from Korean red ginseng. *Planta Medica* 69(3):235–40.

Chu, D. T., W. Wong, and G. Mavligit. 1988. Immunotherapy with Chinese medicinal herbs I. Immune restoration of local xenogeneic graft-versus-host reaction in cancer patients by fractionated *Astragalus membranaceus* in vitro. *Journal of Clinical and Laboratory Immunology* 25(3):119–23.

Chu, D. T., W. L. Wong, and G. Mavligit. 1988. Immunotherapy with Chinese medicinal herbs. II. Reversal of cyclophosphamide-induced immune suppression by administration of fractionated *Astragalus membranaceus* in vivo. *Journal of Clinical and Laboratory Immunology* 25(3):125–29.

Conklin, K. A. 2005. Coenzyme Q10 for prevention of anthracycline-induced cardiotoxicity. *Integrative Cancer Therapies* 4(2):110–30.

Daniele, B., et al. 2001. Oral glutamine in the prevention of fluorouracil induced intestinal toxicity: A double blind, placebo controlled, ramdomised trial. *Gut* 48(1):28–33.

Davis, L., and G. Kuttan. 1998. Suppressive effect of cyclophosphamide-induced toxicity by *Withania somnifera* extract in mice. *Journal of Ethnopharmacology* 62(3):209–14.

Dhanalakshmi, S., et al. 2003. Silibinin sensitizes human prostate carcinoma DU145 cells to cisplatin- and carboplatin-induced growth inhibition and apoptotic death. *International Journal of Cancer* 106(5):699–705.

Dornish, J. M., and E. O. Pettersesn. 1985. Protection from cis-dichlorodiammineplatinum-induced cell inactivation by aldehydes involves cell membrane amino groups. *Cancer Letters* 29(3):235–43.

Drisko, J. A., J. Chapman, and V. J. Hunter. 2003. The use of antioxidants with first-line chemotherapy in two cases of ovarian cancer. *Journal of the American College of Nutrition* 22(2):118–23.

Du, B., et al. 2006. Synergistic inhibitory effects of curcumin and 5-fluorouracil on the growth of the human colon cancer cell line HT-29. *Chemotherapy* 52(1):23–28.

Duan, P., and Z. M. Wang. 2002. Clinical study on effect of astragalus in efficacy enhancing and toxicity reducing of chemotherapy in patients of malignant tumor. [In Chinese.] *Zhongguo Zhong Xi Yi Jie He Za Zhi* [Chinese Journal of Integrated Traditional and Western Medicine] 22(7):515–17.

Ernst, E., and M. H. Pittler. 2000. Efficacy of ginger for nausea and vomiting: A systematic review of randomized clinical trials. *British Journal of Anaesthesia* 84(3):367–71.

Fabian, C. J., et al. 1990. Pyridoxine therapy for palmar-plantar erythrodysesthesia associated with continuous 5-fluorouracil infusion. *Investigational New Drugs* 8(1):57–63.

Fimognari, C., et al. 2006. Sulforaphane increases the efficacy of doxorubicin in mouse fibroblasts characterized by p53 mutations. *Mutation Research* 601(1–2):92–101.

Fukaya, H., and H. Kanno. 1999. Experimental studies of the protective effect of ginkgo biloba extract (GBE) on cisplatin-induced toxicity in rats. [In Japanese.] *Nippon Jibiinkoka Gakkai Kaiho* 102(7):907–17.

Gansauge, F., et al. 2002. NSC-631570 (Ukrain) in the palliative treatment of pancreatic cancer. Results of a phase II trial. *Langenbeck's Archives of Surgery* 386(8):570–74.

Gercel-Taylor, C., A. Feitelson, and D. Taylor. 2004. Inhibitory effect of genistein and daidzein on ovarian cancer cell growth. *Anticancer Research* 24(2B):795–800.

Gomez de Segura, I. A., et al. 2004. Protective effects of dietary enrichment with docosahexaenoic acid plus protein in 5-fluorouracil-induced intestinal injury in the rat. *European Journal of Gastroenterology and Hepatology* 16(5):479–85.

Hanus, B., et al. 2001. Phase II study of combined 5-fluorouracil/ginkgo biloba extract (GBE 761 ONC) therapy in 5-fluorouracil pretreated patients with advanced colorectal cancer. *Phytotherapy Research* 15(1):34–38.

Hardman, W. E. 2004. (n-3) fatty acids and cancer therapy. *Journal of Nutrition* 134(12 Suppl):3427S–3430S.

Hardman, W. E., M. P. Moyer, and I. L. Cameron. 1999. Fish oil supplementation enhanced CPT-11 (irinotecan) efficacy against MCF7 breast carcinoma xenografts and ameliorated intestinal side-effects. *British Journal of Cancer* 81(3):440–48.

Hardman, W. E., M. P. Moyer, and I. L. Cameron. 2002. Consumption of an omega-3 fatty acids product, INCELL AAFA, reduced side-effects of CPT-11 (irinotecan) in mice. *British Journal of Cancer* 86(6):983–88.

Horie, T., et al. 2001. Alleviation by garlic of antitumor drug-induced damage to the intestine. *Journal of Nutrition* 131(3s):1071S–74S.

Hrelia, S., et al. 2004. Nutritional interventions to counteract oxidative stress in cardiac cells. *Italian Journal of Biochemistry* 53(4):157–63.

Husain, K., et al. 2005. Partial protection by lipoic acid against carboplatin-induced ototoxicity in rats. *Biomedical and Environmental Sciences* 18(3):198–206.

Iino, Y., et al. 1995. Immunochemotherapies versus chemotherapy as adjuvant treatment after curative resection of operable breast cancer. *Anticancer Research* 15(6B):2907–11.

Ishikawa, Y., T. Konata, and M. Kitamura. 2000. Spontaneous shift in transcriptional profile of explanted glomeruli via activation of the MAP kinase family. *American Journal of Physiology. Renal Physiology* 279(5): F954–59.

Kalkanis, J. G., C. Whitworth, and L. P. Rybak. 2004. Vitamin E reduces cisplatin ototoxicity. *Laryngoscope* 114(3):538–42.

Karimi, G., M. Ramezani, and Z. Tahoonian. 2005. Cisplatin nephrotoxicity and protection by milk thistle extract in rats. *Evidence-Based Complementary and Alternative Medicine* 2(3):383–86.

Khoo, K. S., and P. T. Ang. 1995. Extract of *Astragalus membranaceus* and *Ligustrum lucidum* does not prevent cyclophosphamide-induced myelosuppression. *Singapore Medical Journal* 36(4):387–90.

Kim, C., et al. 2005. Modulation by melatonin of the cardiotoxic and antitumor activities of adriamycin. *Journal of Cardiovascular Pharmacology* 46(2):200–10.

Kim, S. H., et al. 1998. Suppression of multidrug resistance via inhibition of heat shock factor by quercetin in MDR crells. *Experimental and Molecular Medicine* 30(2):87–92.

Kobayashi, Y., et al. 1994. Enhancement of anti-cancer activity of cisdiaminedichloroplatinum by the protein-bound polysaccharide of *Coriolus versicolor* QUEL (PS-K) in vitro. *Cancer Biotherapy* 9(4):351–58.

Kodama, M., and T. Kodama. 2006. Four problems with the clinical control of interstitial pneumonia, or chronic fatigue syndrome, using the megadose vitamin C infusion system with dehydroepiandrosterone-cortisol annex. *In Vivo* 20(2):285–91.

Kunnumakkara, A. B., et al. 2007. Curcumin potentiates antitumor activity of gemcitabine in an orthotopic model of pancreatic cancer through suppression of proliferation, angiogenesis, and inhibition of nuclear factor kappa B–regulated gene products. *Cancer Research* 67(8):3853–61.

Kurz, E., P. Douglas, and S. P. Lees-Miller. 2004. Doxorubicin activates ATM-dependent phosphorylation of multiple downstream targets in part through the generation of reactive oxygen species. *Journal of Biological Chemistry* 279(51):53272–81.

Leonetti, C., et al. 2003. Alpha-tocopherol protects against cisplatin-induced toxicity without interfering with antitumor efficacy. *International Journal of Cancer* 104(2):243–50.

Lissoni, P., et al. 1999. Decreased toxicity and increased efficacy of cancer chemotherapy using the pineal hormone melatonin in metastatic solid tumour patients with poor clinical status. *European Journal of Cancer* 35(12):1688–92.

Lissoni, P., et al. 2003. Five years survival in metastatic non-small cell lung cancer patients treated with chemotherapy alone or chemotherapy and melatonin: A randomized trial. *Journal of Pineal Research* 35(1):12–15.

Madhavi, N., and U. Das. 1994. Effect of n-6 and n-3 fatty acids on the survival of vincristine sensitive and resistant human cervical carcinoma cells in vitro. *Cancer Letters* 84(1):31–41.

Manusirivithaya, S., et al. 2004. Antiemetic effect of ginger in gynecologic oncology patients receiving cisplatin. *International Journal of Gynecological Cancer* 14(6):1063–69.

Marone, M., et al. 2001. Quercetin abrogates taxol-mediated signaling by inhibiting multiple kinases. *Experimental Cell Research* 270(1):1–12.

Masuda, M., M. Suzui, and I. B. Weinstein. 2001. Effects of epigallocatechin-3-gallate on growth, epidermal growth factor receptor signaling pathways, gene expression, and chemosensitivity in human head and neck squamous cell carcinoma cell lines. *Clinical Cancer Research* 7(12):4220–29.

Masuda, M., et al. 2003. Epigallocatechin-3-gallate inhibits activation of HER-2/neu and downstream signaling pathways in human head and neck and breast carcinoma cells. *Clinical Cancer Research* 9(9):3486–91.

Mathijssen, R. H., et al. 2002. Effects of St. John's wort on irinotecan metabolism. *Journal of the National Cancer Institute* 94(16):1247–49.

McCulloch, M., et al. 2006. Astragalus-based Chinese herbs and platinum-based chemotherapy for advanced non-small-cell lung cancer: Meta-analysis of randomized trials. *Journal of Clinical Oncology* 24(3):419–30.

Menendez, J. A., et al. 2001. Effects of gamma-linolenic acid and oleic acid on paclitaxel cytotoxicity in human breast cancer cells. *European Journal of Cancer* 37(3):402–13.

Menendez, J. A., R. Lupu, and R. Colomer. 2005. Exogenous supplementation with omega-3 polyunsaturated fatty acid docosahexaenoic acid (DHA; 22:6n-3) synergistically enhances taxane cytotoxicity and downregulates Her-2/neu (c-erbB-2) oncogene expression in human breast cancer cells. *European Journal of Cancer Prevention* 14(3):263–70.

Michael, M., et al. 2004. Phase II study of activated charcoal to prevent irinotecan-induced diarrhea. *Journal of Clinical Oncology* 22(21):4410–17.

Mimoto, T., et al. 1992. Randomized controlled study on adjuvant immunochemotherapy with PSK in curatively resected colorectal cancer. The Cooperative Study Group of Surgical Adjuvant Immunochemotherapy for Cancer of Colon and Rectum (Kanagawa). *Diseases of the Colon and Rectum* 35(2):123–30.

Mitsugi, K., et al. 2004. Protection against methotrexate toxicity by a soybean protein– and omega-3 fatty acid–containing diet: Comparative study with a casein-containing diet. *Oncology Reports* 12(1):41–45.

Miyoshi, N., et al. 2005. Alpha-tocopherol-mediated caspase-3 up-regulation enhances susceptibility to apoptotic stimuli. *Biochemical and Biophysical Research Communications* 334(2):466–73.

Mollui, J., et al. 2000. Membrane associated antitumor effects of crocine-, ginsenoside- and cannabinoid derivates. *Anticancer Research* 20(2A):861–67.

Mushiake, H., et al. 2005. Dendritic cells might be one of key factors for eliciting antitumor effect by chemoimmunotherapy in vivo. *Cancer Immunology, Immunotherapy* 54(2):120–28.

Navarro-Peran, E., et al. 2005. The antifolate activity of tea catechins. *Cancer Research* 65(6):2059–64.

Norsa, A., and V. Martino. 2006. Somatostatin, retinoids, melatonin, vitamin D, bromocriptine, and cyclophosphamide in advanced non-small-cell lung cancer patients with low performance status. *Cancer Biotherapy and Radiopharmacology* 21(1):68.

Osmak, M., et al. 1997. Ascorbic acid and 6-deoxy-6-chloro-ascorbic acid: Potential anticancer drugs. *Neoplasma* 44(2):101–7.

Ozturk, G., et al. 2004. The effect of ginkgo extract EGb761 in cisplatin-induced peripheral neuropathy in mice. *Toxicology and Applied Pharmacology* 196(1):169–75.

Pace, A., et al. 2003. Neuroprotective effect of vitamin E supplementation in patients treated with cisplatin chemotherapy. *Journal of Clinical Oncology* 21(5):927–31.

Pathak, A. K., et al. 2002. Potentiation of the effect of paclitaxel and carboplatin by antioxidant mixture on human lung cancer h520 cells. *Journal of the American College of Nutrition* 21(5):416–21.

Plouzek, C. A., et al. 1999. Inhibition of P-glycoprotein activity and reversal of multidrug resistance in vitro by rosemary extract. *European Journal of Cancer* 35(10):1541–45.

Qian, Z. M., M. F. Xu, and P. L. Tang. 1997. Polysaccharide peptide (PSP) restores immunosuppression induced by cyclophosphamide in rats. *American Journal of Chinese Medicine* 25(1):27–35.

Recchia, F., et al. 1999. Chemo-immunotherapy in advanced head and neck cancer. *Anticancer Research* 19(1B):773–77.

Reddy, V., N. Khana, and N. Singh. 2001. Vitamin C augments chemotherapeutic response of cervical carcinoma HeLa cells by stabilizing P53. *Biochemical and Biophysical Research Communications* 282(2):409–15.

Rockwell, S., Y. Liu, and S. A. Higgins. 2005. Alteration of the effects of cancer therapy agents on breast cancer cells by the herbal medicine black cohosh. *Breast Cancer Research and Treatment* 90(3):233–39.

Roffe, L., K. Schmidt, E. Ernest. 2005. A systemic review of guided imagery as an adjuvant cancer therapy. *Psychooncology* 14(8):607–17.

Sadzuka, Y., et al. 2002. Glutamate transporter mediated increase of antitumor activity by theanine, an amino acid in green tea. [In Japanese.] *Yakugaku Zasshi* [Journal of the Pharmaceutical Society of Japan] 122(11):995–99.

Sadzuka, Y., T. Sugiyama, and S. Hirota. 1998. Modulation of cancer chemotherapy by green tea. *Clinical Cancer Research* 4(1):153–56.

Sallman, D.A., et al. 2007. Clusterin mediates TRAIL resistance in prostate tumor cells. *Molecular Cancer Therapy* 6(11):2938–47.

Sato, M., et al. 2000. SAPKs regulation of ischemic preconditioning. *American Journal of Physiology. Heart and Circulatory Physiology* 279(3):H901–7.

Saunders, D. E., et al. 1993. Additive inhibition of RL95-2 endometrial carcinoma cell growth by carboplatin and 1,25 dihydroxyvitamin D3. *Gynecologic Oncology* 51(2):155–59.

Sayed-Ahmed, M. M., et al. 1999. Reversal of doxorubicin-induced cardiac metabolic damage by L-carnitine. *Pharmacological Research* 39(4):289–95.

Sayed-Ahmed, M. M., et al. 2004. Progression of cisplatin-induced nephrotoxicity in a carnitine-depleted rat model. *Chemotherapy* 50(4):162–70.

Scherwitz, L.W., P. McHenry, and R. Herrero. 2005. Interactive guided imagery therapy with medical patients: Predictors of health outcomes. *Journal of Alternative and Complementary Medicine* 11(1):69–83.

Senturker, S., et al. 2002. Induction of apoptosis by chemotherapeutic drugs without generation of reactive oxygen species. *Archives of Biochemistry and Biophysics* 397(2):262–72.

Sharma, S., and Y. Gupta. 1998. Reversal of cisplatin-induced delay in gastric emptying in rats by ginger (*Zingiber officinale*). *Journal of Ethnopharmacology* 62(1):49–55.

Shiroky, J. B. 1997. The use of folates concomitantly with low-dose pulse methotrexate. *Rheumatic Disease Clinics of North America* 23(4):969–80.

Sluitz, G., et al. 1996. Drug resistance against gemcitabine and topotecan mediated by constuitive hsp70 overexpression in vitro: Implication of quercetin as sensitiser in chemotherapy. *British Journal of Cancer* 74(2):172–7.

Sreerama, L., and N. Sladek. 2001. Primary breast tumor levels of suspected molecular determinants of cellular sensitivity to cyclophosphamide, ifosfamide, and certain other anticancer agents as predictors of paired metastatic tumor levels of these determinants: Rational individualization of cancer chemotherapeutic regimens. *Cancer Chemotherapy and Pharmacology* 47(3):255–62.

Suh, S. O., et al. 2002. Effects of red ginseng upon postoperative immunity and survival in patients with stage III gastric cancer. *American Journal of Chinese Medicine* 30(4):483–94.

Takahashi, Y., and M. Mai. 2001. Chemotherapy by combination of low-dose CPT-11 and PSK in an elderly man with liver metastasis from gastric cancer. [In Japanese.] *Gan To Kagaku Ryoho* [Cancer and Chemotherapy] 28(4):531–34.

Teicher, B. A., et al. 1994. In vivo modulation of several anticancer agents by beta-carotene. *Cancer Chemotherapy and Pharmacology* 34(3):235–41.

Tomita, Y., et al. 1982. Combined treatments with vitamin A and 5-fluorouracil and the growth of allotransplantable and syngeneic tumors in mice. *Journal of the National Cancer Institute* 68(5):823–27.

Tyagi, A. K., et al. 2004. Synergistic anti-cancer effects of silibinin with conventional cytotoxic agents doxorubicin, cisplatin and carboplatin against human breast carcinoma MCF-7 and MDA-MB468 cells. *Oncology Reports* 11(2):493–99.

Urayama, S., et al. 2000. Effect of vitamin K2 on osteoblast apoptosis: Vitamin K2 inhibits apoptotic cell death of human osteoblasts induced by Fas, proteasome inhibitor, etoposide, and staurosporine. *Journal of Laboratory and Clinical Medicine* 136(3):181–93.

Vahdat, L., et al. 2001. Reduction of paclitaxel-induced peripheral neuropathy with glutamine. *Clinical Cancer Research* 7(5):1192–97.

Van Rensburg, C., G. Joone, and R. Anderson. 1998. Alpha-tocopherol antagonizes the multidrug-resistance-reversal activity of cyclosporin A, verapamil, GF120918, clofazimine and B669. *Cancer Letters* 127(1–2):107–12.

Von Bultzingslowen, I., et al. 2003. Oral and intestinal microflora in 5-fluorouracil treated rats, translocation to cervical and mesenteric lymph nodes and effects of probiotic bacteria. *Oral Microbiology and Immunology* 18(5):278–84.

Vukelja, S. J., et al. 1993. Pyridoxine therapy for palmar-plantar erythrodysesthesia associated with taxotere. *Journal of the National Cancer Institute* 85(17):1432–33.

Wakui, A., et al. 1986. Randomized study of lentinan on patients with advanced gastric and colorectal cancer. Tohoku lentinan study group. [In Japanese.] *Gan To Kagaku Ryoho* [Cancer and Chemotherapy] 13(4 Pt 1):1050–59.

Walsky, R. L., E. A. Gaman, and R. S. Obach. 2005. Examination of 209 drugs for inhibition of cytochrome P450 2C8. *Journal of Clinical Pharmacology* 45(1):68–78.

Wan, J. M., W. H. Sit, and J. C. Louie. 2008. Polysaccharopeptide enhances the anticancer activity of doxorubicin and etoposide on human breast cancer cells ZR-75-30. *International Journal of Oncology* 32(3):680–99.

Wang, W. S., et al. 2007. Oral glutamine for prevention oxaliplatin-induced neuropathy in colorectal patients. *Oncology* 12(11):1371–2.

Wigington, D. P., et al. 2004. Combination study of 1,24(S)-dihydroxyvitamin D2 and chemotherapeutic agents on human breast and prostate cancer cell lines. *Anticancer Research* 24(5A):2905–12.

Willcox, J. C., et al. 1986. Effects of magnesium supplementation in testicular cancer patients receiving cis-platin: A randomised trial. *British Journal of Cancer* 54(1):19–23.

Yoshida, T., et al. 2003. Apoptosis induction of vitamin K2 in lung carcinoma cell lines: The possibility of vitamin K2 therapy for lung cancer. *International Journal of Oncology* 23(3):627–32.

Yun, J., Tomida, A., Nagata, K., and Tsuruo, T. 1995. Glucose-regulated stresses confer resistance to VP-16 in human cancer cells through a decreased expression of DNA topoisomerase II. *Oncology Research* 7(12):583–90.

Zerourga, M., W. Stillwell, and L. Jenski. 2002. Synthesis of a novel phosphatidylcholine conjugated to docosahexaenoic acid and methotrexate that inhibits cell proliferation. *Anticancer Drugs* 13(3):301–11.

Zhao, K., C. Mancini, and G. Doria. 1990. Enhancement of the immune response in mice by *Astragalus membranaceus* extracts. *Immunopharmacology* 20:225–34.

Radiation

Bairati, I. 2005. Randomized trial of antioxidant vitamins to prevent acute adverse effects of radiation therapy in head and neck cancer patients. *Journal of Clinical Oncology* 23(24):5805–13.

Delia, P., et al. 2007. Use of probiotics for prevention of radiation-induced diarrhea. *World Journal of Gastroenterology* 13(6):912–15.

Jagetia, G. C., and G. K. Rajanikant. 2005. Curcumin treatment enhances the repair and regeneraton of wounds in mice exposed to hemibody gamma radiation. *Plastic Reconstructive Surgery* 115(2):515–28.

Khaff, A., et al. 2005. Curcumin: A new radio-sensitizer of squamous cell carcinoma cells. *Otolaryngology Head Neck Surgery* 132(2):317–21.

Lissoni, P., M. A. Galli, G. Tancini, and S. Barni. 1993. Prevention by L-carnatine of interleukin-2 related cardiac toxicity during cancer immunotherapy. *Tomorii* 79(3):202–204.

Rezvani, M., and G. A. Ross. 2004. Modification of radiation-induced acute oral mucositis in the rat. *International Journal of Radiation Biology* 80(2):177–82.

Hormonal and Targeted Therapies

Almstrup, K., et al. 2002. Dual effects of phytoestrogens result in U-shaped dose-response curves. *Environmental Health Perspectives* 110(8):743–48.

Babu, J. R., et al. 2000. Salubrious effect of vitamin C and vitamin E on tamoxifen-treated women in breast cancer with reference to plasma lipid and lipoprotein levels. *Cancer Letters* 151(1):1–5.

Barton, D. L., et al. 1998. Prospective evaluation of vitamin E for hot flashes in breast cancer survivors. *Journal of Clinical Oncology* 16(2):495–500.

Brooks, J. D., and L. U. Thompson. 2005. Mammalian lignans and genistein decrease the activities of aromatase and 17beta-hydroxysteroid dehydrogenase in MCF-7 cells. *Journal of Steroid Biochemistry and Molecular Biology* 94(5):461–67.

Chen, J., et al. 2004. Dietary flaxseed enhances the inhibitory effect of tamoxifen on the growth of estrogen-dependent human breast cancer (MCF-7) in nude mice. *Clinical Cancer Research* 10(22):7703–11.

Chisolm, K., B. J. Bray, and R. J. Rosengren. 2004. Tamoxifen and epigallocatechin gallate are synergistically cytotoxic to MDA-MB-231 human breast cancer cells. *Anti-cancer Drugs* 15(9):889–97.

Clover, A., and D. Ratsey. 2002. Homeopathic treatment of hot flushes: A pilot study. *Homeopathy* 91(2):75–79.

Constantinou, A. I., et al. 2005. The soy isoflavone daidzein improves the capacity of tamoxifen to prevent mammary tumours. *European Journal of Cancer* 41(4):647–54.

DeGraffenried, L. A., et al. 2003. Eicosapentaenoic acid restores tamoxifen sensitivity in breast cancer cells with high AKT activity. *Annals of Oncology* 14(7):1051–56.

Eddy, S. F., S. E. Kane, and G. E. Sonenshein. 2007. Trastuzumag-resistant HER2-driven breast cancer cells are sensitive to epigallocatechin-3 gallate. *Cancer Res* 67(19):9018–23.

El-Beshbishy, H. A. 2005. Hepatoprotective effect of green tea (*Camellia sinensis*) extract against tamoxifen-induced liver injury in rats. *Journal of Biochemistry and Molecular Biology* 38(5):563–70.

Eng, E. T., et al. 2003. Suppression of estrogen biosynthesis by procyanidin dimers in red wine and grape seeds. *Cancer Research* 63(23):8516–22.

Golden, E. B., et al. 2009. Green tea polyphenols block the anticancer effects of bortezomib and other boronic acid-based proteasome inhibitors. *Blood* 113(23):5927–37.

Hardman, W. E. 2004. (n-3) fatty acids and cancer therapy. *Journal of Nutrition* 134(12 Suppl):3427S–3430S.

Hedlund, T. E., W. U. Johannes, and G. J. Miller. 2003. Soy isoflavonoid equol modulates the growth of benign and malignant prostatic epithelial cells in vitro. *Prostate* 54(1):68–78.

Jacobson, J. S., et al. 2001. Randomized trial of black cohosh for the treatment of hot flashes among women with a history of breast cancer. *Journal of Clinical Oncology* 19(10):2739–45.

Ju, Y. H., et al. 2002. Dietary genistein negates the inhibitory effect of tamoxifen on growth of estrogen-dependent human breast cancer (MCF-7) cells implanted in athymic mice. *Cancer Research* 62(9):2474–77.

Katchamart, S., et al. 2000. Concurrent flavin-containing monooxygenase down-regulation and cytochrome P-450 induction by dietary indoles in rat: Implications for drug-drug interaction. *Drug Metabolism and Disposition* 28(8):930–36.

Katchamart, S., et al. 2001. Indole-3-carbinol modulation of hepatic monooxygenases CYP1A2 and FMO1 in guinea pig, mouse and rabbit. *Comparitive Biochemical and Physiological C Toxicology and Pharmacology* 129(4):377–84.

Kenny, F. S., et al. 2000. Gamma linolenic acid with tamoxifen as primary therapy in breast cancer. *International Journal of Breast Cancer* 85(5):643–48.

Le Bail, J. C., et al. 2001. Chalcones are potent inhibitors of aromatase and 17 beta-hydroxysteroid dehydrogenase activities. *Life Sciences* 68(7):751–61.

Lissoni, P., et al. 1995. Modulation of cancer endocrine therapy by melatonin: A phase II study of tamoxifen plus melatonin in metastatic breast cancer patients progressing under tamoxifen alone. *British Journal of Cancer* 71(4):854–56.

Lissoni, P., et al. 1996. A phase II study of tamoxifen plus melatonin in metastatic solid tumour patients. *British Journal of Cancer* 74(9):1466–68.

Liu, B., et al. 2005. Low-dose dietary phytoestrogen abrogates tamoxifen-associated mammary tumor prevention. *Cancer Research* 65(3):879–86.

Liu, F. T., et al. 2008. Dietary flavonoids inhibit the anticancer effects of the proteasome inhibitor bortezomib. *Blood* 112(9):3835–46.

Mahady, G. B., et al. 2002. Black cohosh: An alternative therapy for menopause? *Nutrition in Clinical Care* 5(6):283–89.

Marcsek, Z., et al. 2004. The efficacy of tamoxifen in estrogen receptor-positive breast cancer cells is enhanced by a medical nutriment. *Cancer Biotherapy and Radiopharmaceuticals* 19(6):746–53.

Menendez, J. A., L. Vellon, R. Colomer, and R. Lupu. 2005. Effect of gamma-linolenic acid on the transcriptional activity of the Her-2/neu (erbB-2) oncogene. *J Natl Cancer Inst* 97(21):1611–5.

Morris, K. T., et al. 2001. High dehydroepiandrosterone-sulfate predicts breast cancer progression during new aromatase inhibitor therapy and stimulates breast cancer cell growth in tissue culture: A renewed role for adrenalectomy. *Surgery* 130(6):947–53.

Nisslein, T., and J. Freudenstein. 2004. Concomitant administration of an iso-propanolic extract of black cohosh and tamoxifen in the in vivo tumor model of implanted RUCA-I rat endometrial adenocarcinoma cells. *Toxicology Letters* 150(3):271–75.

Parkin, D. R., and D. Malejka-Giganti. 2004. Differences in the hepatic P450-dependent metabolism of estrogen and tamoxifen in response to treatment of rats with 3,3'-diindolylmethane and its parent compound indole-3-carbinol. *Cancer Detection and Prevention* 28(1):72–79.

Perumal, S. S., P. Shanthi, and P. Sachdanandam. 2005. Augmented efficacy of tamoxifen in rat breast tumorigenesis when gavaged along with riboflavin, niacin, and CoQ10: Effects on lipid peroxidation and antioxidants in mitochondria. *Chemico-Biological Interactions* 152(1):49–58.

Perumal, S. S., P. Shanthi, and P. Sachdanandam. 2005. Combined efficacy of tamoxifen and coenzyme Q10 on the status of lipid peroxidation and antioxidants in DMBA induced breast cancer. *Molecular and Cellular Biochemistry* 273(1–2):151–60.

Satoh, K., et al. 2002. Inhibition of aromatase activity by green tea extract catechins and their endocrinological effects of oral administration in rats. *Food and Chemical Toxicology* 40(7):925–33.

Shah, Y. M., et al. 2005. Selenium disrupts estrogen receptor (alpha) signaling and potentiates tamoxifen antagonism in endometrial cancer cells and tamoxifen-resistant breast cancer cells. *Molecular Cancer Therapeutics* 4(8):1239–49.

Tamir, S., et al. 2000. Estrogenic and antiproliferative properties of glabridin from licorice in human breast cancer cells. *Cancer Research* 60(20):5704–9.

Thompson, E. A., and D. Reilly. 2003. The homeopathic approach to the treatment of symptoms of oestrogen withdrawal in breast cancer patients. A prospective observational study. *Homeopathy* 92(3):131–34.

Way, T. D., et al. 2004. Black tea polyphenol theaflavins inhibit aromatase activity and attenuate tamoxifen resistance in HER2/neu-transfected human breast cancer cells through tyrosine kinase suppression. *European Journal of Cancer* 40(14):2165–74.

Welsh, J. 1994. Induction of apoptosis in breast cancer cells in response to vitamin D and anti-estrogens. *Biochemistry and Cell Biology* 72(11–12):537–45.

Yuvaraj, S., et al. 2009. Effect of coenzyme Q(10), riboflavin and niacin on tamoxifen treated postmenopausal breast cancer women with special reference to blood chemistry profiles. *Breast Cancer Research and Treatment* 114(2):377–84.

Zeitlin, L., et al. 2003. Effects of long-term administration of N-3 polyunsaturated fatty acids (PUFA) and selective estrogen receptor modulator (SERM) derivatives in ovariectomized (OVX) mice. *Journal of Cellular Biochemistry* 90(2):347–60.

Integrative Cancer Care Supplement Guide
and Questionable Alternatives Charts

Al-Sukhni, W., A. Grunbaum, and N. Fleshner. 2005. Remission of hormone-refractory prostate cancer attributed to Essiac. *Canadian Journal of Urology* 12(5):2841–42.

American Cancer Society. 2002. *Complementary and Alternative Cancer Methods Handbook.* Atlanta, GA: American Cancer Society.

American Cancer Society. 2006. Making treatment decisions: Venus flytrap. www.cancer.org /docroot/ETO/content/ETO_5_3X_Venus_Flytrap.asp (accessed June 14, 2006).

Bennett, M. J., et al. 2005. Hyperbaric oxygenation for tumour sensitisation to radiotherapy. *Cochrane Database of Systematic Reviews* no. 4: CD005007.

Boros, Laszlo G., Michelle Nichelatti, and Yehuda Shoenfeld. 2005. Fermented wheat germ extract (Avemar) in the treatment of cancer and autoimmune diseases. *Annals of the New York Academy of Sciences* 1051:529–42.

Cancer Research UK. 2006. What are cellular zeolites? www.cancerhelp.org.uk/help/default .asp?page=19399 (accessed June 14, 2006).

Cao, G. W., W. G. Yang, and P. Du. 1994. Observation of the effects of LAK/IL-2 therapy combining with *Lycium barbarum* polysaccharides in the treatment of 75 cancer patients. [In Chinese.] *Zhonghua Zhong Liu Za Zhi* [Chinese Journal of Oncology] 16(6):428–31.

Cassileth, B., and C. Lucarelli. 2003. *Herb-Drug Interactions in Oncology.* Hamilton, Ontario: B. C. Decker.

Centano, J. A., et al. 2003. Blood and tissue concentration of cesium after exposure to cesium chloride: A report of two cases. *Biological Trace Element Research* 94(2):97–104.

Cheung, S., K. T. Lim, and J. Tai. 2005. Antioxidant and anti-inflammatory properties of Essiac and Flor-Essence. *Oncology Reports* 14(5):1345–50.

Dabrosin, C., et al. 2002. Flaxseed inhibits metastasis and decreases extracellular vascular endothelial growth factor in human breast cancer xenografts. *Cancer Letters* 185(1):31–37.

Dalal, A. K., J. D. Harding, and R. J. Verdino. 2004. Acquired long QT syndrome and monomorphic ventricular tachycardia after alternative treatment with cesium chloride for brain cancer. *Mayo Clinic Proceedings* 79(8):1065–69.

Dandekar, D. S., et al. 2003. An orally active Amazonian plant extract (BIRM) inhibits prostate cancer growth and metastasis. *Cancer Chemotherapy and Pharmacology* 52(1):59–66.

Ernst, E. 2001. A primer of complementary and alternative medicine commonly used by cancer patients. *Medical Journal of Australia* 174(2):88–92.

Ghoneum, M., and S. Abedi. 2004. Enhancement of natural killer cell activity of aged mice by modified arabinoxylan rice bran (MGN-3/Biobran). *Journal of Pharmacy and Pharmacology* 56(12):1581–88.

Ghoneum, M., and S. Gollapudi. 2005. Modified arabinoxylan rice bran (MGN-3/Biobran) enhances yeast-induced apoptosis in human breast cancer cells in vitro. *Anticancer Research* 25(2A):859–70.

Green, Saul. 2001. Oxygenation therapy: Unproven treatments for cancer and AIDS. *Quackwatch*, June 21. www.quackwatch.org/01QuackeryRelatedTopics/Cancer/oxygen.html (accessed November 15, 2006).

Guns, E. S., et al. 2005. pH modulation using CsCl enhances therapeutic effects of vitamin D in LNCaP tumor bearing mice. *Prostate* 64(3):316–22.

Hainer, M. I., et al. 2000. Fatal hepatorenal failure associated with hydrazine sulfate. *Annals of Internal Medicine* 133(11):877–80.

Hathcock, J., et al. 2007. Risk assessment for vitamin D. *American Journal of Clinical Nutrition* 85(1): 6–18.

Hildenbrand, G. L., et al. 1995. Five-year survival rates of melanoma patients treated by diet therapy after the manner of Gerson: A retrospective review. *Alternative Therapies in Health and Medicine* 1(4):29–37.

Hong, F., et al. 2004. Mechanism by which orally administered b-1,3-glucans enhance the tumoricidal activity of antitumor monoclonal antibodies in murine tumor models. *Journal of Immunology* 173(2):797–806.

Iino, Y., et al. 1995. Immunochemotherapies versus chemotherapy as adjuvant treatment after curative resection of operable breast cancer. *Anticancer Research* 15(6B):2907–11.

Josefson, Deborah. 2000. U.S. Cancer Institute funds trial of complementary therapy. *Western Journal of Medicine* 173(3):153–54.

Jung, K. O., S. Y. Park, and K. Y. Park. 2006. Longer aging time increases the anticancer and antimetastatic properties of doenjang. *Nutrition* 22(5):539–45.

Kaegi, Elizabeth. 1998. Unconventional therapies for cancer: 1. Essiac. *Canadian Medical Association Journal* 158(7):897–902.

Kelly, G. S. 1999. Larch arabinogalactan: Clinical relevance of a novel immune-enhancing polysaccharide. *Alternative Medicine Review* 4(2):96–103.

Kim, L. S., R. F. Waters, and P. M. Burkholder. 2002. Immunological activity of larch arabinogalactan and *Echinacea*: A preliminary, randomized, double-blind, placebo-controlled trial. *Alternative Medicine Review* 7(2):138–49.

Klein, A., et al. 2006. Prolonged stabilization of platinum-resistant ovarian cancer in a single patient consuming a fermented soy therapy. *Gynecologic Oncology* 100(1):205–9.

Kuhlman, M. K., et al. 1998. Reduction of cisplatin toxicity in cultured renal tubular cells by the bioflavonoid quercetin. *Archives of Toxicology* 72(8):536–40.

Kulp, K. S., et al. 2006. Essiac and Flor-Essence herbal tonics stimulate the in vitro growth of human breast cancer cells. *Breast Cancer Research and Treatment* 98(3):249–59.

Leonard, S. S., et al. 2006. Essiac tea: Scavenging of reactive oxygen species and effects on DNA damage. *Journal of Ethnopharmacology* 103(2):288–96.

Levy, R. L., and N. R. Miller. 2006. Hyperbaric oxygen therapy for radiation-induced optic neuropathy. *Annals of the Academy of Medicine, Singapore* 35(30):151–57.

Lissoni, P., et al. 1996. Adjuvant therapy with the pineal hormone melatonin in patients with lymph node relapse due to malignant melanoma. *Journal of Pineal Research* 21(4):239–42.

Lissoni, P., et al. 1997. A randomized study of chemotherapy with cisplatin plus etoposide versus chemoendocrine therapy with cisplatin, etoposide and the pineal hormone melatonin as a first-line treatment of advanced non-small cell lung cancer patients in a poor clinical state. *Journal of Pineal Research* 23(1):15–19.

Loprinzi, C. L., et al. 2005. Evaluation of shark cartilage in patients with advanced cancer: A North Central Cancer Treatment Group trial. *Cancer* 104(1):176–82.

Marcsek, Z., et al. 2004. The efficacy of tamoxifen in estrogen receptor-positive breast cancer cells is enhanced by a medical nutriment. *Cancer Biotherapy and Radiopharmaceuticals* 19(6):746–53.

Marett, R., and J. L. Slavin. 2004. No long-term benefits of supplementation with arabinogalactan on serum lipids and glucose. *Journal of the American Dietetic Association* 104(4):636–39.

Milazzo, S., et al. 2006. Laetrile treatment for cancer. *Cochrane Database of Systematic Reviews* no. 2: CD005476.

Moss, Ralph W. 2003. A friendly skeptic looks at graviola. *Moss Reports*, August 29. (Available at http://chetday.com/gojijuice.htm; accessed November 15, 2006.)

Moss, Ralph W. 2003. A friendly skeptic looks at poly MVA, part two. *Moss Reports*, October 24.

Moss, Ralph W. 2004. A friendly skeptic looks at goji. *Moss Reports*, November 21.

Mueller, B. A., et al. 2000. Noni juice (*Morinda citrifolia*): Hidden potential for hyperkalemia? *American Journal of Kidney Disease* 35(2):330–32.

Murali, P. M., et al. 2006. Plant-based formulation in the management of chronic obstructive pulmonary disease: A randomized double-blind study. *Respiratory Medicine* 100(1):39–45.

Nakazato, H., et al. 1994. Efficacy of immunochemotherapy as adjuvant treatment after curative resection of gastric cancer: Study group of immunochemotherapy with PSK for gastric cancer. *Lancet* 344(8917):274.

National Cancer Institute. 2006. Cancell/Entelev. www.cancernet.nci.nih.gov/cancertopics/pdq/cam/cancell/healthprofessional (accessed June 12, 2006).

National Cancer Institute. 2006. Complementary and alternative medicine. www.cancernet.nci.nih.gov/cancertopics/pdq/cam (accessed May 9, 2006).

National Cancer Institute. 2006. Essiac/Flor-Essence. www.cancernet.nci.nih.gov/cancertopics/pdq/cam/essiac/healthprofessional (accessed June 16, 2006).

National Cancer Institute. 2006. Gonalez regimen. www.cancer.gov/cancertopics/pdq/cam/gonzalez/patient (accessed June 14, 2006).

National Cancer Institute. 2006. Hydrazine sulfate. www.cancernet.nci.nih.gov/cancertopics/pdq/cam/hydrazinesulfate/patient (accessed November 15, 2006).

National Cancer Institute. 2006. Laetrile/amygdalin. www.cancernet.nci.nih.gov/cancertopics/pdq/cam/laetrile (accessed November 15, 2006).

National Center for Complementary and Alternative Medicine. 2004. Consumer advisory: Coral calcium. www.nccam.nih.gov/health/alerts/coral/coral.htm (accessed June, 16, 2006).

Navis, I., P. Sriganth, and B. Premalatha. 1999. Dietary curcumin with cisplatin administration modulates tumour marker indices in experimental fibrosarcoma. *Pharmacological Research* 39(3):175–79.

Neri, B., et al. 1998. Melatonin as biological response modifier in cancer patients. *Anticancer Research* 18(2B):1329–32.

Nicholas, R. L., E. U. Choe, and C. B. Weldon. 2005. Mechanical and antibacterial bowel preparation in colon and rectal surgery. *Chemotherapy* 51(suppl.1):115–21.

Ohuchi, Y., et al. 2005. Decrease in size of azoxymethane induced colon carcinoma in F344 rats by 180-day fermented miso. *Oncology Reports* 14(6):1559–64.

Ottenweller, J., et al. 2004. Inhibition of prostate cancer-cell proliferation by Essiac. *Journal of Alternative and Complementary Medicine* 10(4):687–91.

PDR Health. Larch arabinogalactan. www.pdrhealth.com/drug_info/nmdrugprofiles/nutsupdrugs/lar_0320.shtml (accessed June 16, 2006).

Questionable methods of cancer management: Cancell/Entelev. 1993. *CA: A Cancer Journal for Clinicians* 43(1):57–62.

Reinhold, Vieth, Pak-Cheung R. Chan, and Gordon D. MacFarlane. 2001. Efficacy and safety of vitamin D3 intake exceeding the lowest observed adverse effect level. *American Journal of Clinical Nutrition* 73: 288-94.

Rickard, S. E., et al. 1999. Dose effects of flaxseed and its lignan on N-methyl-N-nitrosourea-induced mammary tumorigenesis in rats. *Nutrition and Cancer* 35(1):50–57.

Robinson, R. R., J. Freitag, and J. L. Slavin. 2001. Effects of dietary arabinogalactan on gastrointestinal and blood parameters in healthy human subjects. *Journal of the American College of Nutrition* 20(4):279–85.

Sartori, H. E. 1984. Cesium therapy in cancer patients. *Pharmacology, Biochemistry, and Behavior* 21(suppl.1):11–13.

Seljelid, R. 1986. A water-soluble aminated beta 1-3D-glucan derivative causes regression of solid tumors in mice. *Bioscience Reports* 6(9):845–51.

Sparreboom, A., et al. 2004. Herbal remedies in the United States: Potential adverse interactions with anticancer agents. *Journal of Clinical Oncology* 22(12):2489–503.

Suchard, J. R., K. L. Wallace, and R. D. Gerkin. 1998. Acute cyanide toxicity caused by apricot kernel ingestion. *Annals of Emergency Medicine* 32(6):742–44.

Tamayo, C., et al. 2000. The chemistry and biological activity of herbs used in Flor-Essence herbal tonic and Essiac. *Phytotherapy Research* 14(1):1–14.

UC Berkeley Wellness Letter. 2006. Can mangosteen juice cure cancer, migraines, and other conditions, as claimed? University of California Berkeley Health Letter, February. www .wellnessletter.com/html/wl/2006/wlAskExperts0206.html (accessed November 16, 2006).

Wilson, H. D., J. R. Wilson, and P. N. Fuchs. 2006. Hyperbaric oxygen treatment decreases inflammation and mechanical hypersensitivity in an animal model of inflammatory pain. *Brain Research* 1098(1):126–28.

Zarkovic, N., et al. 2003. Anticancer and antioxidative effects of micronized zeolite clinoptilolite. *Anticancer Research* 23(2B):1589–95.

Chapter Eight Immune System

Alschuler, Lise. 2002. Pathophysiology of stress: Implications for chronic disease management. Presentation given at the American Academy of Nurse Practitioners annual conference.

American Autoimmune Related Diseases Association. 1999. Autoimmune disease in women—The facts. www.aarda.org/women.html (accessed June 20, 2006).

American Cancer Society. 2005. Cancer vaccines. www.cancer.org/docroot/ETO/content /ETO_1_4X_Cancer_Vaccines_Active_Specific_Immunotherapies.asp?sitearea=ETO (accessed July 4, 2006).

American Cancer Society. 2006. HPV vaccine approved: Prevents cervical cancer. *ACS New Center*, June 8. www.cancer.org/docroot/NWS/content/NWS_1_1x_HPV_Vaccine _Approved_Prevents_Cervical_Cancer.asp (accessed June 23, 2006).

Borghadt, J., et al. 2000. Effects of a spleen peptide preparation as supportive therapy in inoperable head and neck cancer patients. *Arzneimittel-Forschung* 50(2):178–84.

Bouic, P. J., and J. H. Lamprecht. 1999. Plant sterols and sterolins: A review of their immune-modulating properties. *Alternative Medicine Review* 4(3):170–77.

Chiang, B. L., et al. 2001. Enhancing immunity by dietary consumption of a probiotic lactic acid bacterium: Optimization and definition of cellular immune responses—*Bifidobacterium lactis* HN019. *European Journal of Clinical Nutrition* 54(11):849–55.

Gaynor, Mitchell L., Jerry Hickey, and William Fryer. 2000. *Dr. Gaynor's Cancer Prevention Program.* New York: Kensington Publishing.

Hyman, Mark A. 2006. The evolution of research, part 2: The clinician's dilemma—treating systems, not diseases. *Alternative Therapies in Health and Medicine* 12(4):10–13.

Jameison, K., and T. G. Dinan. 2001. Glucocorticoids and cognitive function: From physiology to pathophysiology. *Human Psychopharmacology* 16(4):293–302.

Jeffrey Modell Foundation. 2006. Ten warning signs of primary immunodeficiency. www .info4pi.org/patienttopatient/index.cfm?section=patienttopatient&content=warningsigns (accessed July 4, 2006).

Kiecolt-Glaser, J. K., and R. Glaser. 2002. Depression and immune function: Central pathways to morbidity and mortality. *Journal of Psychosomatic Research* 53(4): 873–76.

Kiecolt-Glaser, J. K., et al. 2002. Psycho-oncology and cancer: Psychoneuroimmunology and cancer. *Annals of Oncology* 13(suppl.4):165–69.

Klotter, Julie. 2006. New autoimmune drugs. *Townsend Letter for Doctors and Patients* 247/248:24.

Liang, B., et al. 2008. Impact of postoperative omega-3 fatty acid-supplemented parenteral nutrition on clinical outcomes and immunomodulations in colorectal cancer patients. *World Journal of Gastroenterology* 14(15):2434–9.

Merck Manual Home Edition. 2003. Autoimmune disorders. www.merck.com/mmhe/sec16
/ch186/ch186a.html (accessed June 20, 2006).

Mustain, Karen H., et al. 2006. A randomized controlled pilot of home-based exercise (HBEX)
versus standard care (SC) among breast (BC) and prostate cancer (PC) patients receiving
radiation therapy (RTH). Paper presented to the annual meeting of the American Society
of Clinical Oncology.

National Cancer Institute. 2006. Cancer vaccine fact sheet. www.cancer.gov/cancertopics
/factsheet/cancervaccine (accessed June 23, 2006)

National Institute of Allergy and Infectious Diseases. 2003. The immune system. www.niaid
.nih.gov/final/immun/immun.htm (accessed June 20, 2006).

National Institute of Arthritis and Musculoskeletal and Skin Diseases. 2002. Questions and
answers about autoimmunity. www.niams.nih.gov/hi/topics/autoimmune/autoimmunity
.htm (accessed June 20, 2006).

National Institutes of Health. 2002. Stress system malfunction could lead to serious, life
threatening disease. *NIH Backgrounder*, September 9. www.nih.gov/news/pr/sep2002
/nichd-09.htm (accessed June 20, 2006).

Norton, Amy. 2003. Immune system may sway ovarian cancer survival. *Reuters Health*, January
15. (Available at www.cancerpage.com/news/article.asp?id=5425; accessed July 4, 2006.)

O'Garra, A., and P. Vieira. 2004. Regulatory T cells and mechanisms of immune system control. *Nature Medicine* 10(8):801–5.

Onuki, J., et al. 2005. Inhibition of 5-aminolevulinic acid-induced DNA damage by melatonin,
N1-acetyl-N2-formyl-5-methoxykynuramine, quercetin or resveratrol. *Journal of Pineal
Research* 38(2):107–15.

Prasad, A. S., and O. Kucuk. 2002. Zinc in cancer prevention. *Cancer Metastasis Reviews* 21(3–
4):291–95.

Ravaglia, G., et al. 2000. Effect of micronutrient status on natural killer cell immune function in healthy free-living subjects aged >/=90 y. *American Journal of Clinical Nutrition*
71(2):590–98.

Reiche, E. M., S. O. Nunes, and H. K. Morimoto. 2004. Stress, depression, the immune system, and cancer. *Lancet Oncology* 5(10):617–25.

Rountree, Robert, and Carol Colman. 2000. *Immunotics: A Revolutionary Way to Fight Infection,
Beat Chronic Illness, and Stay Well.* New York: Putnam Adult.

Shklar, G. 1998. Mechanisms of cancer inhibition by anti-oxidant nutrients. *Oral Oncology*
34(1):24–29.

Vojdani, A., and J. Erde. 2006. Regulatory T cells, a potent immunoregulatory target for CAM
researchers: The ultimate antagonist (I). *Evidence-Based Complementary and Alternative
Medicine* 3(1):25–30.

Weber, B., et al. 2000. Increased diurnal plasma concentrations of cortisone in depressed
patients. *Journal of Clinical Endocrinology and Metabolism* 85(3):1133–36.

Weiger, Wendy A., et al. 2003. Advising patients who seek complementary and alternative
medical therapies for cancer. *Annals of Internal Medicine* 139(2):155.

Zhang, L., et al. 2003. Intratumoral T cells, recurrence, and survival in epithelial ovarian cancer. *New England Journal of Medicine* 348(3):203–13.

Chapter Nine Inflammation

Alschuler, Lise. 2005. Implications of inflammation and cancer development. Lecture given
at the annual conference of the Northwest Association of Naturopathic Physicians.
November.

Alschuler, Lise. 2006. Presentation given at the annual International Complementary and
Alternative Medicine Expo, New York.

Bachelot, T., et al. 2003. Prognostic value of serum levels of interleukin 6 and of serum and
plasma levels of vascular endothelial growth factor in hormone-refractory metastatic breast
cancer patients. *British Journal of Cancer* 88(11):1721–6.

Bellavite, P., et al. 2006. Immunology and homeopathy. 2. Cells of the immune system and
inflammation. *Evidence-Based Complementary and Alternative Medicine* 3(1):13–24.

Bemis, D. L., et al. 2005. Zyflamend, a unique herbal preparation with nonselective COX inhibitory activity, induces apoptosis of prostate cancer cells that lack COX-2 expression. *Nutrition and Cancer* 52(2):202–12.

Block, G., et al. 2004. Plasma C-reactive protein concentrations in active and passive smokers: Influence of antioxidant supplementation. *Journal of the American College of Nutrition* 23(2):141–47.

Chainani-Wu, N. 2003. Safety and anti-inflammatory activity of curcumin: A component of turmeric (*Curcumin longa*). *Journal of Alternative and Complementary Medicine* 9(1):161–68.

Chan, A. T., et al. 2005. Genetic variants in the UGT1A6 enzyme, aspirin use, and the risk of colorectal adenoma. *Journal of the National Cancer Institute* 97(16):1227.

CNN.com. 2003. Can daily aspirin prevent colon cancer? (Available at www.cnn.com/2003/HEALTH/conditions/03/05/aspirin.cancer.reut/index.html; accessed January 29, 2007.)

de Mello, V. D., et al. 2008. Downregulation of genes involved in NFkappaB activation in peripheral blood mononuclear cells after weight loss is associated with the improvement of insulin sensitivity in individuals with the metabolic syndrome: The GENOBIN study. *Diabetologia* 51(11):2060–7.

Donato, A. J., et al. 2008. Aging is associated with greater nuclear NFkappaB, reduced IkappaBalpha, and increased expression of proinflammatory cytokines in vascular endothellal cells of healthy humans. *Aging Cell* 7(6):805–12.

Fichtlscherer, S., et al. 2004. Interleukin-10 serum levels and systemic endothelial vasoreactivity in patients with coronary artery disease. *Journal of the American College of Cardiologists* 44(1):44–49.

Greenwald, P., C. K. Clifford, and J. A. Milner. 2001. Diet and cancer prevention. *European Journal of Cancer Prevention* 37(3):948–65.

Health Media Ltd. 2003. Anti-inflammatory drugs may reduce breast-cancer risk. July 16. (Available at www.cancercompass.com/cancer-news/1,4933,00.htm; accessed August 6, 2006.)

Horstman, Judith. 1999. Ayurvedic herbs. *Arthritis Today*. www.arthritis.org/resources/arthritistoday/1999_archives/1999_05_06explorations.asp (accessed August 6, 2006).

Horstman, Judith. 2000. Acupuncture. *Arthritis Today*. www.arthritis.org/resources/arthritistoday/2000_archives/2000_05_06_acupuncture.asp (accessed August 6, 2006).

Imperiale, T. 2003. Aspirin and the prevention of colorectal cancer. *New England Journal of Medicine* 348(10):879–80.

Isolauri, E., et al. 2001. Probiotics: Effects on immunity. *American Journal of Clinical Nutrition* 73(suppl.2):444S–50S.

Jacobs, E. J., and M. J. Thun. 2005. Low-dose aspirin and vitamin E: Challenges and opportunities in cancer prevention. *Journal of the American Medical Association* 294(1):105–6.

Jauduszus, A., et al. 2005. Cis-9,trans-11-CLA exerts anti-inflammatory effects in human bronchial epithelial cells and eosinophils: Comparison to trans-10,cis-12-CLA and to linoleic acid. *Biochimica et Biophysica Acta* 1737(2–3):111–18.

Kalliomaki, M., et al. 2001. Probiotics in primary prevention of atopic disease: A randomised placebo-controlled trial. *Lancet* 357(9262):1076–79.

Kamhi, Ellen, and Eugene R. Zampieron. 2006. *Alternative Medicine Definitive Guide to Arthritis: Reverse Underlying Causes of Arthritis with Clinically Proven Alternative Therapies.* 2nd edition. Berkeley, CA: Celestial Arts.

Liang, B., et al. 2008. Impact of postoperative omega-3 fatty acid-supplemented parenteral nutrition on clinical outcomes and immunomodulations in colorectal cancer patients. *World Journal of Gastroenterology* 14(15):2434–9.

Lussignoli, S., et al. 1999. Effect of Traumeel S, a homeopathic formulation, on blood-induced inflammation in rats. *Complementary Therapies in Medicine* 7(4):225–30.

National Digestive Diseases Information Clearinghouse. 2004. NSAIDs and peptic ulcers. http://digestive.niddk.nih.gov/ddiseases/pubs/nsaids/index.htm (accessed August 6, 2006).

Natural Standard Research Collaboration. 2005. Bromelain. www.nlm.nih.gov/medlineplus/druginfo/natural/patient-bromelain.html (accessed August 6, 2006).

Ohshima, H., and H. Bartsch. 1994. Chronic infections and inflammatory processes as cancer risk factors: Possible role of nitric oxide in carcinogenesis. *Mutation Research* 305(2):253–64.

Ojewole, J. A. 2006. Analgesic, antiinflammatory and hypoglycaemic effects of ethanol extract of *Zingiber officinale* (Roscoe) rhizomes (Zingiberaceae) in mice and rats. *Phytotherapy Research* 29(4):764–72.

Penna, G., et al. 2009. The vitamin D receptor agonist elocalcitol inhibits IL-8-dependent benign prostatic hyperplasia stromal cell proliferation and inflammatory response by targeting the RhoA/Rho kinase and NF-kappaB pathways. *Prostate* 69(5):480–93.

President and Fellows of Harvard College. 2006. Hidden trans fats exposed. www.hsph .harvard.edu/nutritionsource/transfats.html (accessed August 6, 2006).

Ramos, E. J., et al. 2003. Is obesity an inflammatory disease? *Surgery* 134(2):329–35.

Ross, Mairi R. 2004. Chronic inflammation: Rocking the medical world. *Health Matters Monthy Supplemental Report*, fall issue.

Rountree, Robert, and Carol Colman. 2000. *Immunotics: A Revolutionary Way to Fight Infection, Beat Chronic Illness, and Stay Well.* New York: Putnam Adult.

Ruegg, Curzio. 2006. Leukocytes, inflammation, and angiogenesis in cancer: Fatal attractions. *Journal of Leukocyte Biology* 80(4):682–84.

Schmid-Schonbein, G. W. 2006. Analysis of inflammation. *Annual Review of Biomedical Engineering* 8:93–151.

Shacter, E., and S. A. Weitzman. 2002. Chronic inflammation and cancer. *Oncology* 16(2):217–26.

Siegfried, Donna Rae. 2006. Drug news: In a class by itself. *Arthritis Today*, August. www .arthritis.org/resources/arthritistoday/2005_archives/2005_07_08/2005_07_08_Drug_ News_p1.asp (accessed August 6, 2006).

U.S. Food and Drug Administration Center for Drug Evaluation and Research. 2005. COX-2 selective (includes Bextra, Celebrex, and Vioxx) and non-selective non-steroidal anti-inflammatory drugs (NSAIDs). www.fda.gov/cder/drug/infopage/cox2/ (accessed August 6, 2006).

Vgontzas, A. N., and G. P. Chrousos. 2002. Sleep, the hypothalamic-pituitary-adrenal axis, and cytokines: Multiple interactions and disturbances in sleep disorders. *Endocrinology and Metabolism Clinics of North America* 31(1):15–36.

Walter, M., et al. 2009. Interleukin 6 secreted from adipose stromal cells promotes migration and invasion of breast cancer cells. *Oncogene* [Epub ahead of print].

Wang, X. L., et al. 2004. Cosupplementation with vitamin E and coenzyme Q10 reduces circulating markers of inflammation in baboons. *American Journal of Clinical Nutrition* 80(3):649–55.

Yuan, A., J. J. Chen, P. L. Yao, and P. C. Yang. 2005. The role of interleukin-8 in cancer cells and microenvironment interaction. 10:853–65.

Zittermann, A., et al. 2009. Vitamin D supplementation enhances he beneficial effects of weight loss on cardiovascular disease risk markers. *American Journal of Clinical Nutrition* 89(5):321–7.

Zulet, M. A., et al. 2005. Inflammation and conjugated linoleic acid: Mechanisms of action and implications for human health. *Journal of Physiology and Biochemistry* 61(3):483–94.

Chapter Ten Hormonal Influences

Alkner, S., et al. 2009. Tamoxifen reduces the risk of contralateral breast cancer in premenopausal women: Results from a controlled randomised trial. *European Journal of Cancer* [Epub ahead of print].

Anderson, G. L., et al. 2004. Effects of conjugated equine estrogen in postmenopausal women with hysterectomy: The Women's Health Initiative randomized controlled trial. *Journal of the American Medical Association* 291(14):1701–12.

Bakalar, Nicholas. 2006. Survey finds use of herbs for menopause is common. *New York Times*, June 20.

Banks, E., et al. 2006. Hormone replacement therapy and false positive recall in the Million Women Study: Patterns of use, hormonal constituents and consistency of effect. *Breast Cancer Research* 8(1):R8.

Barrett-Connor, E., et al. 2006. Effects of raloxifene on cardiovascular events and breast cancer in postmenopausal women. *New England Journal of Medicine* 355(2):190–92.

Barton, Debra, et al. 2002. Venlaxafine for the control of hot flashes: Results of a longitudinal continuation study. *Oncology Nursing Forum* 29(1):33–40.

Beral, V., D. Bull, and G. Reeves. 2005. Endometrial cancer and hormone-replacement therapy in the Million Women Study. *Lancet* 365(9470):1543–51.

Beral, V., et al. 1999. Use of HRT and the subsequent risk of cancer. *Journal of Epidemiology and Biostatistics* 4(3):191–210.

Blask, D. E., R. T. Dauchy, and L. A. Sauer. 2005. Putting cancer to sleep at night: The neuro-endocrine/circadian melatonin signal. *Endocrine* 27(2):179–88.

Bouic, P. J. D. 2001. The role of phytosterols and phytosterolins in immune modulation: A review of the past 10 years. *Current Opinion in Clinical Nutrition and Metabolic Care* 4(6):471–75.

Bouic, P. J. D. 2002. Sterols and sterolins: New drugs for the immune system? *Drug Discovery Today* 7(14):775–78.

Breastcancer.org. 2005. Facing menopause and its symptoms. www.breastcancer.org/bey_cope_meno_fcSympt.html (accessed July 7, 2006).

Breastcancer.org. 2006. What role do hormones play in breast cancer treatment? www.breastcancer.org/tre_sys_hrt_role.html (accessed July 3, 2006).

Cassidy, A., et al. 2006. Factors affecting the bioavailability of soy isoflavones in humans after ingestion of physiologically relevant levels from different soy foods. *Journal of Nutrition* 136(1):45–51.

Chen, J., et al. 2004. Dietary flaxseed enhances the inhibitory effect of tamoxifen on the growth of estrogen-dependent human breast cancer (MCF-7) in nude mice. *Clinical Cancer Research* 10(22):7703–11.

Chen, S., et al. 2006. Anti-aromatase activity of phytochemicals in white button mushrooms (Agaricus bisporus). *Cancer Research* 66(24):12026–34.

Choi, J. Y., et al. 2003. Role of alcohol and genetic polymorphisms of CYP2E1 and ALDH2 in breast cancer development. *Pharmacogenetics* 13(2):67–72.

Conklin, C. M., et al. 2006. Genistein and quercetin increase connexin43 and suppress growth of breast cancer cells. *Carcinogenesis*, June 15 (advance release copy).

Cowley, Geoffrey, and Karen Springen. 2002. The end of the age of estrogen? *Newsweek* 139(4):38–41.

De Lemos, M. L. 2001. Effects of phytoestrogens genistein and daidzein on breast cancer growth. *Annals of Pharmacotherapy* 35(9):1118–21.

Guha, N., et al. 2009. Soy isoflavones and risk of cancer recurrence in a cohort of breast cancer survivors: The Life After Cancer Epidemiology study. *Breast Cancer Research and Treatment* [Epub ahead of print].

Hays, J., et al. 2003. Effects of estrogen plus progestin on health-related quality of life. *New England Journal of Medicine* 348(19):1839–54.

Hill, D. A., et al. 2000. Continuous combined hormone replacement therapy and risk of endometrial cancer. *American Journal of Obstetrics and Gynecology* 183(6):1456–61.

Hrushesky, William J. M., David Blask, and Paolo Lissoni. 2003. Melatonin, chronobiology, and cancer. Paper presented at the National Cancer Institute Office of Cancer Complementary and Alternative Medicine Invited Speaker Series, February 28.

Hyman, Mark A. 2006. The evolution of research, part 2: The clinician's dilemma—treating systems, not diseases. *Alternative Therapies in Health and Medicine* 12(4):10–13.

Lee, S. A., et al. 2009. Adolescent and adult soy food intake and breast cancer risk: Results from the Shanghai Women's Health Study. *American Journal of Clinical Nutrition* 89(6):1920–6.

Limer, J. L., A. T. Parkes, and V. Speirs. 2006. Differential response to phyto-estrogens in endocrine sensitive and resistant breast cancer cells in vitro. *International Journal of Cancer* 119(3):515–21.

Lissoni, P., et al. 1995. Modulation of cancer endocrine therapy by melatonin: A phase II study of tamoxifen plus melatonin in metastatic breast cancer patients progressing under tamoxifen alone. *British Journal of Cancer* 71(4):854–6.

Lupu, R., et al. 2003. Black cohosh, a menopausal remedy, does not have estrogenic activity and does not promote breast cancer cell growth. *International Journal of Oncology* 23(5):1407–12.

Medical Economics. 2005. *Physician's Desk Reference*. 59th edition. Stamford, CT: Thomson Healthcare.

Messina, M., and Wu, A.H. 2009. Perspectives on the soy-breast cancer relation. *American Journal of Clinical Nutrition* 89(5):1673S–1679S.

Miquel, J., et al. 2006. Menopause: A review on the role of oxygen stress and favorable effects of dietary antioxidants. *Archives of Gerontology and Geriatrics* 42(3):289–306.

National Cancer Institute. 2006. Aromatase inhibitors. www.cancer.gov/clinicaltrials /developments/aromatase-inhibitors digest (accessed May 7, 2006).

Nelson, H. D., et al. 2006. Nonhormonal therapies for menopausal hot flashes: Systematic review and meta-analysis. *Journal of the American Medical Association* 295(17):2057–71.

Osmers, R., et al. 2005. Efficacy and safety of isopropanolic black cohosh extract for climacteric symptoms. *Obstetrics and Gynecology* 105(5 pt 1):1074–83.

Parkin, D. R., and D. Malejka-Giganti. 2004. Differences in the hepatic P450-dependent metabolism of estrogen and tamoxifen in response to treatment of rats with 3,3'-diindolylmethane and its parent compound indole-3-carbinol. *Cancer Detection and Prevention.* 28(1):72–79.

Pawlickikowski, M., M. Kolomecha, A. Wojtczak, M. Karasek. 2002. Effects of six months of melatonin treatment on sleep quality and serum concentrations of estradiol, cortisol, dehydroepaindrosterone sulfate, and somatomedin C in elderly women. Neuro Endocrinol Lett 23 Supp 1:17–19.

Petrelli, J. M., et al. 2002. Body mass index, height, and postmenopausal breast cancer mortality in a prospective cohort of U.S. women. *Cancer Causes and Control* 13(4):325–32.

Poclaj, B. A., et al. 2006. Phase III double-blind, randomized, placebo-controlled crossover trial of black cohosh in the management of hot flashes: NCCTG Trial N01CC1. *Journal of Clinical Oncology* 24(18):2836–41.

Qin, W., et al. 2009. Soy isoflavones have an antiestrogenic effect and alter mammary promoter hypermethylation in healthy premenopausal women. *Nutrition and Cancer* 61(2):238–44.

Rodriguez, C., et al. 2001. Body mass index, height and prostate cancer mortality in two large cohorts of adult men in the United States. *Cancer Epidemiology, Biomarkers, and Prevention* 10(4):345–53.

Rodriguez, C., et al. 2002. Body mass index, height, and the risk of ovarian cancer mortality in a prospective cohort of postmenopausal women. *Cancer Epidemiology, Biomarkers, and Prevention* 11(9):822–28.

Rogan, Eleanor, et al. 2003. Relative imbalances in estrogen metabolism and conjugation in breast tissue of women with carcinoma: Potential biomarkers of susceptibility to cancer. *Carcinogenesis* 24(4):697–702.

RxList Staff. 2005: RxList, the Internet drug index: Femara oral. www.rxlist.com/drugs /drug-4363-Femara+Oral.aspx?drugid=4363&drugname=Femara+Oral (accessed July 25, 2006).

RxList Staff. 2005. RxList, the Internet drug index: Raloxifene oral. www.rxlist.com/drugs /drug-5191-Raloxifene+Oral.aspx?drugid=5191&drugname=Raloxifene+Oral (accessed July 25, 2006).

RxList Staff. 2005. RxList, the Internet drug index: Tamoxifen oral. www.rxlist.com/drugs /drug-4497-Tamoxifen+Oral.aspx?drugid=4497&drugname=Tamoxifen+Oral (accessed July 25, 2006).

Saarinen, N. M., et al. 2006. Flaxseed attenuates the tumor growth stimulating effect of soy protein in ovariectomized athymic mice with MCF-7 human breast cancer xenografts. *International Journal of Cancer* 119(4):925–31.

Suzuki, R., et al. 2005. Alcohol and postmenopausal breast cancer risk defined by estrogen and progesterone receptor status: A prospective cohort study. *Journal of the National Cancer Institute* 97(21):1601–8.

Thompson, L. U., et al. 2005. Dietary flaxseed alters tumor biological markers in postmenopausal breast cancer. *Clinical Cancer Research* 11(10):3828–35.

Wang, Y., et al. 2006. Prostate cancer treatment is enhanced by genistein in vitro and in vivo in a syngeneic orthotopic tumor model. *Radiation Research* 166(1):73–80.

Wood, C. E., et al. 2006. Dietary soy isoflavones inhibit estrogen effects in the postmeno-pausal breast. *Cancer Research* 66(2):1241–49.

Yokoe, T., et al. 1997. Changes in cytokines and thyroid function in patients with recurrent breast cancer. *Anticancer Research* 17(1B):695–99.

Chapter Eleven Insulin Resistance

Al Sarakbi, W., M. Salhab, and K. Mokbel. 2005. Dairy products and breast cancer risk: A review of the literature. *International Journal of Fertility and Women's Medicine* 50(6):244–49.

Augustin, L. S., et al. 2003. Glycemic index and glycemic load in endometrial cancer. *International Journal of Cancer* 105(3):404–7.

Barbaglio, M., and L. J. Dominguez. 2006. Magnesium metabolism in type 2 diabetes mellitus, metabolic syndrome and insulin resistance. *Archives of Biochemistry and Biophysics* June 12 [Epub ahead of print].

Blum, C., et al. 2005. Low-grade inflammation and estimates of insulin resistance during the menstrual cycle in lean and overweight women. *Journal of Clinical Endocrinology and Metabolism* 90(6):3230–35.

Brown, J. M., and M. K. McIntosh. 2003. Conjugated linoleic acid in humans: Regulation of adiposity and insulin sensitivity. *Journal of Nutrition* 133(10):3041–46.

Bruning, P. F., et al. 1992. Insulin resistance and breast-cancer risk. *International Journal of Cancer* 52(4):511–16.

Bui, T., and C. B. Thompson. 2006. Cancer's sweet tooth. *Cancer Cell* 9(6):419–20.

Chen, J., P. M. Stavro, and L. U. Thompson. 2002. Dietary flaxseed inhibits human breast cancer growth and metastasis and downregulates expression of insulin-like growth factor and epidermal growth factor receptor. *Nutrition and Cancer* 43(2):187–92.

Chong, Y. M., et al. 2006. The relationship between the insulin-like growth factor-1 system and the oestrogen metabolising enzymes in breast cancer tissue and its adjacent non-cancerous tissue. *Breast Cancer Research and Treatment* 99(3):275–88.

Evans, J. L., B. A. Maddux, and I. D. Goldfine. 2005. The molecular basis for oxidative stress-induced insulin resistance. *Antioxidants and Redox Signaling* 7(7-8):1040–52.

Fantin, Valeria R., Julie St-Pierre, and Philip Leder. 2006. Attenuation of LDH-A expression uncovers a link between glycolysis, mitochondrial physiology, and tumor maintenance. *Cancer Cell* 9(6):425–34.

Fox, Maggie. 2006. Half of Americans will have pre-diabetic condition. *Reuters Health,* June 13, 2006. (Available at www.mainehealthforum.org/SearchResults.asp?cid=450; accessed November 21, 2006.)

Fukino, Y., et al. 2005. Randomized controlled trial for an effect of green tea consumption on insulin resistance and inflammation markers. *Journal of Nutritional Science and Vitaminology* 51(5):335–42.

Furstenberger, G., and H. J. Senn. 2002. Insulin-like growth factors and cancer. *Lancet Oncology* 3(5):298–302.

Furstenberger, G., R. Morant, and H. J. Senn. 2003. Insulin-like growth factors and cancer. *Onkologie* 26(3):290–94.

Giovannucci, Edward L. 2005. Obesity, insulin resistance, and cancer risk. *Cancer Prevention: A National Newsletter and Web Site from New York-Presbyterian Hospital*, Spring (5). www.nypcancerprevention.com/issue/5/con/features/pre_ear-2.shtml (accessed August 4, 2006).

Gunter, M. J., et al. 2009. Insulin, insulin-like growth factor-I, and risk of breast cancer in postmenopausal women. *Journal of the National Cancer Institute* 101(1):48–60.

Hodgson, J. M., et al. 2002. Coenzyme Q10 improves blood pressure and glycaemic control: A controlled trial in subjects with type 2 diabetes. *European Journal of Clinical Nutrition* 56(11):1137–42.

Hoppe, C., C. Molgaard, and K. F. Michaelsen. 2006. Cow's milk and linear growth in industrialized and developing countries. *Annual Review of Nutrition* 26:131–73.

Hsu, C. H., et al. 2007. The mushroom Agaricus Blazel Murill in combination with metformin and gliclazide improves insulin resistance in type 2 diabetes; a randomized, double-blinded, and placebo-controlled clinical trial. *Journal of Alternative Complementary Medicine* 13(1):97–102.

Huerta, M. G., et al. 2005. Magnesium deficiency is associated with insulin resistance in obese children. *Diabetes Care* 20(5):1175–81.

Kahan, Z., et al. 2006. Elevated levels of circulating insulin-like growth factor-I, IGF-binding globulin-3 and testosterone predict hormone-dependent breast cancer in postmenopausal women: A case-control study. *International Journal of Oncology* 29(1):193–200.

Konrad, D. 2005. Utilization of the insulin-signaling network in the metabolic actions of alpha-lipoic acid—Reduction or oxidation? *Antioxidants and Redox Signaling* (7–8):1032–39.

Kunimoto, M., et al. 2008. Benficial effect of coenzyme Q10 on increased oxidative and nitrative stress and inflammation and individual metabolic components developing in a rat model of metabolic syndrome. *Journal of Pharmaceutical Science* 107(2):128–37.

Larsson, S., C. L. Bergkvist, and A. Wolk. 2006. Glycemic load, glycemic index and carbohydrate intake in relation to risk of stomach cancer: A prospective study. *International Journal of Cancer* 118(12):3167–69.

Larsson, S., C. N. Orsini, and A. Wolk. 2005. Diabetes mellitus and risk of colorectal cancer: A meta-analysis. *Journal of the National Cancer Institute* 97(22):1679–87.

Lissoni, P., et al. 1995. Modulation of cancer endocrine therapy by melatonin: A phase II study of tamoxifen plus melatonin in metastatic breast cancer patients progressing under tamoxifen alone. *British Journal of Cancer* 71(4):854–6.

Lofgren, I. E., et al. 2005. Weight loss favorably modifies anthropometrics and reverses the metabolic syndrome in premenopausal women. *Journal of the American College of Nutrition* 24(6):486–93.

Lopez, S., et al. 2008. Distinctive postprandial modulation of beta cell function and insulin sensitivity by dietary fats: Monounsaturated compared with saturated fatty acids. *American Journal of Clinical Nutrition* 88(3):638–44.

Ma, X., Hua, J., and Li, Z. 2008. Probiotics improve high fat diet-induced hepatic steatosis and insulin resistance by increasing hepatic NKT cells. *Journal of Heptology* 49(5):821–30.

Marlett, J. A., M. I. McBurney, and J. L. Slavin. 2002. Position of the American Dietetic Association: Health implications of dietary fiber. *Journal of the American Dietetic Association* 102(7):993–1000.

Mauro, L., et al. 2003. Role of the IGF-I receptor in the regulation of cell-cell adhesion: Implications in cancer development and progression. *Journal of Cell Physiology* 194(2):108–16.

McCarty, M. F. 2004. Elevated sympathetic activity may promote insulin resistance syndrome by activating alpha-1 adrenergic receptors on adipocytes. *Medical Hypotheses* 62(5):830–38.

Medical Economics. 2004. *PDR for Herbal Medicines.* 3rd edition. Boston, MA: Thomson Healthcare.

Michaud, D. S., et al. 2005. Dietary glycemic load, carbohydrate, sugar, and colo-rectal cancer risk in men and women. *Cancer Epidemiology, Biomarkers, and Prevention* 14(1):138–47.

Michels, K. B., et al. 2003. Type 2 diabetes and subsequent incidence of breast cancer in the Nurses' Health Study. *Diabetes Care* 26(6):1752–58.

Moschos, S. J., and C. S. Mantzoros. 2002. The role of the IGF system in cancer: From basic to clinical studies and clinical applications. *Oncology* 63(4):317–32.

Murray, Michael T. 1996. *Encyclopedia of Nutritional Supplements: The Essential Guide for Improving Your Health Naturally.* New York: Three Rivers Press.

Muti, P., et al. 2002. Fasting glucose is a risk factor for breast cancer: A prospective study. *Cancer Epidemiology, Biomarkers, and Prevention* 11(11):1361–68.

Naqpal, J., J. N. Pande, and A. Bhartia. 2009. A double-blind, randomized, placebo-controlled trial of the short-term effect of vitamin D3 supplementation on insulin sensitivity in apparently healthy, middle-aged, centrally obese men. *Diabetes Medicine* 26(1):19–27.

Nishiyama, Y., et al. 2006. Effect of physical training on insulin resistance in patients with chronic heart failure. *Circulation Journal* 70(7):864–67.

Olatunji, L. A., I. P. Oyeyipo, I. P. Michael, and A. O. Soladoye. 2008. Effect of dietary magnesium on glucose tolerance and plasma lipid during oral contraceptive administration in female rats. *African Journal of Medicine and Medicinal Sciences* 37(2):135–9.

Ouellet, V., et al. 2008. Dietary cod protein reduces plasma C-reactive protein in insulin-resistant men and women. *Journal of Nutrition* 138(12):2386–91.

Pasanisi, P., et al. 2006. Metabolic syndrome as a prognostic factor for breast cancer recurrences. *International Journal of Cancer* 119(1):236–38.

Patterson, S., et al. 2006. Detrimental actions of metabolic syndrome risk factor, homocysteine, on pancreatic beta-cell glucose metabolism and insulin secretion. *Journal of Endocrinology* 189(2):301–10.

Pereira, M. A., et al. 2002. Effect of whole grains on insulin sensitivity in overweight hyperinsulinemic adults. *American Journal of Clinical Nutrition* 75(5):848–55.

Rickard, S. E., Y. V. Yuan, and L. U. Thompson. 2000. Plasma insulin-like growth factor I levels in rats are reduced by dietary supplementation of flaxseed or its lignan secoisolariciresinol diglycoside. *Cancer Letters* 161(1):47–55.

Sandhu, J. G., et al. 2006. Timing of puberty determines serum insulin-like growth factor-1 in late adulthood. *Journal of Clinical Endocrinology and Metabolism* 91(8):3150–57.

Saydah, S. H., et al. 2003. Abnormal glucose tolerance and the risk of cancer death in the United States. *American Journal of Epidemiology* 157(12):1092–100.

Shaibi, G. Q., et al. 2006. Effects of resistance training on insulin sensitivity in overweight Latino adolescent males. *Medicine and Science in Sports and Exercise* 38(7):1208–15.

Soilini, A., E. Santini, and E. Ferrannini. 2006. Effect of short-term folic acid supplementation on insulin sensitivity and inflammatory markers in overweight subjects. *International Journal of Obesity (London)* 30(8):1197–202.

Sola, S., et al. 2005. Irbesartan and lipoic acid improve endothelial function and reduce markers of inflammation in the metabolic syndrome: Results of the irbesartan and lipoic acid in endothelial dysfunction (ISLAND) study. *Circulation* 111(3):343–48.

Soliman, P. T., et al. 2006. Association between adiponectin, insulin resistance, and endometrial cancer. *Cancer* 106(11):2376–81.

Stolzenberg-Solomon, R. Z., et al. 2005. Insulin, glucose, insulin resistance, and pancreatic cancer in male smokers. *Journal of the American Medical Association* 294(22):2872–78.

Viadeva, S. V., D. D. Terzieva, and D. T. Arabadjiiska. 2005. Effect of chromium on the insulin resistance in patients with type II diabetes mellitus. *Folia Medica* 47(3):59–62.

Wei, E. K., et al. 2005. A prospective study of C-peptide, insulin-like growth factor-1, insulin-like growth factor binding protein-1, and the risk of colorectal cancer in women. *Cancer Epidemiology, Biomarkers, and Prevention* 14(4):850–55.

Wu, L. Y., et al. 2004. Green tea supplementation ameliorates insulin resistance and increases glucose transporter IV content in a fructose-fed rat model. *European Journal of Nutrition* 43(2):116–24.

Xie, J. T., et al. 2003. Anti-diabetic effects of *Gymnema yunnanense* extract. *Pharmacological Research* 47(4):323–29.

Ziegler, D. 2004. Thioctic acid for patients with symptomatic diabetic polyneuropathy: A critical review. *Treatments in Endocrinology* 3(3):173–89.

Chapter Twelve Digestion and Detoxification

Amakura, Y., et al. 2003. Screening of the inhibitory effect of vegetable constituents on the aryl hydrocarbon receptor-mediated activity induced by 2,3,7,8-tetra-chlorodibenzo-p-dioxin. *Biological and Pharmaceutical Bulletin* 26(12):1754–60.

American Academy of Family Physicians. Antacids and acid reducers: OTC relief for heartburn and acid reflux. http://familydoctor.org/854.xml (accessed August 1, 2006).

American Cancer Society. 2005. Liver flush. www.cancer.org/docroot/ETO/content/ETO_5_3x_Liver_Flush.asp (accessed August 1, 2006).

American Gastroenterological Association. Take the core quiz. www.gastro.org/wmspage.cfm?parm1=671 (accessed August 1, 2006).

Bengmark, S., and B. Jeppsson. 1995. Gastrointestinal surface protection and mucosa reconditioning. *Journal of Parenteral and Enteral Nutrition* 19(5):410–15.

Bottiglieri, T., et al. 2000. Homocysteine, folate, methylation, and monoamine metabolism in depression. *Journal of Neurology, Neurosurgery and Psychiatry* 69(2):228–32.

Cuzzocrea, S., et al. 2000. Role of free radicals and poly(ADP-ribose) synthetase in intestinal tight junction permeability. *Molecular Medicine* 6(9):766–78.

Fiander, H., and H. Schneider. 2000. Dietary ortho phenols that induce glutathione S-transferase and increase the resistance of cells to hydrogen peroxide are potential cancer chemopreventives that act by two mechanisms: The alleviation of oxidative stress and the detoxification of mutagenic xenobiotics. *Cancer Letters* 156(2):117–24.

Fryer, A. A., and P. W. Jones. 1999. Interactions between detoxifying enzyme polymorphisms and susceptibility to cancer. *IARC Scientific Publications* (148):303–22.

Fukudo, S., T. Nomura, and M. Hongo. 1998. Impact of corticotropin-releasing hormone on gastrointestinal motility and adrenocorticotropic hormone in normal controls and patients with irritable bowel syndrome. *Gut* 42(6):845–49.

Gaynor, Mitchell L. 2005. *Nurture Nature, Nurture Health: Your Health and the Environment.* New York: Nurture Nature Press.

Heymann, M., and J. F. Desjeux. 2000. Cytokine-induced alteration of the epithelial barrier to food antigens in disease. *Annals of the New York Academy of Sciences* 915:304–11.

Khayyal, M. T., et al. 2001. Antiulcerogenic effect of some gastrointestinally acting plant extracts and their combination. *Arzneimittel-Forschung* 51(7):545–53.

Kleiner, S. M. 1999. Water: An essential but overlooked nutrient. *Journal of the American Dietetic Association* 99(2):200–6.

Ledowchowski, M., et al. 2001. Increased serum amylase and lipase in fructose malabsorbers. *Clinica Chimica Acta* 311(2):119–23.

Lee, I. P., et al. 1997. Chemopreventive effect of green tea *(Camellia sinensis)* against cigarette smoke-induced mutations (SCE) in humans. *Journal of Cellular Biochemistry. Supplement* 27:68–75.

Lu, W. Z., G. H. Song, K. A. Gwee, and K. Y. Ho. 2008. The effects of melatonin on colonic transit time in normal controls and IBS patients. *Digestive Disease and Sciences* 54(5):1087–93.

Mayo Clinic Staff. 2005. Over the counter laxatives: Use them with caution. www.mayoclinic .com/health/laxatives/HQ00088 (accessed August 1, 2006).

Murray, Michael, et al. 2002. *How to Prevent and Treat Cancer with Natural Medicine.* New York: Riverhead Books.

National Digestive Diseases Information Clearinghouse (NDDIC). 2003. Heartburn, hiatal hernia, and gastroesophageal reflux disease (GERD). http://digestive.niddk.nih.gov/ddiseases/pubs/gerd/ (accessed August 1, 2006).

National Digestive Diseases Information Clearinghouse (NDDIC). 2004. Your digestive system and how it works. http://digestive.niddk.nih.gov/ddiseases/pubs/yrdd/ (accessed August 8, 2006).

Patel, A. B., et al. 2001. Glutamine is the major precursor for GABA synthesis in rat neocortex in vivo following acute GABA-transaminase inhibition. *Brain Research* 919(2):207–20.

Playford, R. J., et al. 2001. Co-administration of the health food supplement, bovine colostrum, reduces the acute non-steroidal anti-inflammatory drug-induced increase in intestinal permeability. *Clinical Science (London)* 100(6):627–33.

Poonia, B., et al. 2006. Intestinal lymphocyte subsets and turnover are affected by chronic alcohol consumption: Implications for SIV/HIV infection. *Journal of Acquired Immune Deficiency Syndromes* 41(5):537–47.

Pritchard, D. M., and A. J. Watson. 1996. Apoptosis and gastrointestinal pharma-cology. *Pharmacology and Therapeutics* 72(2):149–69.

Rafi, M. M., et al. 2002. Novel polyphenol molecule isolated from licorice root *(Glycrrhiza glabra)* induces apoptosis, G2/M cell cycle arrest, and Bcl-2 phosphorylation in tumor cell lines. *Journal of Agricultural and Food Chemistry* 50(4):677–84.

Ringer, Y., A. D. Sperber, and D. A. Drossman. 2001. Irritable bowel syndrome. *Annual Review of Medicine* 52:319–38.

Rouse, K., et al. 1995. Glutamine enhances selectivity of chemotherapy through changes in glutathione metabolism. *Annals of Surgery* 221(4):420–26.

Sandler, R. S., et al. 2000. Abdominal pain, bloating, and diarrhea in the United States: Prevalence and impact. *Digestive Diseases and Science* 45(6):1166–71.

Sotolo-Felix, J. I., et al. 2002. Evaluation of the effectiveness of *Rosmarinus officinalis* (Lamiaceae) in the alleviation of carbon tetrachloride-induced acute hepatotoxicity in the rat. *Journal of Ethnopharmacology* 81(2):145–54.

Thor, P. J., et al. 2007. Melatonin and seratonin effecs on gastrointestinal motility. *Journal of Physiology and Pharmacology* 58(suppl.6):97–103.

Wollowski, I., G. Rechkemmer, and B. L. Pool-Zobel. 2001. Protective role of probiotics and prebiotics in colon cancer. *American Journal of Clinical Nutrition* 73(suppl.2):451S–55S.

Yoshida, S., et al. 1998. Effects of glutamine supplements and radiochemotherapy on systemic immune and gut barrier function in patients with advanced esophageal cancer. *Annals of Surgery* 227(4):485–91.

Zhao, B., et al. 2000. Correlation between acetylation phenotype and genotype in Chinese women. *European Journal of Clinical Pharmacology* 56(9–10):689–92.

Chapter Fourteen Bladder Cancer

American Urological Association Education and Research. 2003. Bladder cancer. www.urologyhealth.org/adult/index.cfm?cat=04&topic=37 (accessed June 12, 2006).

Boggs, Will. 2006. Delayed surgery decreases bladder cancer survival. *Reuters Health*, April 13. (Available at www.cancerpage.com/news/article.asp?id=9614; accessed November 21, 2006.)

Elasser-Beile, U., et al. 2005. Adjuvant intravesical treatment with a standardized mistletoe extract to prevent recurrence of superficial urinary bladder cancer. *Anticancer Research* 25(6C):4733–36.

Goebell, P. J., et al. 2002. Evaluation of an unconventional treatment modality with mistletoe lectin to prevent recurrence of superficial bladder cancer: A randomized phase II trial. *Journal of Urology* 168(1):72–75.

Hoesl, C. E., and J. E. Altwein. 2005. The probiotic approach: An alternative treatment option in urology. *European Urology* 47(3):288–96.

Kemberling, J. K., et al. 2003. Inhibition of bladder tumor growth by the green tea derivative epigallocatechin-3-gallate. *Journal of Urology* 170(3):773–76.

Kuno, T., et al. 2006. Chemoprevention of mouse urinary bladder carcinogenesis by fermented brown rice and rice bran. *Oncology Reports* 15(3):533–38.

Kurashige, S., Y. Akuzawa, and F. Endo. 1999. Effects of astragali radix extract on carcinogenesis, cytokine production, and cytotoxicity in mice treated with a carcinogen, N-butyl-N'-butanolnitrosoamine. *Cancer Investigation* 17(1):30–35.

Lamm, D. L., et al. 1994. Megadose vitamins in bladder cancer: A double-blind clinical trial. *Journal of Urology* 151(1):21–26.

Lehmann, J., et al. 2006. Complete long-term survival data from a trial of adjuvant chemotherapy vs. control after radical cystectomy for locally advanced bladder cancer. *BJU International* 97(1):42–47.

Lin, J. G., et al. 2006. Aloe-emodin induces apoptosis in T24 human bladder cells through the p53 apoptotic pathway. *Journal of Urology* 175(1):343–47.

Nagano, J., et al. 2000. Bladder-cancer incidence in relation to vegetable and fruit consumption: A prospective study of atomic-bomb survivors. *International Journal of Cancer* 86(1):132–38.

Naito, S., et al. 2008. Prevention of recurrence with epirubicin and lactobacillus casei after transurethral resection of bladder cancer. *Journal of Urology* 179(2):485–90.

Park, C., et al. 2006. Induction of G2/M arrest and inhibition of cyclooxy-genase-2 activity by curcumin in human bladder cancer T24 cells. *Oncology Reports* 15(5):1225–31.

Pazdur, Richard, et al., eds. 2004. *Cancer Management: A Multidisciplinary Approach; Medical, Surgical, and Radiation Oncology.* 8th edition. Philadelphia, PA: F. A. Davis Company.

Sato, D., and M. Matsushima. 2003. Preventive effects of urinary bladder tumors induced by N-butyl-N-(4-hydroxybutyl)-nitrosamine in rats by green tea leaves. *International Journal of Urology* 10(3):160–66.

Singh, A. V., et al. 2006. Soy phytochemicals prevent orthotopic growth and metastasis of bladder cancer in mice by alterations of cancer cell proliferation and apoptosis and tumor angiogenesis. *Cancer Research* 66(3):1851–58.

Skalkos, D., et al. 2005. The lipophilic extract of *Hypericum perforatum* exerts significant cytotoxic activity against T24 and NBT-II urinary bladder tumor cells. *Planta Medica* 71(11):1030–35.

Stavropoulos, N. E., et al. 2006. *Hypericum perforatum* L. extract: Novel photosensitizer against human bladder cancer cells. *Journal of Photochemistry and Photobiology* 84(1):64–69.

Sun, M., et al. 2004. The effect of curcumin on bladder cancer cell line EJ in vitro. [In Chinese.] *Zhong Yao Cai* [Journal of Chinese Medicinal Materials] 27(11):848–50.

Tong, Q. S., et al. 2006. Apoptosis-inducing effects of curcumin derivatives in human bladder cancer cells. *Anticancer Drugs* 17(3):279–87.

Totterman, T. H., A. Loskog, and M. Essand. 2005. The immunotherapy of prostate and bladder cancer. *BJU International* 96(5):728–35.

Wakai, K., et al. 2004. Foods and beverages in relation to urothelial cancer: Case-control study in Japan. *International Journal of Urology* 11(1):11–19.

Zi, X., and A. R. Simoneau. 2005. Flavokawain A, a novel chalcone from kava extract, induces apoptosis in bladder cancer cells by involvement of Bax protein-dependent and mitochondria-dependent apoptotic pathway and suppresses tumor growth in mice. *Cancer Research* 65(8):3479–86.

Chapter Fifteen Bone Cancer

Altundaq, O., et al. 2004. Calcium and vitamin D supplementation during bisphosphonate administration may increase osteoclastic activity in patients with bone metastasis. *Medical Hypotheses* 63(6):1010–13.

American Cancer Society. 2006. Detailed guide: Bone cancer. www.cancer.org/docroot/CRI /CRI_2_3x.asp?rnav=cridg&dt=2 (accessed July 20, 2006).

Hiraoka, K., et al. 2001. Osteosarcoma cell apoptosis induced by selenium. *Journal of Orthopaedic Research* 19(5):809–14.

Jelinek, G. G., and R. H. Gawler. 2008. Thirty-year follow-up at pneumonectomy of a 58-year-old survivor of disseminated osteosarcoma. *Medical Journal of Australia* 189(11–12):663–5.

Li, B. B., S. F. Yu, and S. Z. Pang. 2005. Effect of genistein on the proliferation, differentiation and apoptosis of the osteoblasts. [In Chinese.] *Zhongou Kou Qiang Yi Xue Za Zhi* [Chinese Journal of Stomatology] 40(3):237–40.

National Cancer Institute. 2002. Bone cancer: Questions and answers. www.cancer.gov /cancertopics/factsheet/Sites-Types/bone (accessed July 20, 2006).

Roomi, M. W., et al. 2006. In vivo and in vitro antitumor effect of ascorbic acid, lysine, proline, arginine, and green tea extract on human fibrosarcoma cells HT-1080. *Medical Oncology* 23(1):105–11.

Sloan-Kettering Memorial Cancer Center. 2006. Bone cancer: Symptoms. www.mskcc.org /mskcc/html/11606.cfm (accessed July 20, 2006).

Chapter Sixteen Brain Cancer

American Cancer Society. 2006. What are the risk factors for brain and spinal cord tumors in adults? www.cancer.org/docroot/CRI/content/CRI_2_4_2X_What_are_the_risk_factors _for_brain_and_spinal_cord_tumors_3.asp?sitearea (accessed July 20, 2006).

Annabi, B., et al. 2005. Probing the infiltrating character of brain tumors: Inhibition of RhoA/ ROK-mediated CD44 cell surface shedding from glioma cells by the green tea catechin EGCG. *Journal of Neurochemistry* 94(4):906–16.

Burzynski, S. R., et al. 2004. Phase II study of antineoplaston A10 and AS2-1 in children with recurrent and progressive multicentric glioma: A preliminary report. *Drugs in R & D* 5(6):315–26.

Burzynski, S. R., T. J. Janicki, R. A. Weaver, and B. Burzynski. 2006. Targeted therapy with antineoplastons A10 and AS2-1 of high-grade, recurrent, and progressive brainstem glioma. *Integrated Cancer Therapies* 5(1):40–7.

Jung, S. H., et al. 2006. Ginseng saponin metabolite suppresses phorbol ester-induced matrix metalloproteinase-9 expression through inhibition of activator protein-1 and mitogen-activated protein kinase signaling pathways in human astroglioma cells. *International Journal of Cancer* 118(2):490–97.

Karmakar, S., N. L. Banik, and S. K. Ray. 2007. Curcumin suppressed anti-apoptic signals and activated cysteine protease for apoptosis in human malignant glioblastoma U87MG cells. *Neurochemical Research* 32(12):2103–13.

Kim, S. Y., S. H. Jung, and H. S. Kim. 2005. Curcumin is a potent broad spectrum inhibitor of matrix metalloproteinase gene expression in human astroglioma cells. *Biochemical and Biophysical Research Communications* 337(2):510–16.

Lee, W. J., et al. 2005. Agricultural pesticide use and risk of glioma in Nebraska, United States. *Occupational and Environmental Medicine* 62(11):786–92.

National Cancer Institute. 2005. Adult brain tumors: Treatment. www.cancer.gov/cancerinfo /pdq/treatment/adultbrain/patient/ (accessed July 20, 2006).

Purkayastha, S., et al. 2009. Curcumin blocks brain tumor formation. *Brain Research* [Epub ahead of print].

Rooprai, H. K., M. Christidou, and G. J. Pilkington. 2003. The potential for strategies using micronutrients and heterocyclic drugs to treat invasive gliomas. *Acta Neurochirurgica* 145(8):683–90.

Tsai, N. M., et al. 2005. The antitumor effects of *Angelica sinensis* on malignant brain tumors in vitro and in vivo. *Clinical Cancer Research* 11(9):3475–84.

Chapter Seventeen Breast Cancer

American Cancer Society. 2006. What causes breast cancer? www.cancer.org/docroot/CRI /content/CRI_2_2_2X_What_causes_breast_cancer_5.asp (accessed July 20, 2006).

Arroyo-Helguera, O., Rojas, E., Delgado, G., and Aceves, C. 2008. Signaling pathways involved in the antiproliferative effect of molecular iodine in normal and tumoral breast cells: Evidence that 6-iodolactone mediates apoptic effects. *Endocrine-Related Cancer* 15(4):1003–11.

Baglietto, L., et al. 2005. Does dietary folate intake modify effect of alcohol consumption on breast cancer risk? Prospective cohort study. *British Medical Journal* 331(7520):807.

Barton, M. B., et al. 2005. Complications following bilateral prophylactic mastectomy. *Journal of the National Cancer Institute. Monographs* (35):61–66.

Berry, D., et al. 2006. Decline in breast cancer cases likely linked to reduced use of hormone replacement (as featured on www.mdanderson.org and presented at the 29th Annual San Antonio Breast Cancer Symposium).

Beuth, J., B. Schneider, and J.M. Schierholz. 2008. Impact of complementary treatment of breast cancer patients with standardized mistletoe extract during aftercare: A controlled multicenter comparative epidemiological cohort study. *Anticancer Research* 28(1B):523–7.

Bradshaw, P. T., et al. 2009. Consumption of sweet foods and breast cancer risk: A case-control study of women on Long Island, New York. *Cancer Causes Controlled* [Epub ahead of print].

Chamras, H., et al. 2005. Novel interactions of vitamin E and estrogen in breast cancer. *Nutrition and Cancer* 52(1):43–48.

Dai, Q., et al. 2009. Oxidative stress, obesity, and breast cancer risk: Results from the Shanghai Women's Health Study. *Journal of Clinical Oncology* 27(15):2482–8.

Diglianni, L. M., et al. 2006. Complementary medicine use before and 1 year following genetic testing for BRCA1/2 mutations. *Cancer Epidemiology, Biomarkers, and Prevention* 15(1): 70–75.

Duda, R. B., et al. 1999. American ginseng and breast cancer therapeutic agents synergistically inhibit MCF-7 breast cancer cell growth. *Journal of Surgical Oncology* 72(4):230–39.

Early Breast Cancer Trialists' Collaborative Group (EBCTCG). 1998. Tamoxifen for early breast cancer: An overview of the randomised trials. *Lancet* 351(9114):1451–67.

Early Breast Cancer Trialists' Collaborative Group (EBCTCG). 2005. Effects of chemotherapy and hormonal therapy for early breast cancer on recurrence and 15-year survival: An overview of the randomised trials. *Lancet* 365(9472):1687–717.

Fan, S., et al. 2006. BRCA1 and BRCA2 as molecular targets for phytochemicals indole-3-carbinol and genistein in breast and prostate cancer cells. *British Journal of Cancer* 94(3):407–26.

Fisher, B., et al. 1999. Lumpectomy and radiation therapy for the treatment of intraductal breast cancer: Findings from National Surgical Adjuvant Breast and Bowel Project B-17. *Journal of Clinical Oncology* 16(2):441–52.

Fisher, B., et al. 1999. Tamoxifen in treatment of intraductal breast cancer: National Surgical Adjuvant Breast and Bowel Project B-24 randomised controlled trial. *Lancet* 353(9169):1993–2000.

Fisher, B., et al. 2001. Five versus more than five years of tamoxifen for lymph node-negative breast cancer: Updated findings from the National Surgical Adjuvant Breast and Bowel Project B-14 randomized trial. *Journal of the National Cancer Institute* 93(9):684–90.

Freudenheim, J. L., et al. 2004. Diet and alcohol consumption in relation to p53 mutations in breast tumors. *Carcinogenesis* 25(6):931–39.

Gennatas, C., et al. 2006. Third-line hormonal treatment with exemestane in postmenopausal patients with advanced breast cancer progressing on letrozole or anastrozole. A phase II trial conducted by the Hellenic Group of Oncology (HELGO). *Tumori* 92(1):13–17.

Habel, L. A., et al. 2006. A population-based study of tumor gene expression and risk of breast cancer death among lymph node-negative patients. *Breast Cancer Research* 8(3):R25.

Hsu, E. L., et al. 2008. CXCR4 and CXCL12 down-regulation: A novel mechanism for the chemoprotection of 3,3'-diindolylmethane for breast and ovarian cancers. *Cancer Letters* 265(1):113–23.

Imaginis. 2006. Breast cancer diagnosis. www.imaginis.com/breasthealth/menu-diagnosis.asp (accessed July 20, 2006).

Inano, H., et al. 1999. Chemoprevention by curcumin during the promotion stage of tumorigenesis of mammary gland in rats irradiated with gamma-rays. *Carcinogenesis* 20(6):1011–18.

Irwin, M. L., et al. 2005. Relationship of obesity and physical activity with C-peptide, leptin, and insulin-like growth factors in breast cancer survivors. *Cancer, Epidemiology, Biomarkers, and Prevention* 14(12):2881–88.

Jaiswal-McEligot, A., J. Largent, A. Ziogas, D. Peel, and H. Anton-Culver. 2006. Dietary fat, fiber, vegetables, and micronutrients are associated with overall survival in postmenopausal women diagnosed with breast cancer. *Nutrition and Cancer* 55(2):132–40.

Jo, E. H., et al. 2004. Modulations of the BCL-2/Bax family were involved in the chemopreventive effects of licorice root (*Glycyrrhiza uralensis* Fisch) in MCF-7 human breast cancer cell. *Journal of Agricultural and Food Chemistry* 52(6):1715–19.

Jolliet, P., et al. 1998. Plasma coenzyme Q10 concentrations in breast cancer: Prognosis and therapeutic consequences. *International Journal of Clinical Pharmacology and Therapeutics* 36(9):506–9.

Jonat, W., K. I. Pritchard, R. Sainsbury, and J. G. Klijn. 2006. Trends in endocrine therapy and chemotherapy for early breast cancer: A focus on the premenopausal patient. *Journal of Cancer Research in Clinical Oncology* 132(5):275–86.

Jones, D. T., I. S. Trowbridge, and A. L. Harris. 2006. Effects of transferring receptor blockage on cancer cell proliferation and hypoxi-inducible factor function and their differential regulation by ascorbate. *Cancer Research* 66(5):2749–56.

Kaklamani, V. G., and W. J. Gradishar. 2006. Gene expression in breast cancer. *Current Treatment Options in Oncology* 7(2):123–8.

Kavanagh, K. T., et al. 2001. Green tea extracts decrease carcinogen-induced mammary tumor burden in rats and rate of breast cancer cell proliferation in culture. *Journal of Cellular Biochemistry* 82(3):387–98.

Khanzode, S. S., et al. 2004. Antioxidant enzyme and lipid peroxidation in different stages of breast cancer. *Free Radical Research* 38(1):81–5.

Kim, K. N., et al. 2006. Retinoic acid and ascorbic acid act synergistically in inhibiting human breast cancer cell proliferation. *Journal of Nutritional Biochemistry* 17(7):454–62.

Kulp, K. S., et al. 2006. Essiac and Flor-Essence herbal tonics stimulate the in vitro growth of human breast cancer cells. *Breast Cancer Research and Treatment* 98(3):249–59.

Larsson, S. C., L. Bergkvist, and A. Wolk. 2009. Glycemic load, glycemic index and breast cancer risk in a prospective cohort of Swedish women. *International Journal of Cancer* 125(1)153–7.

Lockwood, K., et al. 1994. Apparent partial remission of breast cancer in "high risk" patients supplemented with nutritional antioxidants, essential fatty acids and coenzyme Q10. *Molecular Aspects of Medicine* 15(suppl.):S231–40.

Lostumbo, L., et al. 2004. Prophylactic mastectomy for the prevention of breast cancer. *Cochrane Database of Systematic Reviews* no. 4: CD002748.

Lowe, L. C., et al. 2005. Plasma 25-hydroxy vitamin D concentrations, vitamin D receptor genotype and breast cancer risk in a UK Caucasian population. *European Journal of Cancer* 41(8):1164–69.

Marcsek, Z. et al. 2004. The efficacy of tamoxifen in estrogen receptor-positive breast cancer cells is enhanced by a medical nutriment. *Cancer Biotherapy Radiopharmacology* 19(6):746–53.

Martinez, M. E., C. A. Thompson, and S. A. Smith-Warner. 2006. Soy and breast cancer: The controversy continues. *Journal of the National Cancer Institute* 98(7):430–31.

Mayo Clinic Staff. 2006. Breast cancer. www.mayoclinic.com/health/breast-cancer/DS00328/DSECTION=3 (accessed July 20, 2006).

Melkinow, J., et al. 2006. Chemoprevention: Drug pricing and mortality: The case of tamoxifen. *Cancer* 107(5):950–58.

Morimoto, T. et al. 1996. Postoperative adjuvant randomised trial comparing chemoendocrine therapy, chemotherapy and immunotherapy for patients with stage II breast cancer: 5-year results from the Nishinihon Cooperative Study Group of Adjuvant Chemoendocrine Therapy for Breast Cancer (ACETBC) of Japan. *European Journal of Cancer* 32A(2):235–42.

Mumber, Matthew P., ed. 2006. *Integrative Oncology: Principles and Practice*. Abingdon, Oxon, UK: Taylor and Francis.

Nackerdien, Z. E. 2008. Perspectives on microbes as oncogenic infectious agents and implications for breast cancer. *Medical Hypotheses* 71(2):302–6.

Nakachi, K., et al. 1998. Influence of drinking green tea on breast cancer malignancy among Japanese patients. *Japanese Journal of Cancer Research* 89(3):254–61.

National Cancer Institute. 2005. Breast cancer: Treatment. www.cancer.gov/cancerinfo/pdq/treatment/breast/patient/ (accessed July 20, 2006).

Neuhouser, M. L., et al. 2008. Vitamin D insufficiency in a multiethnic cohort of breast cancer survivors. *American Journal of Clinical Nutrition* 88(1):133–9.

Nunez-Anita, R. E., et al. 2009. A complex between 6-iodolactone and the peroxisome proliferators-activated receptor type gamma may mediate the antineoplastic effect of iodine in mammary cancer. *Prostaglandins Other Lipid Mediations* 89(1–2):34–42.

Paik, S., et al. 2006. Gene expression and benefit of chemotherapy in women with node-negative, estrogen receptor-positive breast cancer. *Journal of Clinical Oncology* 24(23):3726–34.

Pierce, J. P., et al. 1997. Feasibility of a randomized trial of high-vegetable diet to prevent breast cancer recurrence. *Nutrition and Cancer* 28(3):282–8.

Pierce, J. P., et al. 2007. Greater survival after breast cancer in physically active women with high vegetable-fruit intake regardless of obesity. *Journal of Clinical OncologyJournal of Clinical Oncology* 25(17):2345–51.

Ravdin, P. M., et al. 2006. Reduced hormone therapy use might be cause of steep decline in breast cancer cases. *North American Menopause Society Newsletter*, December 20.

Rebbeck, T. R., et al. 2007. A rerospective case-control study of the use of hormone-related supplements and association with breast cancer. *International Journal of Cancer* 120(7):1523–8.

Ronco, A. L., et al. 2006. Food patterns and risk of breast cancer: A factor analysis study in Uruguay. *International Journal of Cancer* 119(7):1672–78.

Schernhammer, E. S., and S. E. Hankinson. 2005. Urinary melatonin levels and breast cancer risk. *Journal of the National Cancer Institute* 97(14):1084–87.

Senie, R. T., et al. 1991. Timing of breast cancer excision during the menstrual cycle influences duration of disease-free survival. *Annals of Internal Medicine* 115(5):337–42.

Slivova, V., et al. 2005. Green tea polyphenols modulate secretion of urokinase plasminogen activator (uPA) and inhibit invasive behavior of breast cancer cells. *Nutrition and Cancer* 52(1):66–73.

Smith-Warner, S. A., et al. 1998. Alcohol and breast cancer in women: A pooled analysis of cohort studies. *Journal of the American Medical Association* 279(7):535–40.

Stan, S. D., E. R. Hahm, R. Warin, and S. V. Singh. 2008. Withaferin A causes FOXO3a- and Bim-dependent apoptosis and inhibits growth of human breast cancer cells in vivo. *Cancer Research* 68(18):7661–9.

Stoddard, F. R. 2nd, A. D. Brooks, B. A. Eskin, and G. J. Johannes. 2008. Iodine alters gene expression in the MCF7 breast cancer cell line: Evidence for an anti-estrogen effect of iodine. *International Journal of Medical Sciences* 5(4):189–96.

Thangapazham, R. L., et al. 2006. Green tea polyphenols and its constituent epigallocatechin gallate inhibits proliferation of human breast cancer cells in vitro and in vivo. *Cancer Letters*, March 3 (advance release copy).

Thompson, L. U., et al. 1996. Flaxseed and its lignan and oil components reduce mammary tumor growth at a late stage of carcinogenisis. *Carcinogenesis* 17(6):1373–76.

Todorova, V. K., et al. 2006. Modulation of p53 and c-myc in DMBA-induced mammary tumors by oral glutamine. *Nutrition and Cancer* 54(2):263–73.

Velentzis, L. S., et al. 2009. Lignans and breast cancer risk in pre- and postmenopausal women: Meta-analyses of observational studies. *British Journal of Cancer* 100(9):1492–8.

Wang, L., J. Chen, and L. U. Thompson. 2005. The inhibitory effect of flaxseed on the growth and metastasis of estrogen receptor negative human breast cancer xenograftsis attributed to both its lignan and oil components. *International Journal of Cancer* 116(5):793–8.

WebMD. 2006. Breast cancer symptoms. www.webmd.com/hw/breast_cancer/tv3621.asp (accessed July 20, 2006).

Weiss, L. K., et al. 2002. Hormone replacement therapy regimens and breast cancer risk(1). *Obstetrics and Gynecology* 100(6):1148–58.

Wood, C. E., et al. 2006. Dietary soy isoflavones inhibit estrogen effects in the postmenopausal breast. *Cancer Research* 66(20):1241–49.

Wu, A. H., D. O. Stram, and M. C. Pike. 1999. Response: Re: Meta-analysis: Dietary fat intake, serum estrogen levels, and the risk of breast cancer. *Journal of the National Cancer Institute* 91(17):1512.

Zepelin, H. H., et al. 2007. Isopropanolic black cohosh extract and recurrence-free survival after breast cancer. *International Journal of Clinical Pharmacological Therapies* 45(3):143–54.

Chapter Eighteen Cervical Cancer

Basu, J., et al. 2005. Plasma uric acid levels in women with cervical intraepithelial neoplasia. *Nutrition and Cancer* 51(1):25–31.

Gagandeep, et al. 2003. Chemopreventive effects of *Cuminum cyminum* in chemically induced forestomach and uterine cervix tumors in murine model systems. *Nutrition and Cancer* 47(2):171–80.

Ho, G. Y., et al. 1998. Viral characteristics of human papillomavirus infection and antioxidant levels as risk factors for cervical dysplasia. *International Journal of Cancer* 78(5):594–99.

Lacey, J. V., et al. 2003. Obesity as a potential risk factor for adenocarcinomas and squamous cell carcinomas of the uterine cervix. *Cancer* 98(4):814–21.

McDougal, G. J., H. A. Ross, M. Ikeji, and D. Stewart. 2008. Berry extracts exert different antiproliferative effects against cervical and colon cancer cells grown in vitro. *Journal of Agricultural and Food Chemistry* 56(9):3016–23.

National Cancer Institute. 2005. What you need to know about cancer of the cervix. www.cancer.gov/cancertopics/wyntk/cervix/ (accessed July 20, 2006).

National Cancer Institute. 2006. Cervical cancer treatment. www.cancer.gov/cancerinfo/pdq/treatment/cervical/patient/ (accessed July 20, 2006).

Palan, P. R., et al. 2003. Plasma concentrations of coenzyme Q10 and tocopherols in cervical intraepithelial neoplasia and cervical cancer. *European Journal of Cancer Prevention* 12(4):321–26.

Pazdur, Richard, et al., eds. 2004. *Cancer Management: A Multidisciplinary Approach; Medical, Surgical, and Radiation Oncology.* 8th edition. Philadelphia, PA: F. A. Davis Company.

Chapter Nineteen Colon Cancer

American Cancer Society. 2006. How is colorectal cancer found? www.cancer.org/docroot /CRI/content/CRI_2_2_3X_How_is_colorectal_cancer_found.asp (accessed July 20, 2006).

American Cancer Society. 2006. What causes colorectal cancer? www.cancer.org/docroot /CRI/content/CRI_2_2_2X_What_causes_colorectal_cancer.asp (accessed July 20, 2006).

American Cancer Society. 2006. What is colorectal cancer? www.cancer.org/docroot/CRI /content/CRI_2_2_1X_What_is_colon_and_rectum_cancer_10.asp (accessed July 20, 2006).

Arbiser, J. L., et al. 1998. Curcumin is an in vivo inhibitor of angiogenesis. *Molecular Medicine* 4(6):376-83.

Balavenkatraman, K. K., et al. 2006. DEP-1 protein tyrosine phosphatase inhibits proliferation and migration of colon carcinoma cells and is upregulated by protective nutrients. *Oncogene* 25(47):6319–24.

Bobe, G., et al. 2008. Dietary flavonoids and colorectal adenoma recurrence in the Polyp Prevention Trial. *Cancer Epidemiological Biomarkers Preview* 17(6):1344–53.

Bommareddy, A., et al. 2006. Chemopreventive effects of dietary flaxseed on colon tumor development. *Nutrition and Cancer* 54(2):216–22.

Brose, Marcia. 2004. MedlinePlus Medical Encyclopedia: Colon cancer. www.nlm.nih.gov /medlineplus/ency/article/000262.htm#Symptoms (accessed July 20, 2006).

Cerea, G., et al. 2003. Biomodulation of cancer chemotherapy for metastatic colo-rectal cancer: A randomized study of weekly low-dose irinotecan alone versus irinotecan plus the oncostatic pineal hormone melatonin in metastatic colorectal cancer patients progressing on 5-fluorouracil-containing combinations. *Anticancer Research* 23(2C):1951–54.

Chan, A. T., et al. 2005. Long-term use of aspirin and nonsteroidal anti-inflammatory drugs and risk of colorectal cancer. *Journal of the American Medical Association* 294(8):914–23.

Fleischauer, A. T., and L. Arab. 2001. Garlic and cancer: A critical review of the epidemiologic literature. *Journal of Nutrition* 131(3s):1032S–40S.

Fleischauer, A. T., C. Poole, and L. Arab. 2000. Garlic consumption and cancer prevention: Meta-analyses of colorectal and stomach cancers. *American Journal of Clinical Nutrition* 72(4):1047–52.

Frydoonfar, H. R., D. R. McGrath, and A. D. Spigelman. 2002. Inhibition of proliferation of a colon cancer cell line by indole-3-carbinol. *Colorectal Disease* 4(3):205–7.

Fung, T., et al. 2003. Major dietary patterns and the risk of colorectal cancer in women. *Archives of Internal Medicine* 163(3):309–14.

Gonder, U., and N. Worm. 2005. Re: Meat, fish, and colorectal cancer risk: The European prospective investigation into cancer and nutrition. *Journal of the National Cancer Institute* 97(23):1788.

Gonzalez, C. A. 2006. The European prospective investigation into cancer and nutrition (EPIC). *Public Health Nutrition* 9(1A):124–26.

Hanson, M. G., et al. 2007. A short-term dietary supplementation with high doses of vitamin E increases NK cell cytolic activity in advanced colorectal cancer patients. *Cancer Immunology and Immunotherapy* 56(7):973–84.

Haqmar, B., W. Ryd, and H. Skomedal. 1991. Arabinogalactan blockade of experimental metastases to liver by murine hepatoma. *Invasion and Metastasis* 11(6):348–55.

Jacobs, E. J., et al. 2001. Multivitamin use and colon cancer mortality in the Cancer Prevention Study II cohort (United States). *Cancer Causes and Control* 12(10):927–34.

Kabat, G. C., et al. Dietary carbohydrate, glycemic index, and glycemic load in relation to colorectal cancer risk in the Women's Health Initiative. *Cancer Causes Control* 19(10):1291–8.

Kossoy, G., et al. 2000. Melatonin and colon carcinogenesis. IV. Effect of melatonin on proliferative activity and expression of apoptosis-related proteins in the spleen of rats exposed to 1,2-dimethylhydrazine. *Oncology Reports* 7(6):1401–15.

Lala, G., et al. 2006. Anthocyanin-rich extracts inhibit multiple biomarkers of colon cancer in rats. *Nutrition and Cancer* 54(1):84–93.

Lewin, M. H., et al. 2006. Red meat enhances the colonic formation of the DNA adduct O6-carboxymethyl guanine: Implications for colorectal cancer risk. *Cancer Research* 66(3):1859–65.

Lieberman, D. A., et al. 2003. Risk factors for advanced colonic neoplasia and hyperplastic polyps in asymptomatic individuals. *Journal of the American Medical Association* 290(22):2959–67.

Matsuura, N., et al. 2006. Aged garlic extract inhibits angiogenesis and proliferation of colorectal carcinoma cells. *Journal of Nutrition* 136(suppl.3):842S–46S.

Meyerhardt, J. A., et al. 2006. Physical activity and survival after colorectal cancer diagnosis. *Journal of Clinical Oncology* 24(22):3527–34.

Murtaza, I., et al. 2006. A preliminary investigation demonstrating the effect of quercetin on the expression of genes related to cell-cycle arrest, apoptosis and xenobiotic metabolism in human CO115 colon-adenocarcinoma cells using DNA microarray. *Biotechnology and Applied Biochemistry* 45(Pt 1):29–36.

Roller, M., et al. 2007. Consumption of prebiotic insulin enriched with oligofructose in combination with the probiotics *Lactobacillus rhamnosus* and *Bifidobacterium lactis* has minor effects on selected immune parameters in polypectomised and colon cancer patients. *British Journal of Nutrition* 97(4):676–84.

Schink, M., et al. 2007. Mistletoe extract reduces the surgical suppression of natural killer cell activity in cancer patients: A randomized phase III trial. *Forsch Komplementmed* 14(1):9–17.

Sengottuvelan, M., and N. Nalini. 2006. Dietary supplementation of resveratrol suppresses colonic tumour incidence in 1,2-dimethylhydrazine-treated rats by modulating biotransforming enzymes and aberrant crypt foci development. *British Journal of Nutrition* 96(1):145–53.

Su, L. J., and L. Arab. 2004. Alcohol consumption and risk of colon cancer: Evidence from the National Health and Nutrition Examination Survey I epidemiologic follow-up study. *Nutrition and Cancer* 50(2):111–19.

Sun, C. L., et al. 2006. Green tea, black tea and colorectal cancer risk: A meta-analysis of epidemiologic studies. *Carcinogenesis* 27(7):1301–19.

van Duijnhoven, F. J., et al. 2009. Fruit, vegetable, and colorectal cancer risk: The European Prospective Investigation into Cancer and Nutrition. *American Journal of Clinical Nutrition* 89(5):1441–52.

Vician, M., et al. 1999. Melatonin content in plasma and large intestine of patients with colorectal carcinoma before and after surgery. *Journal of Pineal Research* 27(3):164–69.

Wenzel, U., A. Nickel, and H. Daniel. 2005. Melatonin potentiates flavone-induced apoptosis in human colon cancer cells by increasing the level of glycolytic end products. *International Journal of Cancer* 116(2):236–42.

Winczyk, K., M. Pawlikowski, and M. Karasek. 2001. Melatonin and RZR/ROR receptor ligand CGP 52608 induce apoptosis in the murine colonic cancer. *Journal of Pineal Research* 31(2):179–82.

Chapter Twenty Esophageal Cancer

Abnet, C. C., et al. 2008. A prospective study of BMI and risk of oesophageal and gastric adenocarcinoma. *European Journal of Cancer* 44(3):465–71.

Graham, A. J., et al. 2007. Defining the optimal treatment of locally advanced esophageal cancer: A systematic review and decision analysis. *Annals of Thoracic Surgery* 83:1257–1264.

Lagiou, P., et al. 2009. Diet and upper-aerodigestive tract cancer in Europe: The ARCAGE study. *International Journal of Cancer* 124(11):2671–6.

Singh, N., and Verma, K. 2002. Case report of a laryngeal squamous cell carcinoma treated with artensunate. *Archive of Oncology* 10(4):279–80.

Ryan, A. M., et al. Enteral nutrition enriched with eicosapentaenoic acid (EPA) preserves lean body mass following esophageal cancer surgery: Results of a double-blinded randomized controlled trial. *Annals of Surgery* 249(3):355–63.

Taylor, P. R., et al. 2003. Prospective study of serum Vitamin E levels and esophageal and gastric cancers. *Journal of National Cancer Institute* 95(18):1414–6.

Yoshida, S., A. Kaibara, N. Ishibashi, and K. Shirouzu. 2001. Glutamine supplementation in cancer patients. *Nutrition* 17(9):766–8.

Chapter Twenty-One Gastric Cancer

Bjelakovic, G., et al. 2004. Antioxidant supplements for preventing gastrointestinal cancers. *Cochrane Database of Systematic Reviews* no. 4: CD004183.

Chen, A. L., et al. 2001. Phase I clinical trial of curcumin, a chemopreventive agent, in patients with high-risk or pre-malignant lesions. *Anticancer Research* 21(4B):2895–900.

Chen, H. S., et al. 2003. Clinical study on treatment of patients with upper digestive tract malignant tumors of middle and late stage with ginkgo biloba exocarp polysaccharides capsule preparation. [In Chinese.] *Zhong Xi Yi Jie He Xue Bao* [Journal of Chinese Integrative Medicine] 1(3):189–91.

Duan, P., and Z. M. Wang. 2002. Clinical study on effect of astragalus in efficacy enhancing and toxicity reducing of chemotherapy in patients of malignant tumor. [In Chinese.] *Zhonguo Zhong Xi Yi Jie He Za Zhi* [Chinese Journal of Modern Developments in Traditional Medicine] 22(7):515–17.

Fleischauer, A. T., and L. Arab. 2001. Garlic and cancer: A critical review of the epidemiologic literature. *Journal of Nutrition* 131(3s):1032S–40S.

Fleischauer, A. T., C. Poole, and L. Arab. 2000. Garlic consumption and cancer prevention: Meta-analyses of colorectal and stomach cancers. *American Journal of Clinical Nutrition* 72(4):1047–52.

Gonzalez, C. A., et al. 2006. Fruit and vegetable intake and the risk of stomach and oesophagus adenocarcinoma in the European prospective investigation into cancer and nutrition (EPIC-EURGAST). *International Journal of Cancer* 118(10):2559–66.

Hibasami, H., et al. 1998. Induction of apoptosis in human stomach cancer cells by green tea catechins. *Oncology Reports* 5(2):527–29.

Hibasami, H., et al. 2004. Induction of apoptosis by three types of procyanidin isolated from apple (Rosaceae *Malus pumila*) in human stomach cancer KATO III cells. *International Journal of Molecular Medicine* 13(6):795–99.

Kim, H. J., et al. 2005. Effect of nutrient intake and *Helicobacter pylori* infection on gastric cancer in Korea: A case-control study. *Nutrition and Cancer* 52(2):138–46.

Koo, J. Y., et al. Curcumin inhibits the growth of AGS human gastric carcinoma cells in vitro and shows synergism with 5-fluorouracil. *Journal of Medicinal Food* 7(2):117–21.

Leitzmann, M. F., et al. 2009. Physical activity and esophageal and gastric carcinoma in a large prospective study. *American Journal of Preventive Medicine* 36(2):112–9.

Li, H., et al. 2004. An intervention study to prevent gastric cancer by micro-selenium and large dose of allitridum. *Chinese Medical Journal (English)* 117(8):1155–60.

Lin, J., et al. 2003. Effects of astragali radix on the growth of different cancer cell lines. *World Journal of Gastroenterology* 9(4):670–73.

Linblad, M., L. A. Rodriguez, and J. Lagergren. 2005. Body mass, tobacco and alcohol and risk of esophageal, gastric cardia, and gastric non-cardia adenocarcinoma among men and women in a nested case-control study. *Cancer Causes and Control* 16(3):285–94.

Liu, H. K., et al. 2009. Inhibitory effects of gamma-tocotrienol on invasion and metastasis of human gastric adenocarcinoma SGC-7901 cells. *Journal of Nutritional Biochemistry* [Epub ahead of print].

Liu, J. R., et al. 2002. Effect of apoptosis on gastric adenocarcinoma cell line SGC-7901 induced by cis-9, trans-11-conjugated linoleic acid. *World Journal of Gastroenterology* 8(6):999–1004.

Macdonald, J. S., et al. 2001. Chemoradiotherapy after surgery compared with surgery alone for adenocarcinoma of the stomach or gastroesophageal junction. *New England Journal of Medicine* 345(10):725–30.

MacInnis, R. J., et al. 2006. Body size and composition and the risk of gastric and oesophageal adenocarcinoma. *International Journal of Cancer* 118(10):2628–31.

Mark, S. D., et al. 2000. Prospective study of serum selenium levels and incident esophageal and gastric cancers. *Journal of the National Cancer Institute* 92(21):1753–63.

Moragoda, L., R. Jaszewski, and A. P. Majumdar. 2001. Curcumin induced modulation of cell cycle and apoptosis in gastric and colon cancer cells. *Anticancer Research* 21(2A):873–8.

Mu, L. N., et al. 2005. Green tea drinking and multigenetic index on the risk of stomach cancer in a Chinese population. *International Journal of Cancer* 116(6):972–83.

Nagata, C., et al. 2002. A prospective cohort study of soy product intake and stomach cancer death. *British Journal of Cancer* 87(1):31–36.

Nakazato, H., et al. 1994. Efficacy of immunochemotherapy as adjuvant treatment after curative resection of gastric cancer. *Lancet* 343:1122–26.

Nanda, Rita. 2006. MedlinePlus Medical Encyclopedia: Gastric cancer. www.nlm.nih.gov /medlineplus/ency/article/000223.htm (accessed July 20, 2006).

National Cancer Institute. 2005. What you need to know about stomach cancer. www.cancer .gov/cancertopics/wyntk/stomach/page6 (accessed July 6, 2006).

Nouarie, M., et al. 2004. Ecologic study of serum selenium and upper gastro-intestinal cancers in Iran. *World Journal of Gastroenterology* 10(17):2544–6.

Orlando, A., et al. 2009. Effects of *Lactobacillus rhamnosus* GG on proliferation and polyamine metabolism in HGC-27 human gastric and DLD-1 colonic cancer cell lines. *Immunopharmacology and Immunotoxicology* 31(1):108–16.

Pazdur, Richard, et al., eds. 2004. *Cancer Management: A Multidisciplinary Approach; Medical, Surgical, and Radiation Oncology.* 8th edition. Philadelphia, PA: F. A. Davis Company.

Qiao, Y. L., et al. 2009. Total and cancer mortality after supplementation with vitamins and minerals: Follow-up of the Linxian General Population Nutrition Intervention Trial. *Journal of the National Cancer Institute* 101(7):507–18.

Roth, J., and S. Mobarhan. 2001. Preventive role of dietary fiber in gastric cardia cancers. *Nutrition Review* 59(11):372–74.

Setiawan, V. W., et al. 2001. Protective effect of green tea on the risks of chronic gastritis and stomach cancer. *International Journal of Cancer* 92(4):600–4.

Setiawan, V. W., et al. 2005. Allium vegetables and stomach cancer risk in China. *Asian Pacific Journal of Cancer Prevention* 6(3):387–95.

Stoicov, C., Saffari, R., and Houghton, J. 2009. Green tea inhibits Helicobacter growth in vivo and in vitro. *International Journal of Antimicrobial Agents* 33(5):473–8.

Suh, S. O., et al. 2002. Effects of red ginseng upon postoperative immunity and survival in patients with stage III gastric cancer. *American Journal of Chinese Medicine* 30(4):483–94.

Velmurugan, B., A. Mani, and S. Nagini. 2005. Combination of S-allylcysteine and lycopene induces apoptosis by modulating Bcl-2, Bax, Bim and caspases during experimental gastric carcinogenesis. *European Journal of Cancer Prevention* 14(4):387–93.

Velmurugan, B., and S. Nagini. 2005. Combination chemoprevention of experimental gastric carcinogenesis by S-allylcysteine and lycopene: Modulatory effects on glutathione redox cycle antioxidants. *Journal of Medicinal Food* 8(4):494–501.

Xu, A. H., et al. 2003. Therapeutic mechanism of ginkgo biloba exocarp polysaccharides on gastric cancer. *World Journal of Gastroenterology* 9(11):2424–27.

Chapter Twenty-Two Head and Neck Cancer

Bairati, I., et al. 2006. Antioxidant vitamins supplementation and mortality: A randomized trial in head and neck cancer patients. *International Journal of Cancer* 119(9):2221–4.

Kato, K., et al. 2008. Effects of green tea polyphenol on methylation status of RECK gene and cancer cell invasion in oral squamous cell carcinoma cells. *British Journal of Cancer* 99(4):647–54.

Meyer, F., et al. 2008. Interaction between antioxidant vitamin supplementation and cigarette smoking during radiation therapy in relation to long-term effects on recurrence and mortality: A randomized trial among head and neck cancer patients. *International Journal of Cancer* 122(7):1679–83.

Nam, W., et al. 2007. Effects of artemisinin and its derivatives on growth inhibition and apoptosis of oral cancer cells. *Head and Neck* 29(4):335–40.

Pelucchi, C., et al. 2003. Fiber intake and laryngeal cancer risk. *Annals of Oncology* 14(1):162–7.

Pisters, K. M., et al. 2001. Phase I trial of oral green tea extract in adult patients with solid tumors. *Journal of Clinical Oncology* 19(6):1830–8.

Rashad, U. M., Al-Gezawy, S. M., El-Gezawhy, E., and Azzaz, A. N. 2009. Honey as topical prophylaxis against radiochemotherapy-induced mucositis in head and neck cancer. *Journal of Larygology and Otolaryngology* 123(2):223–8.

Rogers, L. O., et al. 2006. Physical activity and quality of life in head and neck cancer survivors. *Support Care Cancer* 14(10):1012–9.

Zhang, X., et al. 2008. Synergistic inhibition of head and neck tumor growth by green tea—Epigallocate-3-gallate and EGFR tyrosine kinase inhibitor. *International Journal of Cancer* 123(5):1005–14.

Chapter Twenty-Three Kidney Cancer

American Cancer Society. 2005. How is kidney cancer (renal cell carcinoma) diagnosed? www.cancer.org/docroot/cri/content/cri_2_4_3x_how_is_kidney_cancer_diagnosed_22.asp (accessed July 20, 2006).

Batist, G., et al. 2002. Neovasttat (AE-941) in refractory renal cell carcinoma patients: Report of a phase II trial with two dose levels. *Annals of Oncology* 13(8):1259–63.

Canadian Cancer Society. 2006. What causes kidney cancer? www.cancer.ca/ccs/internet/standard/0,3182,3172_10175_269991_langId-en,00.html (accessed July 20, 2006).

Cancer Treatment Centers of America. 2006. Kidney cancer symptoms. www.cancercenter.com/kidney-cancer-symptoms.htm (accessed July 20, 2006).

Escudier, B., et al. 2007. Prognostic factors of metastatic renal cell carcinoma after failure of immunotherapy: New paradigm from a large phase III trial with shark cartilage extract AE 941. *Journal of Urology* 178(5):1901–5.

Han, H. J., et al. 2002. Ginsenosides inhibit EGF-induced proliferation of renal proximal tubule cells via decrease of c-fos and c-jun gene expression in vitro. *Planta Medica* 68(11):971–74.

Handa, K., and N. Kreiger. 2002. Diet patterns and the risk of renal cell carcinoma. *Public Health Nutrition* 5(6):757–67.

Kadiroglu, A. K., et al. 2005. The evaluation of postdialysis L-carnitine administration and its effect on weekly requiring doses of rHuEPO in hemodialysis patients. *Renal Failure* 27(4):367–72.

Mayo Clinic Staff. 2006. Kidney cancer. www.mayoclinic.com/health/kidney-cancer/DS00360 (accessed July 20, 2006).

Moore, S. C., et al. 2008. Physical activity during adulthood and adolescence in relation to renal cell cancer. *American Journal of Epidemiology* 168(2):149–57.

Murray, Michael. 1996. *Encyclopedia of Nutritional Supplements: The Essential Guide for Improving Your Health Naturally.* New York: Three Rivers Press.

Neri, B., et al. 1994. Modulation of human lymphoblastoid interferon activity by melatonin in metastatic renal cell carcinoma. A phase II study. *Cancer* 73(12):3015–19.

Obara, W., et al. 2008. Prospective study of combined treatment with interferon-alpha and active vitamin D3 for Japanese patients with metastatic renal cell carcinoma. *International Journal of Urology* 15(9):794–9.

Pischon, T., et al. 2006. Body size and risk of renal cell carcinoma in the European prospective investigation into cancer and nutrition (EPIC). *International Journal of Cancer* 118(3):728–38.

Sohn, J., et al. 1998. Effect of petroleum ether extract of Panax ginseng roots on proliferation and cell cycle progression of human renal cell carcinoma cells. *Experimental and Molecular Medicine* 30(1):47–51.

Weikert, S., et al. 2006. Fruits and vegetables and renal cell carcinoma: Findings from the European Prospective Investigation into Cancer and Nutrition (EPIC). *International Journal of Cancer* 118(12):3133–39.

Wu, X. X., et al. 2009. Induction of apoptosis in human renal cell carcinoma cells by vitamin E succinate in caspase-independent manner. *Urology* 73(1):193–9.

Chapter Twenty-Four Leukemia, Lymphoma, and Myeloma

Aquayo, A., et al. 2000. Angiogenesis in acute and chronic leukemias and myelodysplastic syndromes. *Blood* 96(6):2240–45.

Aquino, V. M., et al. 2005. A double-blind randomized placebo-controlled study of oral glutamine in the prevention of mucositis in children undergoing hematopoietic stem cell transplantation: A pediatric blood and marrow transplant consortium study. *Bone Marrow Transplant* 36(7):611–6.

Aratanechemuge, Y., et al. 2002. Selective induction of apoptosis by ar-turmerone isolated from turmeric (*Curcuma longa* L) in two human leukemia cell lines, but not in human stomach cancer cell line. *International Journal of Molecular Medicine* 9(5):481–84.

Asou, H., et al. 2002. Resveratrol, a natural product derived from grapes, is a new inducer of differentiation in human myeloid leukemias. *International Journal of Hepatology* 75(5):528–33.

Baxa, D. M., X. Luo, and F. K. Yoshimura. 2005. Genistein induces apoptosis in T lymphoma cells via mitochondrial damage. *Nutrition and Cancer* 51(1):93–101.

Chen, D., et al. 2005. Dietary flavonoids as proteasome inhibitors and apoptosis inducers in human leukemia cells. *Biochemical Pharmacology* 69(10):1421–32.

Cipak, L., et al. 2003. Effects of flavonoids on cisplatin-induced apoptosis of HL-60 and L1210 leukemia cells. *Leukemia Research* 27(1):65–72.

Clark, C. S., J. E. Konyer, and K. A. Meckling. 2004. 1-alpha,25-dihydroxyvitamin D3 and bryostatin-1 synergize to induce monocytic differentiation of NB4 acute promyelocytic leukemia cells by modulating cell cycle progression. *Experimental Cell Research* 294(1):301–11.

Coleman, E. A., et al. 2008. Effects of exercise in combination with epoetin alfa during high-dose chemotherapy and autologous peripheral blood stem cell transplantation for multiple myeloma. *Oncology Nurse Forum* 35(3):E53–61.

Currier, N. L., and S. C. Miller. 2001. *Echinacea purpurea* and melatonin augment natural-killer cells in leukemic mice and prolong life span. *Journal of Alternative and Complementary Medicine* 7(3):241–51.

Dong, J., et al. 2005. Effects of large dose of *Astragalus membranaceus* on the dendritic cell induction of peripheral mononuclear cell and antigen presenting ability of dendritic cells in children with acute leukemia. *Zhongguo Zhong Xi Yi Jie He Za Zhi* 25(10):872–5.

Kovacs, E., and J. J. Kuehn. 2002. Measurements of IL-6, soluble IL-6 receptor and soluble gp1130 in sera of B-cell lymphoma patients. Does viscum album treatment affect these parameters? *Biomedical Pharmacotherapy* 56(3):152–8.

Kovacs, E., S. Link, and U. Toffol-Schmidt. 2006. Cytostatic and cytocidal effects of mistletoe (Viscum album L.) quercus extract Iscador. *Arzneimittelforschung* 56(6A):467–73.

Krasteva, I. N., R. A. Toshkova, and S. D. Nikolov. 2004. Protective effect of *Astragalus corniculatus* saponins against myeloid graffi tumour in hamsters. *Phytotherapy Research* 18(3):255–57.

Kuskonmaz, B., et al. 2008. The effect of glutamine supplementation on hematopoietic stem cell transplant outcome in children: A case-control study. *Pediatric Transplant* 12(1):47–51.

Lee, Y. K., et al. 2004. VEGF receptor phosphorylation status and apoptosis is modulated by a green tea component, epigallocatechin-3-gallate (EGCG), in B-cell chronic lymphocytic leukemia. *Blood* 104(3):788–94.

Leukemia and Lymphoma Society. 2006. Disease information: Leukemia. www.leukemia-lymphoma.org/all_page?item_id=7026 (accessed July 7, 2006).

Leukemia and Lymphoma Society. 2006. Disease information: Lymphoma. www.leukemia-lymphoma.org/all_page?item_id=7030 (accessed July 20, 2006).

Leukemia and Lymphoma Society. 2006. Disease information: Myeloma. www.leukemia-lymphoma.org/all_page?item_id=7032 (accessed July 20, 2006).

Li, H. C., et al. 2000. Green tea polyphenols induce apoptosis in vitro in peripheral blood T lymphocytes of adult T-cell leukemia patients. *Japanese Journal of Cancer Research* 91(1):34–40.

Lissoni, P., et al. 2000. A phase II study of neuroimmunotherapy with subcutaneous low-dose IL-2 plus the pineal hormone melatonin in untreatable advanced hematologic malignancies. *Anticancer Research* 20(3B):2103–5.

Liu, C. Y., et al. 2009. Cured meat, vegetables, and bean-curd foods in relation to childhood acute leukemia risk: A population based case-control study. *BMC Cancer* 9:15.

Monasterio, A., et al. 2004. Flavonoids induce apoptosis in human leukemia U937 cells through caspase- and caspase-calpain-dependent pathways. *Nutrition and Cancer* 50(1):90–100.

Moyer-Mileur, L. J., Ransdell, L., and Bruggers, C. S. 2009. Fitness of children with standard-risk acute lymphoblastic leukemia during maintenance therapy: Response to a home-based exercise and nutrition program. *Journal of Pediatric Hematology and Oncology* 31(4):259–66.

Pan, S. Y., Y. Mao, and A. M. Ugnat. 2005. Physical activity, obesity, energy intake, and the risk of non-Hodgkin's lymphoma: A population-based case-control study. *American Journal of Epidemiology* 162(12):1162–73.

Persengiev, S. P., and S. Kyurkchiev. 1993. Selective effect of melatonin on the proliferation of lymphoid cells. *International Journal of Biochemistry* 25(3):441–44.

Pryme, I. F., et al. 2004. A mistletoe lectin (ML-1)-containing diet reduces the viability of a murine non-Hodgkin lymphoma tumor. *Cancer Detection and Prevention* 28(1):52–56.

Rajasingh, J., et al. 2006. Curcumin induces growth-arrest and apoptosis in association with the inhibition of constitutively active JAK-STAT pathway in T cell leukemia. *Biochemical and Biophysical Research Communications* 340(2):359–68.

Seifert, G., et al. 2008. Molecular mechanisms of mistletoe plant extract-induced apoptosis in acute lymphoblastic leukemia in vivo and in vitro. *Cancer Letters* 264(2):218–28.

Smith, D. M., and Q. P. Dou. 2001. Green tea polyphenol epigallocatechin inhibits DNA replication and consequently induces leukemia cell apoptosis. *International Journal of Molecular Medicine* 7(6):645–52.

Stumpf, C., et al. 2000. Mistletoe extracts in the therapy of malignant, hematological and lymphatic diseases—A monocentric, retrospective analysis over 16 years. [In German.] *Forschende Komplementärmedizin und Klassische Naturheilkunde* [Research in Complementary and Natural Classical Medicine] 7(3):139–46.

Tomita, M., et al. 2006. Curcumin targets AKT cell survival signaling pathway in HTLV-I-infected T-cell lines. *Cancer Science* 97(4):322–27.

Vassiliadis, S., et al. 2002. The role of L-carnitine on a restricted number of myeloid leukemia progenitor cells: Generation of atypical cell types. *Haematologia* 32(4):341–53.

Yoon, T. J., et al. 2003. Antitumor activity of the Korean mistletoe lectin is attributed to activation of macrophages and NK cells. *Archives of Pharmaceutical Research* 26(10):861–67.

Chapter Twenty-Five Liver Cancer

American Cancer Society. 2006. Do we know what causes liver cancer? www.cancer.org/docroot/CRI/content/CRI_2_4_2X_Do_we_know_what_causes_liver_cancer_25.asp (accessed July 20, 2006).

American Cancer Society. 2006. What is liver cancer? www.cancer.org/docroot/cri/content/cri_2_2_1x_what_is_liver_cancer_25.asp (accessed July 20, 2006).

Biswas, S. J., et al. 2005. Efficacy of the potentized homeopathic drug, Carcinosin 200, fed alone and in combination with another drug, Chelidonium 200, in amelioration of p-dimethylaminoazobenzene-induced hepatocarcinogenesis in mice. *Journal of Alternative and Complementary Medicine* 11(5):839–54.

Cowawintaweewat, S., et al. 2006. Prognostic improvement of patients with advanced liver cancer after active hexose correlated compound (AHCC) treatment. *Asian Pacific Journal of Allergy Immunology* 24(1):33–45.

Cui, W., Gu, F., and Hu, K.Q. 2009. Effects and mechanisms of silibinin on human hepatocellular carcinoma xenografts in nude mice. *World Journal of Gastroenterology* 15(16):1943–50.

Cui, Y., H. Xie, and J. Wang. 2005. Potential biomedical properties of *Pinus massoniana* bark extract. *Phytotherapy Research* 19(1):34–38.

Giri, R. K., T. Parija, and B. R. Das. 1999. D-limonene chemoprevention of hepatocarcinogenesis in AKR mice: Inhibition of c-jun and c-myc. *Oncology Reports* 6(5):1123–27.

Habib, S. H., et al. 2008. Ginger extract (*Zingiber officinale*) has anti-cancer and anti-inflammatory effects on ethionine-induced hepatoma rats. *Clinics (Sao Paulo)* 63(6):807–13.

Hagmar, B., W. Ryd, and H. Skomedal. 1991. Arabinogalactan blockade of experimental mtas-tases to liver by murine hepatoma. *Invasion Metastasis* 11(6):348–55.

Hwang, E. S., and E. H. Jeffery. 2005. Induction of quinone reductase by sulforaphane and sulforaphane N-acetylcysteine conjugate in murine hepatoma cells. *Journal of Medicinal Food* 8(2):198–203.

Komatsu, W., Y. Miura, and K. Yagasaki. 2002. Induction of tumor necrosis factor production and antitumor effect by cabbage extract. *Nutrition and Cancer* 43(1):82–89.

Li, X., et al. 2005. Anticarcinogenic effect of 20(R) ginsenoside Rg3 on induced hepatocellu-lar carcinoma in rats. [In Chinese.] *Sichuan Da Xue Xue Bao Yi Xue Ban* [Journal of Sichuan University. Medical Science Edition] 36(2):217–20.

Matsui, Y., et al. 2002. Improved prognosis of postoperative hepatocellular carcinoma patients when treated with functional foods: A prospective cohort study. *Journal of Hepatology* 37(1):78–86.

Nanda, Rita. 2006. MedlinePlus Medical Encyclopedia: Hepatocellular carcinoma. www.nlm.nih.gov/medlineplus/ency/article/000280.htm (accessed July 20, 2006).

Nishikawa, T., et al. 2006. A green tea polyphenol, epigallocatechin-3-gallate, induces apop-tosis of human hepatocellular carcinoma, possibly through inhibition of Bcl-2 family pro-teins. *Journal of Hepatology* 44(6):1074–82.

Parija, T., and B. R. Das. 2003. Involvement of YY1 and its correlation with c-myc in NDEA induced hepatocarcinogenesis, its prevention by d-limonene. *Molecular Biology Reports* 30(1):41–46.

Pathak, S., et al. 2006. Protective potentials of a potentized homeopathic drug, Lycopo-dium-30, in ameliorating azo dye induced hepatocarcinogenesis in mice. *Molecular and Cel-lular Biochemistry* 285(1–2):121–31.

Surjyo, B., and K. B. Anisur. 2004. Protective action of an anti-oxidant (L-ascorbic acid) against genotoxicity and cytotoxicity in mice during p-DAB-induced hepatocarcinogen-esis. *Indian Journal of Cancer* 41(2):72–80.

Varghese, L., et al. 2005. Silibinin efficacy against human hepatocellular carcinoma. *Clinical Cancer Research* 11(23):8441–48.

Vijaya, P. V., D. C. S. Arul, and K. M. Ramkuma. 2007. Induction of apoptosis by ginger in HEp-2 cell line is mediated by reactive oxygen species. *Basic Clinical Pharmacology and Toxi-cology* 100(5):302–7.

Chapter Twenty-Six Lung Cancer

Alexander, S., et al. 1999. Phase I/II study of stage III and IV non-small cell lung cancer patients taking a specific dietary supplement. *Nutrition and Cancer* 34(1):62–69.

Balcerek, M., and I. Matlawska. 2005. Preventive role of curcumin in lung cancer. [In Polish.] *Przegla Lekarski* 62(10):1180–81.

Bezjak, A., et al. 2006. Symptom improvement in lung cancer patients treated with erlotinib: Quality of life analysis of the National Cancer Institute of Canada clinical trials group study BR.21. *Journal of Clinical Oncology* 24(24):3831–37.

Clark, J., and M. You. 2006. Chemoprevention of lung cancer by tea. *Molecular Nutrition and Food Research* 50(2):144–51.

Hidvegi, M., et al. 1999. MSC, a new benzoquinone-containing natural product with antimet-astatic effect. *Cancer Biotherapy and Radiopharmacology* 14(4):277–89.

Jakab, F., A. Mayer, A. Hoffman, and M. Hidvegi. 2000. First clinical data of a natural immu-nomodulator in colorectal cancer. *Hepatogastroenterology* 47(32):393–5.

Latreille, J., et al. 2003. Phase I/II trial of the safety and efficacy of AE-941 (Neovastat) in the treatment of non-small-cell lung cancer. *Clinical Lung Cancer* 4(4):231–6.

Laurie, S. A., et al. 2005. Phase I study of green tea extract in patients with advanced lung can-cer. *Cancer Chemotherapy and Pharmacology* 55(1):33–8.

Lissoni, P., et al. 2003. Five years survival in metastatic non-small cell lung cancer patients treated with chemotherapy alone or chemotherapy and melatonin: A randomized trial. *Journal of Pineal Research* 35(1):12–15.

Lu, Y., et al. 2006. A gene expression signature that can predict green tea exposure and chemopreventive efficacy of lung cancer in mice. *Cancer Research* 66(4):1956–63.

McCulloch, M., et al. 2006. Astragalus-based Chinese herbs and platinum-based chemotherapy for advanced non-small-cell lung cancer: Meta-analysis of randomized trials. *Journal of Clinical Oncology* 24(3):419–30.

National Cancer Institute. 2002. What you need to know about lung cancer. www.cancer.gov /cancertopics/wyntk/lung/ (accessed July 20, 2006).

Norsa, A., and V. Martino. 2006. Somatostatin, retinoids, melatonin, vitamin D, bromocriptine, and cyclophosphamide in advanced non-small-cell lung cancer patients with low performance status. *Cancer Biotherapy and Radiopharmaceuticals* 21(1):68–73.

Patel, J. D., P. B. Bach, and M. G. Kris. 2004. Lung cancer in U.S. women: A contemporary epidemic. *Journal of the American Medical Association* 291(14):1763–68.

Pazdur, Richard, et al., eds. 2004. *Cancer Management: A Multidisciplinary Approach; Medical, Surgical, and Radiation Oncology.* 8th edition. Philadelphia, PA: F. A. Davis Company.

Senthilnathan, P., et al. 2006. Chemotherapeutic efficacy of paclitaxel in combination with *Withania somnifera* on benzo(a)pyrene-induced experimental lung cancer. *Cancer Science* 97(7):658–64.

Senthilnathan, P., et al. 2006. Enhancement of antitumor effect of paclitaxel in combination with immunomodulatory *Withania somnifera* on benzo(a)pyrene induced experimental lung cancer. *Chemico-Biological Interactions* 159(3):180–85.

Singh, R. P., et al. 2006. Effect of silibinin on the growth and progression of primary lung tumors in mice. *Journal of the National Cancer Institute* 98(12):846–55.

Sun, A. S., et al. 1999. Phase I/II study of stage III and IV non-small cell lung cancer patients taking a specific dietary supplement. *Nutrition and Cancer* 34(1):62–9.

Wright, M. E., et al. 2004. Development of a comprehensive dietary antioxidant index and application to lung cancer risk in a cohort of male smokers. *American Journal of Epidemiology* 160(1):68–76.

Zhou, W., et al. 2007. Circulating 25-hydroxyvitamin D levels predict survival in early-stage non-small-cell lung cancer patients. *Journal of Clinical Oncology* 25(5):479–85.

Chapter Twenty-Seven Ovarian Cancer

Ahonen, M. H., et al. 2000. Androgen receptor and vitamin D receptor in human ovarian cancer: Growth stimulation and inhibition by ligands. *International Journal of Cancer* 86(1):40–46.

American Cancer Society. 2006. How is ovarian cancer diagnosed? www.cancer.org/docroot /CRI/content/CRI_2_4_3X_How_is_ovarian_cancer_diagnosed_33.asp (accessed July 20, 2006).

American Cancer Society. 2006. What is ovarian cancer? www.cancer.org/docroot/cri/content /cri_2_4_1x_what_is_ovarian_cancer_33.asp (accessed July 20, 2006).

Chan, M. M., et al. 2003. Inhibition of growth and sensitization to cisplatin-mediated killing of ovarian cancer cells by polyphenolic chemopreventive agents. *Journal of Cell Physiology* 194(1):63–70.

Chan, M. M., et al. 2006. Epigallocatechin-3-gallate delivers hydrogen peroxide to induce death of ovarian cancer cells and enhances their cisplatin susceptibility. *Journal of Cell Physiology* 207(2):389–96.

Chen, O., et al. Pharmacologic doses of ascorbate act as a prooxidant and decrease growth of aggressive tumor xenografts in mice. *Proceedings of the National Academy of Sciences in the U.S.A.* 105(32):1105–9.

Chen, X., and J. J. Anderson. 2001. Isoflavones inhibit proliferation of ovarian cancer cells in vitro via an estrogen receptor-dependent pathway. *Nutrition and Cancer* 41(1–2):165–71.

Drisko, J. A., J. Chapman, and V. J. Hunter. 2003. The use of antioxidants with first-line chemotherapy in two cases of ovarian cancer. *Journal of the American College of Nutrition* 22(2):118–23.

Futugami, M., et al. 2001. Effects of melatonin on the proliferation and cisdiamminedichloro-platinum (CDDP) sensitivity of cultured human ovarian cancer cells. *Gynecologic Oncology* 82(3):544–49.

Ganmaa, D., and A. Sato. 2005. The possible role of female sex hormones in milk from pregnant cows in the development of breast, ovarian and corpus uteri cancers. *Medical Hypotheses* 65(6):1028–37.

Klein, A., et al. 2006. Prolonged stabilization of platinum-resistant ovarian cancer in a single patient consuming a fermented soy therapy. *Gynecological Oncology* 100(1):205–9.

Larsson, S. C., and A. Wolk. 2005. Tea consumption and ovarian risk in a population-based cohort. *Archives of Internal Medicine* 165(22):2683–86.

Pan, S. Y., A. M. Ugnat, and Y. Mao. 2005. Physical activity and the risk of ovarian cancer: A case-control study in Canada. *International Journal of Cancer* 117(2):300–7.

Rezk, Y. A., et al. 2006. Use of resveratrol to improve the effectiveness of cisplatin and doxorubicin: Study in human gynecologic cancer cell lines and in rodent heart. *American Journal of Obstetrics and Gynecology* 194(5):e23–e26.

Roomi, M. W., et al. 2006. Inhibition of matrix metalloproteinase-2 secretion and invasion by human ovarian cancer cell line SK-OV-3 with lysine, proline, arginine, ascorbic acid and green tea extract. *Journal of Obstetrics and Gynecology Research* 32(2):148–54.

Shen, F., M. Herenyiova, and G. Weber. 1999. Synergistic down-regulation of signal transduction and cytotoxicity by tiazofurin and quercetin in human ovarian carcinoma cells. *Life Sciences* 64(21):1869–76.

Shi, M., et al. 2006. Antiproliferation and apoptosis induced by curcumin in human ovarian cancer cells. *Cell Biology International* 30(3):221–26.

Tung, K. H., et al. 2005. Association of dietary vitamin A, carotenoids, and other antioxidants with the risk of ovarian cancer. *Cancer Epidemiology, Biomarkers, and Prevention* 14(3):669–76.

Weber, G., et al. 2000. Signal transduction and biological targeting of ovarian carcinoma. *European Journal of Gynaecological Oncology* 21(3):231–36.

Xu, M. J., et al. 2005. Effects of retinoic acid on proliferation and differentiation of a human ovarian carcinoma cell line: 3AO. *Chinese Medical Sciences Journal* 20(1):51–54.

Zheng, L., Q. Tong, and C. Wu. 2004. Growth-inhibitory effects of curcumin on ovary cancer cells and its mechanisms. *Journal of Huazhong University of Science and Technology, Medical Sciences* 24(1):55–58.

Chapter Twenty-Eight Pancreatic Cancer

Banerjee, S., et al. 2005. Molecular evidence for increased antitumor activity of gemcitabine by genistein in vitro and in vivo using an orthotopic model of pancreatic cancer. *Cancer Research* 65(19):9064–72.

Berkson, B. M., D. M. Rubin, and A. J. Berkson. 2006. The long-term survival of a patient with pancreatic cancer with metastases to the liver after treatment with the intravenous alpha-lipoic acid/low-dose naltrexone protocol. *Integrative Cancer Therapies* 5(1):83–89.

Berrington de Gonzalez, A., et al. 2006. Anthropometry, physical activity, and the risk of pancreatic cancer in the European prospective investigation into cancer and nutrition. *Cancer Epidemiology, Biomarkers, and Prevention* 15(5):879–85.

Burney, P. G., G. W. Comstock, and J. S. Morris. 1989. Serologic precursors of cancer: Serum micronutrients and the subsequent risk of pancreatic cancer. *American Journal of Clinical Nutrition* 49(5):895–900.

Chen, X., et al. 1999. Inhibition of farnesyl protein transferase and P21ras membrane association by d-limonene in human pancreas tumor cells in vitro. *Chinese Medical Sciences Journal* 14(3):138–44.

Dhillon, N., et al. Phase II trial of curcumin in patients with advanced pancreatic cancer. *Clinical Cancer Research* 14(14):4491–9.

Larsson, S. C., et al. 2006. Folate intake and pancreatic cancer incidence: A prospective study of Swedish women and men. *Journal of the National Cancer Institute* 98(6):407–13.

Larsson, S. C., et al. 2006. Fruit and vegetable consumption in relation to pancreatic cancer risk: A prospective study. *Cancer Epidemiology, Biomarkers, and Prevention* 15(2):301–15.

Larsson, S. C., et al. 2006. Meat, fish, poultry and egg consumption in relation to risk of pancreatic cancer: A prospective study. *International Journal of Cancer* 118(11):2866–70.

Li, L., F. S. Braiteh, and R. Kurzrock. 2005. Liposome-encapsulated curcumin: In vitro and in vivo effects on proliferation, apoptosis, signaling, and angiogenesis. *Cancer* 104(6):1322–31.

Li, L., et al. 2004. Nuclear factor-kappaB and IkappaB kinase are constitutively active in human pancreatic cells, and their down-regulation by curcumin (diferuloylmethane) is associated with the suppression of proliferation and the induction of apoptosis. *Cancer* 101(10):2351–62.

Lin, Y., et al. 2005. Nutritional factors and risk of pancreatic cancer: A population-based case-control study based on direct interview in Japan. *Journal of Gastroenterology* 40(3):297–301.

Mayo Clinic Staff. 2006. Pancreatic cancer. www.mayoclinic.com/health/pancreatic-cancer /DS00357 (accessed July 20, 2006).

Merendino, N., et al. 2005. Docosahexaenoic acid induces apoptosis in the human PaCa-44 pancreatic cancer cell line by active reduced glutathione extrusion and lipid peroxidation. *Nutrition and Cancer* 52(2):225–33.

National Cancer Institute. 2002. What you need to know about cancer of the pancreas. www .cancer.gov/cancertopics/wyntk/pancreas/ (accessed July 20, 2006).

Nomura, T., et al. 2007. Probiotics reduce infectious complications after pancreaticoduodenectomy. *Hepatogastroenterology* 54(75):661–3.

Roginsky, A. B., et al. 2005. On the potential use of flavonoids in the treatment and prevention of pancreatic cancer. *In Vivo* 19(1):61–67.

Roomi, M. W., et al. 2005. Antitumor effect of a combination of lysine, proline, arginine, ascorbic acid, and green tea extract on pancreatic cancer cell line MIA PaCa-2. *International Journal of Gastrointestinal Cancer* 35(2):97–102.

Rostock, M., et al. 2005. Anticancer activity of a lectin-rich mistletoe extract injected intratumorally into human pancreatic cancer xenografts. *Anticancer Research* 25(3B):1969–75.

Ruiz-Rabelo, J. F., et al. 2007. Beneficial properties of melatonin in an experimental model of pancreatic cancer. *Journal of Pineal Research* 43(3):270–5.

Shirota, T., et al. 2005. Apoptosis in human pancreatic cancer cells induced by eicosapentaenoic acid. *Nutrition* 21(10):1010–17.

Stolzenberg-Solomon, R. Z., et al. 2009. Serium vitamin D and risk of pancreatic cancer in the prostate, lung, colorectal, and ovarian screening trial. *Cancer Research* 69(4):1439–47.

Suzuki, Y. J., B. B. Aggarwal, and L. Packer. 1992. Alpha-lipoic acid is a potent inhibitor of NF-kappa B activation in human T cells. *Biochemical and Biophysical Research Communications* 189(3):1709–15.

Takada, M., et al. 2002. Suppression of human pancreatic carcinoma cell growth and invasion by epigallocatechin-3-gallate. *Pancreas* 25(1):45–48.

Van de Mark, K., et al. 2003. Alpha-lipoic acid induces p27Kip-dependent cell cycle arrest in non-transformed cell lines and apoptosis in tumor cell lines. *Journal of Cell Physiology* 194(3):325–40.

Wang, Z., et al. 2006. Inhibition of nuclear factor kappa B activity by genistein is mediated via Notch-1 signaling pathway in pancreatic cancer cells. *International Journal of Cancer* 118(8):1930–36.

Chapter Twenty-Nine Prostate Cancer

American Cancer Society. 2006. How is prostate cancer diagnosed? www.cancer.org/docroot /CRI/content/CRI_2_4_3X_How_is_prostate_cancer_diagnosed_36.asp (accessed July 20, 2006).

American Cancer Society. 2006. What are the risk factors for prostate cancer? www.cancer .org/docroot/CRI/content/CRI_2_4_2X_What_are_the_risk_factors_for_prostate _cancer_36.asp (accessed July 20, 2006).

American Cancer Society. 2006. What is prostate cancer? www.cancer.org/docroot/CRI /content/CRI_2_2_1X_What_is_prostate_cancer_36.asp (accessed July 20, 2006).

Beer, T. M., A. Myrthue, and K. M. Eilers. 2005. Rationale for the development and current status of calcitriol in androgen-independent prostate cancer. *World Journal of Urology* 23(1):28–32.

Bettuzzi, S., et al. 2006. Chemoprevention of human prostate cancer by oral administration of green tea catechins in volunteers with high-grade prostate intraepithelial neoplasia: A preliminary report from a one-year proof-of-principle study. *Cancer Research* 66(2):1234–40.

Carmody, J., et al. 2008. A dietary intervention for recurrent prostate cancer after definitive primary treatment: Results of a randomized pilot trial. *Urology* 72(6):1324–8.

Daubenmier, J. J., et al. 2006. Lifestyle and health-related quality of life of men with prostate cancer managed with active surveillance. *Urology* 67(1):125–30.

Giordano, S. H., et al. 2006. Late gastrointestinal toxicity after radiation for prostate cancer. *Cancer* 107(2):423–32.

Giovannucci, E. L., et al. 2005. A prospective study of physical activity and incident and fatal prostate cancer. *Archives of Internal Medicine* 165(9):1005–10.

Hafeez, B. B., et al. A dietary anthocyanidin delphinidin induces apoptosis of human prostate cancer PC3 cells in vitro and in vivo: Involvement of nuclear factor-kappaB signaling. *Cancer Research* 68(20):8564–72.

Hedelin, M., et al. 2006. Dietary phytoestrogen, serum enterolactone and risk of prostate cancer: The cancer prostate Sweden study (Sweden). *Cancer Causes and Control* 17(2):169–80.

Jani, A. B., et al. 2006. Role of external beam radiotherapy with low-dose-rate brachytherapy in treatment of prostate cancer. *Urology* 67(5):1007–11.

Kelavkar, U. P., et al. 2006. Prostate tumor growth and recurrence can be modulated by the omega-6:omega-3 ratio in diet: Athymic mouse xenograft model simulating radical prostatectomy. *Neoplasia* 8(2):112–24.

Khor, T. O., et al. 2006. Combined inhibitory effects of curcumin and phenethyl isothiocyanate on the growth of human PC-3 prostate xenografts in immunodeficient mice. *Cancer Research* 66(2):613–21.

Lee, A. H., et al. 2006. Protective effects of green tea against prostate cancer. *Expert Review of Anticancer Therapy* 6(4):507–13.

Maghell, A., et al. Impact of body mass index on biochemical recurrence rates after radical prostatectomy: An analysis utilizing propensity score matching. *Urology* 72(6):1246–51.

McLarty, J., et al. 2009. Tea polyphenols decrease serum levels of prostate-specific antigen, hepatocyte growth factor, and vascular endothelial growth factor in prostate cancer patients and inhibit production of hepatocyte growth factor and vascular endothelial growth factor in vitro [Epub ahed of print].

McLeod, N., C. C. Huynh, and P. Rashid. 2006. Osteoporosis from androgen deprivation therapy in prostate cancer treatment. *Australian Family Physician* 35(4):243–45.

Meyer, F., et al. 2005. Antioxidant vitamin and mineral supplementation and prostate cancer prevention in the SU.VI.MAX trial. *International Journal of Cancer* 116(2):182–86.

Paine, M. J., et al. 1992. Gene expression in *Echis carinatus* (carpet viper) venom glands following milking. *Toxicon* 30(4):379–86.

Pantuck, A. J., et al. 2006. Phase II study of pomegranate juice for men with rising prostate-specific antigen following surgery or radiation for prostate cancer. *Clinical Cancer Research* 12(13):4018–26.

Pinski, J., et al. 2006. Genistein-induced neuroendocrine differentiation of prostate cancer cells. *Prostate* 66(11):1136–43.

Posner, G. H., et al. 2004. Anticancer and antimalarial efficacy and safety of artemisinin-derived trioxane dimmers in rodents. *Journal of Medicinal Chemistry* 47(5):1299–301.

Prostate Cancer Institute. 2006. Prostate cancer tests and staging. www.prostate-cancer-institute.org/about-prostate-cancer/prostate-cancer-tests.html (accessed July 20, 2006).

Quiles, J. L., et al. 2003. Coenzyme Q differentially modulates phospholipid hydroperoxide glutathione peroxidase gene expression and free radicals production in malignant and nonmalignant prostate cells. *Biofactors* 18(1–4):265–70.

Rimler, A., et al. 2002. Nuclear exclusion of the androgen receptor by melatonin. *Journal of Steroid Biochemistry and Molecular Biology* 81(1):77–84.

Singh, R. P., and R. Agarwal. 2006. Prostate cancer chemoprevention by silibinin: Bench to bedside. *Molecular Carcinogenesis* 45(6):436–42.

Siu, S. W., et al. 2002. Melatonin and prostate cancer cell proliferation: Interplay with castration, epidermal growth factor, and androgen sensitivity. *Prostate* 52(2):106–22.

Strom, S. S., et al. 2006. Influence of obesity on biochemical and clinical failure after external-beam radiotherapy for localized prostate cancer. *Cancer* 107(3):631–39.

Tiszlavicz, L. 1991. Multiple primary malignant tumors involving the liver. [In Hungarian.] *Orvosi Hetilap* 132(46):2527–30.

Traka, M., et al. 2008. Broccoli consumption interacts with GSTM1 to perturb oncogenic signaling pathways in the prostate. *PLoS One* 3(7):e2568.

Woo, T. C., et al. 2005. Pilot study: Potential role of vitamin D (cholecalciferol) in patients with PSA relapse after definitive therapy. *Nutrition and Cancer* 51(1):32–36.

Xing, N., et al. 2001. Quercetin inhibits the expression and function of the androgen receptor in LNCaP prostate cancer cells. *Carcinogenesis* 22(3):409–14.

Chapter Thirty Sarcoma (Soft Tissue)

Albini, A., et al. 2001. Inhibition of angiogenesis-driven Kaposi's sarcoma tumor growth in nude mice by oral N-acetylcysteine. *Cancer Research* 61(22):8171–8.

Barlow, J. W., et al. 2005. Differentiation of rhabdomyosarcoma cell lines using retinoic acid. *Pediatric Blood Cancer* 47(6):773–84.

Beuth, J., et al. 1987. Inhibition of liver metastasis in mice by blocking hepatocyte lectins with arabinogalactan infusions and D-galactose. *Journal of Cancer Research and Clinical Oncology* 113(1):51–5.

Beuth, J., et al. 1988. Inhibition of liver tumor cell colonization in two animal tumor models by lectin blocking with D-galactose or arabinogalactan. *Clinical & Experimental Metastasis* 6(2):115–120.

Dauchy, R. T., et al. 2009. Antineoplastic effects of melatonin on a rare malignancy of mesenchymal origin: Melatonin receptor-mediated inhibition of signal transduction, linoleic acid metabolism and growth in tissue-isolated human leiomyosarcoma xenografts. *Journal of Pineal Research* [Epub ahead of print].

Huang, S. L., C. L. Hsu, and G. C. Yen. 2006. Growth inhibitory effect of quercetin on SW 872 human liposarcoma cells. *Life Sciences* 79(2):203–9.

Landau, J. M., et al. 1998. Inhibition of spontaneous formation of lun tumors and rhabdomyosarcomas in A/J mice by black and green tea. *Carcinogenesis* 19(3):501–7.

Yoshida, S., A. Kaibara, N. Ishibashi, and K. Shirouzu. 2001. Glutamine supplementation in cancer patients. *Nutrition* 17(9):766–8.

Chapter Thirty-One Skin Cancer and Melanoma

Arbiser, J. L., et al. 1998. Curcumin is an in vivo inhibitor of angiogenesis. *Molecular Medicine* 4(6):376–83.

Cos, S., A. Garcia-Bolardo, and E. J. Sanchez-Barcelo. 2001. Direct antiproliferative effects of melatonin on two metastatic cell sublines of mouse melanoma (B16BL6 and PG19). *Melanoma Research* 11(2):197–201.

Demidov, L.V., et al. 2008. Adjuvant fermented wheat germ extract (Avemar) nutraceutical improves survival of high-risk skin melanoma patients: A randomized, pilot, phase II clinical study with a 7-year-old follow-up. *Cancer Biotherapy and Radiopharmaceuticals* 23(4):477–82.

Hakim, I. A., and R. B. Harris. 2001. Joint effects of citrus peel use and black tea intake on the risk of squamous cell carcinoma of the skin. *BMC Dermatology* 1:3.

Hakim, I. A., R. B. Harris, and U. M. Weisgerber. 2000. Tea intake and squamous cell carcinoma of the skin: Influence of type of tea beverages. *Cancer Epidemiology, Biomarkers, and Prevention* 9(7):727–31.

Harris, R. B., et al. 2005. Fatty acid composition of red blood cell membranes and risk of squamous cell carcinoma of the skin. *Cancer Epidemiology, Biomarkers, and Prevention* 14(4): 906–12.

Hasegawa, H., et al. 2002. Prevention of growth and metastasis of murine melanoma through enhanced natural-killer cytotoxicity by fatty acid-conjugate of protopanaxatriol. *Biological and Pharmaceutical Bulletin* 25(7):861–66.

Huang, S. C., et al. 2005. Carnosol inhibits the invasion of B16/F10 mouse melanoma cells by suppressing metalloproteinase-9 through down-regulating nuclear factor-kappa B and c-Jun. *Biochemical Pharmacology* 69(2):221–32.

Inohara, H., and A. Raz. 1994. Effects of natural complex carbohydrate (citrus pectin) on murine melanoma cell properties related to galectin 3 functions. *Glycoconjugate Journal* 11(6):527–32.

Liu, J. D., et al. 2001. Inhibition of melanoma growth and metastasis by combination with (-)-epigallocatechin-3-gallate and dacarbazine in mice. *Journal of Cellular Biochemistry* 83(4):631–42.

Millien, A. E., et al. 2004. Diet and melanoma in a case-control study. *Cancer Epidemiology, Biomarkers, and Prevention* 13(6):1042–51. National Cancer Institute. 2003. What you need to know about melanoma. www.cancer.gov/cancertopics/wyntk/melanoma (accessed July 20, 2006).

Rusciani, L., et al. 2006. Low plasma coenzyme Q10 levels as an independent prognostic factor for melanoma progression. *Journal of the American Academy of Dermatology* 54(2):234–41.

Saul, A. N., et al. 2005. Chronic stress and susceptibility to skin cancer. *Journal of the National Cancer Institute* 97(23):1760–67.

Seifert, M., et al. 2004. Differential biological effects of 1,25-dihydroxyVitamin D3 on melanoma cell lines in vitro. *Journal of Steroid Biochemistry and Molecular Biology* 89–90(1-5):375–79.

Skin Cancer Foundation. 2006. About melanoma. www.skincancer.org/melanoma/index.php (accessed July 20, 2006).

WebMD. 2005. Skin cancer, melanoma: Cause. www.webmd.com/hw/melanoma/hw206559.asp (accessed July 21, 2006).

Wright, T. I., J. M. Spencer, and F. P. Flowers. 2006. Chemoprevention of nonmelanoma skin cancer. *Journal of the American Academy of Dermatology* 54(6):933–46.

Yerneni, L. K., and S. Jayaraman. 2003. Pharmacological action of high doses of melatonin on B16 murine melanoma cells depends on cell number at time of exposure. *Melanoma Research* 13(2):113–17.

Yoon, T. J., et al. 2003. Antitumor activity of the Korean mistletoe lectin is attributed to activation of macrophages and NK cells. *Archives of Pharmaceutical Research* 26(10):861–67.

Zhang, X., Q. Xu, and I. Saiki. 2000. Quercetin inhibits the invasion and mobility of murine melanoma B16–BL6 cells through inducing apoptosis via decreasing Bcl-2 expression. *Clinical and Experimental Metastasis* 18(5):415–21.

Chapter Thirty-Two Testicular Cancer

American Cancer Society. 2006. How is testicular cancer diagnosed? www.cancer.org/docroot/cri/content/cri_2_4_3x_how_is_testicular_cancer_diagnosed_41.asp (accessed July 20, 2006).

American Cancer Society. 2006. What are the risk factors for testicular cancer? www.cancer.org/docroot/CRI/content/CRI_2_4_2X_What_are_the_risk_factors_for_testicular_cancer_41.asp (accessed July 20, 2006).

Chang, S. S., et al. 2005. Performance-enhancing supplement use in patients with testicular cancer. *Urology* 66(2):242–45.

Chapple, A., S. Ziebland, and A. McPherson. 2004. Qualitative study of men's perceptions of why treatment delays occur in the UK for those with testicular cancer. *British Journal of General Practice* 54(498):25–32.

Coffey, D. S., R. H. Getzenberg, and T. L. DeWeese. 2006. Hyperthermic biology and cancer therapies: A hypothesis for the "Lance Armstrong effect." *Journal of the American Medical Association* 296(4):445–48.

Mayo Clinic Staff. 2006. Testicular cancer: Signs and symptoms. www.mayoclinic.com/health/testicular-cancer/DS00046/DSECTION=2 (accessed July 20, 2006).

Sharpe, R. M., and D. S. Irvine. 2004. How strong is the evidence of a link between environmental chemicals and adverse effects on human reproductive health? *British Medical Journal* 328(7437):447–51.

Walcott, F. L., et al. 2002. A case-control study of dietary phytoestrogens and testicular cancer risk. *Nutrition and Cancer* 44(1):44–51.

Chapter Thirty-Three Thyroid Cancer

Al-Brahim, N., and S. L. Asa. 2006. Papillary thyroid carcinoma: An overview. *Archive of Pathology and Laboratory Medicine* 130:1057–1062.

Divi, R. L., and D. R. Doerge. 1996. Inhibition of thyroid peroxidase by dietary flavonoids. *Chemical Research in Toxicology* 9(1):16–23.

Eigelberger, M. S., et al. 2001. Phenylacetate enhances the antiproliferative effect of retinoic acid in follicular thyroid cancer. *Surgery* 130(6):931–5.

Johns Hopkins Thyroid Tumor Center. How are thyroid nodules discovered? Available at www.thyroid-cancer.net/topics/how+are+thyroid+nodules+discovered (accessed January 4, 2006).

Karavitaki, N., et al. 2002. Recurrent and/or metastatic thyroid cancer: Therapeutic options. *Expert Opinion on Pharmacotherapy* 3(7):939–47.

Karbownik, M., and A. Lewinski. 2003. The role of oxidative stress in physiological and pathological processes in the thyroid gland; possible involvement in pineal-thyroid interactions. *Neuro Endocrinol Lett* 24(5):293–303.

Kent, L., et al. 2006. Increased risk of papillary thyroid cancer in celiac disease. *Digestive Disease and Science* 51(10):1875–7.

Lewinski, A., M. Pawlikowski, and D. P. Cardinali. 1993. Thyroid growth-stimulating and growth-inhibiting factors. *Biological Signals* 2(6):313–51.

Mano, T., et al. 1998. Vitamin E and coenzyme Q concentrations in the thyroid tissues of patients with various thyroid disorders. *American Journal of Medical Sciences* 315(4):230–2.

Mayo Clinic Staff. Mayo Clinic thyroid cancer screening and diagnosis webpage. www.mayoclinic.com/health/thyroid-cancer/DS00492/DSECTION=6 (accessed January 4, 2007).

Mayo Clinic Staff. Mayo Clinic thyroid cancer signs and symptoms webpage. www.mayoclinic.com/health/thyroid-cancer/DS00492/DSECTION=2 (accessed January 4, 2007).

Mayo Clinic Staff. Mayo Clinic thyroid cancer webpage. www.mayoclinic.com/health/thyroid-cancer/DS00492. (accessed January 4, 2007).

Murray, Michael T. *Encyclopedia of Nutritional Supplements.* 1996. New York, NY: Prima Publishing.

National Cancer Institute. Thyroid cancer—Who's at risk? webpage. www.cancer.gov/cancertopics/wyntk/thyroid/page4 (Accessed January 4, 2007).

National Cancer Institute. What you need to know about thyroid cancer diagnosis webpage. www.cancer.gov/cancertopics/wyntk/thyroid/page6 (accessed January 4, 2007).

Nishikawa, A., et al. 2005. Pronounced synergistic promotion of N-bis (2-hydroxy-propyl) nitrosamine-initiated thyroid tumorigenesis in rats treated with excess soybean and iodine-deficient diets. *Toxicological Sciences* 86(2):258–63.

Norman Endocrine Surgery Clinic. Thyroid nodule ultrasound: What is it, what does it tell me? Webpage. www.endocrineweb.com/noduleus.html (accessed January 4, 2007).

Sanders, L. E., and B. Cady. 1998. Differentiated thyroid cancer: Reexamination of risk groups and outcome of treatment. *Archives of Surgery* 133(4):419–25.

Shih, A., et al. 2002. Resveratrol induces apoptosis in thyroid cancer cell lines via a MAPK- and p53-dependent mechanism. *Journal of Clinical Endocrinology & Metabolism* 87(3):1223–32.

Chapter Thirty-Four Uterine Cancer

Ahn, W. S., et al. 2004. Natural killer cell activity and quality of life were improved by consumption of a mushroom extract, *Agaricus blazei* Murill Kyowa, in gynecological cancer patients undergoing chemotherapy. *International Journal of Gynecological Cancer* 14(4):589–94.

Bhat, K. P., and J. M. Pezzuto. 2001. Resveratrol exhibits cytostatic and antiestrogenic properties with human endometrial adenocarcinoma (Ishikawa) cells. *Cancer Research* 61(16):6137–44.

Dann, J. M., P. H. Sykes, D. R. Mason, and J. J. Evans. 2009. Regulation of vascular endothelial growth factor in endometrial tumour cells by resveratrol and EGCG. *Gynecologic Oncology* 113(3):374–8.

Friedenreich, C. M., and M. R. Orenstein. 2002. Physical activity and cancer prevention: Etiologic evidence and biological mechanisms. *Journal of Nutrition* 132(suppl.11):3456S–64S.

Iatrakis, G., et al. 2006. Women younger than 50 years with endometrial cancer. *European Journal of Gynaecological Oncology* 27(4):399–400.

Kobayashi, Y., et al. 2003. Melatonin binding sites in estrogen receptor-positive cells derived from human endometrial cancer. *Journal of Pineal Research* 35(2):71–74.

Lian, Z., et al. 2004. Soybean isoflavones inhibit estrogen-stimulated gene expression in mouse uteri. *European Journal of Gynaecological Oncology* 25(3):311–14.

Matthews, C. E., et al. 2005. Physical activity and risk of endometrial cancer: A report from the Shanghai endometrial cancer study. *Cancer Epidemiology, Biomarkers, and Prevention* 14(4):779–85.

Niwa, K., et al. 1999. Preventive effects of Glycyrrhizae radix extract on estrogen-related endometrial carcinogenesis in mice. *Japanese Journal of Cancer Research* 90(7):726–32.

Yeh, M., et al. 2009. Higher intakes of vegetables and vegetable-related nutrients are associated with lower endometrial cancer risks. *Journal of Nutrition* 139(2):317–22.

Conclusion: The Future of Cancer Care

Smith, B. D., et al. 2009. Future of cancer incidence in the United States: Burdens upon an aging changing nation. *Journal of Clinical Oncology* 27(17):2758–65.

Index

Stress
cancer prevention and, 50–51, 137
cancer treatment and, 71–73
herbs/nutrients for, 191
hormone balance and, 211
immune system and, 185–188
massage therapy, 79–80
meditation as medicine, 80–81
movement as medicine, 73–80
reduction, 71–73
skin cancer and, 357
Studies
on cancer, 247
statistical chances, 88, 89
types of, 112, 113
Sugar
avoidance of, 44, 66
breast cancer and, 273
feeds cancer theory, 108–109
hidden, 226
insulin resistance and, 219–222, 223, 225
Sulforaphane, 60
Sunitinib, 159
Supplements. *See also* Nutrients/herbs
antioxidants, 182–183
for cancer prevention, 45, 48, 137–138
chemotherapy drugs and, 140–154
for chemotherapy support, 126–128
with conventional treatment, 119–124
for digestion, 240–242
for esophageal cancer, 291–292
for hormone balance, 210–211
hormone drugs and, 156–157
immune-enhancing, 188–192
for inflammation, 197–198, 200–201
for insulin resistance reversal, 225–229
integrative cancer care supplement guide, 161–172
in integrative medicine plan, 116–117
as integrative therapy, 102
radiation and, 129, 155
safety of, 104
for side effects, 130–132
for stress reduction, 191
surgery and, 124–126

targeted therapies and, 158–159
for treatment recovery, 134
Support, 114, 138
Supportive, use of term, 247
Surgery. *See also* individual cancers
description of, 87
diagnosis by, 36, 38
dismissal of, 120
support before/after, 124–126
Survival, 88–89, 337
Synthetic colors, 41

T

Tai chi, 76
Tamoxifen, 122, 208, 212–213, 216, 270
Target therapies, 94–96, 158–159
Taste changes, 131
T cells
function of, 10
immune system process, 179–182
inflammation and, 193–194
meditation and, 50
stress and, 185, 187
in thymus, 11
Tea, 355, 357. *See also* Green tea
Telomerase, 6, 15
Testes, 206
Testicular cancer
causes, symptoms, diagnosis, 362–363
complementary approaches, 364–365
conventional treatment for, 363–364
environmental toxins and, 27
self-exam, 37
Testicular dysgenesis syndrome, 364
Tests, 28–38. *See also* Diagnosis
THMs (trihalomethanes), 21
Thorneley, Roger, 122
Thymus, 11, 206
Thyroid cancer
causes, symptoms, diagnosis, 367
complementary approaches, 368–370
conventional treatment for, 367–368
overview of, 366
Thyroid gland, 206, 299
TNF (tumor necrosis factor), 184

TNM system, 12
Tobacco. *See* Smoking
Tomatoes, 43, 47
Tomotherapy, 91
Topoisomerase inhibitors, 92
Topotecan, 152
Toxins
causes of cancer, 20–23
evaluation of exposure to, 24–27
kidney cancer and, 305
liver cancer and, 320–321
lung cancer and, 323–324
testicular cancer and, 364
Trans fats, 44–45, 63–64, 199–200
Transplant, stem cell, 313, 316
Trastuzumab, 158
Treatment. *See also* Conventional treatment; Integrative medicine
alternative cancer cures, questionable, 173–176
creative activities, 81–82
emotional expression, 82–85
fats, 62–65
food as medicine, 57–59
food, basics of, 59–60
future of cancer care, 375–378
hormonal cancer treatments, 212–217
lifestyle factors, 69–71
macrobiotic diet, 67
meditation as medicine, 80–81
movement as medicine, 73–80
nutrition, getting adequate, 68–69
protein, 65–66
rating system, 160–161
spirituality and health, 82, 83, 85
stress reduction, 71–73
unhealthy foods, avoiding, 66
vegetables/fruits, 60–61
whole grains, 61–62
Treatment approach overview
alternative cancer treatment theories, 108–110
chemotherapy, 90–93
clinical trials, 96
conventional, 86
drug developments, 94
information gathering, 104, 105–107, 110–112
integrative medicine, choice of, 96–98